Telepractice in Speech-Language Pathology

Telepractice in Speech-Language Pathology

K. Todd Houston, PhD, CCC-SLP, LSLS Cert. AVT

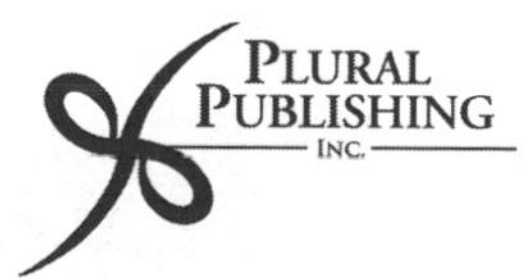

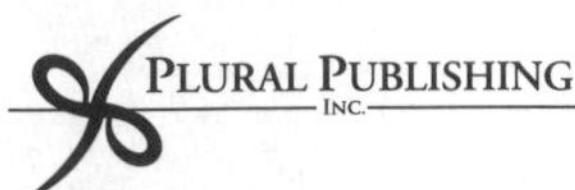

5521 Ruffin Road
San Diego, CA 92123

e-mail: info@pluralpublishing.com
Web site: http://www.pluralpublishing.com

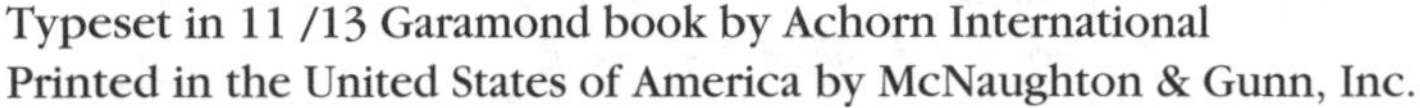

Typeset in 11 /13 Garamond book by Achorn International
Printed in the United States of America by McNaughton & Gunn, Inc.

Library of Congress Cataloging-in-Publication Data

Telepractice in speech-language pathology / [edited by] K. Todd Houston.
p. ; cm.
Includes bibliographical references and index.
ISBN-13: 978-1-59756-479-3 (alk. paper)
ISBN-10: 1-59756-479-6 (alk. paper)
I. Houston, K. Todd, editor of compilation.
[DNLM: 1. Language Disorders—therapy. 2. Speech Disorders—therapy. 3. Speech-Language Pathology—methods. 4. Telemedicine—methods. WL 340.2]
RC427
616.85'506—dc23

2013027154

Contents

Preface

As telecommunication and distance technology continue to evolve, new opportunities to provide comprehensive telepractice services to meet the speech, language, communication, and rehabilitative needs of children and adults are increasing. From high-end dedicated telecommunication systems typically used in medical centers or universities to notebook and tablet computers and smartphones that utilize encrypted software with secure broadband Internet connections, a range of telepractice service delivery models are being rapidly adopted within speech-language pathology.

Speech-language pathologists are embracing the potential of these new technologies to shape service delivery and to raise standards of care. Patients need access to well-qualified practitioners regardless of where they live, and these technologies can ensure that treatment is delivered efficiently, effectively, and with greater consistency. In turn, as technology use becomes more ubiquitous in all of our lives, consumers of speech and language interventions are demanding that these services be delivered at a distance. Telepractice service delivery models are increasingly consumer-driven and are currently outpacing the knowledge and skills of many speech-language pathologists. Similarly, although more training is needed at the undergraduate and graduate levels in university training programs, practitioners in the field need professional development opportunities to enhance and refine their skills in telepractice service delivery.

As speech-language pathologists explore telepractice to meet rising consumer demands, more efforts are needed to ensure that regulatory agencies and federal and state legislation supports its use in speech-language pathology. Likewise, licensure issues, especially at the state level, must be resolved in all 50 states and U.S. territories. The challenge of establishing licensure portability so that practitioners can serve consumers across state lines also must be resolved. Although not an easy task, considerable effort on this issue is being waged by national professional associations, state governments and local agencies, individual practitioners, and consumer-related organizations. Similarly, obtaining reimbursement for telepractice services continues to be a challenge for most speech-language pathologists, and like insurance portability, this issue continues to be addressed by professional associations through policy advocacy and by ensuring that states include telepractice as a billable service in new insurance policies or legislation that is adopted.

This work, *Telepractice in Speech-Language Pathology*, represents the first book devoted entirely to the delivery of speech, language, communication, and rehabilitative services at a distance. The contributing authors are themselves practitioners and continue to pioneer unique ways in which distance technology can meet the needs of the consumers being served. The patient populations, practitioners, and settings profiled in the following chapters represent a vibrant cross-section of telepractice applications, technology, and service delivery models. Because telepractice is expanding and evolving as new technology becomes available, it is impossible to capture all of its manifestations within the field in a single publication. However, whether you are a beginning telepractitioner or someone who is more seasoned, you will find valuable insights, step-by-step guidelines, and readily applicable information that will improve your telepractice service delivery.

Speech-language pathology, as a profession, has arrived at an important intersection of societal and cultural changes that will continue to shape service delivery. New technological trends are shaping how all of us connect, communicate, and interact. Consumers are increasing their demands for technology-based solutions that support service delivery. Through distance technology, notebook or tablet computers, and smartphones coupled to broadband Internet connections, more patients have access to the speech, language, and rehabilitative services they need to improve the quality of their lives. As a speech-language pathologist, I embrace the opportunities that this technology brings to our profession, and I hope you find *Telepractice in Speech-Language Pathology* a useful guide as you navigate these exciting possibilities for your own practice.

K. Todd Houston, PhD
Wadsworth, OH

Acknowledgments

Sincere thanks to the talented editors and staff at Plural Publishing for their patience, guidance, and support through the development process of this book. Your encouragement during the writing and editing processes and your unwavering enthusiasm for this book was inspiring.

I also wish to thank my outstanding graduate students in the School of Speech-Language Pathology and Audiology at The University of Akron: Anne M. Fleming, Kelly J. Brown, Kami Zeckzer Walters, Tali R. Weinberg, and Jessica M. Nafe. You set a new standard for future graduate students, and I deeply appreciate your long hours throughout every step of the book's production.

And finally, I wish to thank each of the contributing authors who so willingly shared their expertise about telepractice service delivery models. Because you were so open to participating, others will now gain from your knowledge and experience. Thank you for your generous colleagueship!

Contributors

Robin L. Alvares, PhD, CCC-SLP
eSLP/Project Coordinator
OMNIE/KSU Telepractice in Speech-Language Pathology Project
School of Health Sciences
Kent State University
Kent, OH
Chapter 3

Marnee Brick, MSc, RSLP, S-LP
Cofounder, Director
TinyEYE Therapy Services
http://www.TinyEYE.com
Chapter 10

Kelly J. Brown, MA
School of Speech-Language Pathology and Audiology
College of Health Professions
The University of Akron
Akron, OH
Chapters 1 and 12

Jessica M. Nafe, MA
School of Speech-Language Pathology and Audiology
College of Health Professions
The University of Akron
Akron, OH
Chapter 1

Michael F. Campbell, MS, MBA, CCC-SLP
Assistant Chief
Audiology and Speech Pathology Service (126)
Gulf Coast Veterans Health Care System
Biloxi, MS
Chapter 3

Charles H. Carlin, PhD, CCC-SLP
Assistant Professor of Speech-Language Pathology
School of Speech-Language Pathology and Audiology
College of Health Professions
The University of Akron
Akron, OH
Chapter 9

Emily L. Carlin, MA, CCC-SLP
Speech-Language Pathologist
School of Speech-Language Pathology and Audiology
College of Health Professions
The University of Akron
Akron, OH
Chapter 9

Gabriella Constantinescu, PhD, BSpPath (Hons)
Lead Researcher
Hear and Say
Queensland, Australia
Chapter 11

Sena Crutchley, MS, CCC-SLP
Speech-Language Pathologist
The University of North Carolina at Greensboro
Greensboro, NC
Avanté at Reidsville Rehabilitation and Nursing
Reidsville, NC
Chapter 3

Dimity Dornan, AM, Associate Professor UQ HonDUniv USQ, BSpTHy, FSPAA, CpSp, LSLS Cert AVT.
Executive Director and Founder
Hear and Say
Queensland, Australia
Chapter 11

Anne M. Fleming, MA
School of Speech-Language Pathology and Audiology
College of Health Professions
The University of Akron
Akron, OH
Chapters 1 and 12

Rodney Gabel, PhD, CCC-SLP, BRS-FD
Department of Rehabilitation Sciences, Speech-Language Pathology
Judith Herb College of Education, Health Sciences, and Human Services
University of Toledo
Toledo, OH
Chapter 6

Sue Grogan-Johnson, PhD, CCC-SLP
Assistant Professor of Speech-Language Pathology
School of Health Sciences
Kent State University
Kent, OH
Chapter 5

K. Todd Houston, PhD, CCC-SLP, LSLS Cert. AVT
Director, Telepractice & eLearning Laboratory (TeLL)
Associate Professor of Speech-Language Pathology
School of Speech-Language Pathology and Audiology
College of Health Professions
The University of Akron
Akron, OH
Chapters 1, 4, and 12

Farzan Irani, PhD, CCC-SLP
Assistant Professor of Speech-Language Pathology
Department of Communication Disorders
Texas State University
San Marcos, TX
Chapters 6 and 8

Jennifer L. Milam, PhD
Assistant Professor
Early Childhood and Curriculum Studies
The University of Akron
Akron, OH
Chapter 9

Scott T. Palasik, PhD, CCC-SLP
Assistant Professor of Speech-Language Pathology
School of Speech-Language Pathology and Audiology
The University of Akron
Akron, OH
Chapter 8

Arlene Stredler-Brown, CCC-SLP, CED
Co-Investigator, TACIT: Therapy After Cochlear Implantation Using Telemedicine
University of Colorado
Boulder, CO
Adjunct Faculty
Department of Speech, Language, and Hearing Sciences
University of British Columbia
Vancouver, British Columbia
Chapters 2 and 4

Lyn R. Tindall, PhD, CCC-SLP
Speech-Language Pathologist
Department of Veterans Affairs Medical Center
Assistant Professor
Physical Medicine and Rehabilitation
University of Kentucky
Lexington, KY
Chapter 7

Kami Zeckzer Walters, MA
Principal
Little Hearts Preschool
Jerusalem, Israel
Chapter 4

Tali R. Weinberg, BA
School of Speech-Language Pathology and Audiology
College of Health Professions
The University of Akron
Akron, OH
Chapters 1 and 9

This book is dedicated to the many families, children, and adults who continue to teach me as I try to serve them through telepractice. You all are a constant inspiration to me, both professionally and personally.

I also dedicate this book to my family: Maria, Kaitlyn, Jordan, Floyd, and Lily. Without your support, this work would not have been possible.

1

History, Definitions, and Overview of Telepractice Models

K. Todd Houston, Anne M. Fleming, Kelly J. Brown, Tali R. Weinberg, and Jessica M. Nafe

Introduction

Throughout history, individuals have created and utilized forms of communication technology to relay or transmit health-related information over a distance (Bashshur & Shannon, 2009). Innovation has led to technological advancements and the development of various forms of "tele" communication. The prefix "tele," the Greek root word for distant or remote (Darkins & Cary, 2000), is used to describe the transfer of information over a distance, such as the telegraph and telephone. Although today's telecommunication applications are quite advanced and allow for relatively seamless audio and video transmission in real time, the origins of this technology can be traced back over centuries—when various methods were used to communicate health information over a range of distances. From the simple messenger who ran to relay critical information, to the telegraph and the telephone, through the present-day use of the Internet, a technological evolution has occurred to support this desire to communicate health care information over long distances.

Today, an increasing number of health care providers are adapting their practices to support models of telehealth, which is rapidly becoming the preferred term across disciplines. Telemedicine, however, continues to be used to describe those diagnostic and treatment services delivered over distance by a physician, nurse, or related professional (Fong, Fong, & Li, 2011). Likewise, speech-language pathologists are using models of telepractice through online videoconferencing software, distance learning technology, and other dedicated telecommunication systems to provide diagnostic and treatment services to a range of patients with speech, language, and hearing disorders or delays. The American Speech-Language-Hearing Association (ASHA) describes this service delivery model as telepractice for practitioners in audiology and speech-language pathology (ASHA, 2005e, 2005f, 2010), and it is defined as "the application of telecommunications technology to deliver professional services at a distance by linking clinician to client, or clinician to clinician for assessment, intervention, and/or consultation." By understanding the past, key definitions, and various service delivery models, practitioners can fully realize the potential of telepractice applications.

History of "Tele" Communication

The Telegraph: The Beginning of Modern Distance Communication

Disagreement among scholars continues to foster considerable discussion and research about early origins of distance communication for health or medical purposes. Some scholars have proposed that the earliest form of distance communication involved the simple messenger who walked or ran from point to point delivering the news of sickness, war casualties, and even famine. However, this was inefficient even when sending messengers by horseback proved to be faster. Although rather crude, one of the earliest but effective means of communication was the lighting of bonfires to signal information about the bubonic plague during the Middle Ages.

By the 1700s, various postal systems were used but were soon deemed unreliable. In the early 1800s, the heliograph, a mirrored device that could reflect sunlight, was used widely in Europe to signal information about death rates as a result of war or famine (Zundel, 1996).

Interestingly, a health-related incident led Samuel Morse to invent the single-wire telegraph, which also enabled the widespread use of Morse code (Bellis, 2009a, 2009b). In 1825, Morse, a respected painter, was in Washington, DC when he received word by horse messenger that his wife, Lucretia, was suffering through a difficult pregnancy. Terrified at the thought of losing his wife, Morse left Washington immediately to return to his home in New Haven, CT. Unfortunately, by the time Morse arrived, Lucretia had died in childbirth and was already buried. During his time in Washington, Morse was unaware that his wife had been sick for quite some time. Feeling deep remorse over his wife's death, Morse abandoned painting to devote the rest of his live in pursuit of a device that could provide long distance communication, the telegraph. On May 24, 1844, using the code that he and his colleagues had developed, Morse sent the message, "What hath God wrought," from the U.S. Capitol to a receiver in Baltimore.

The telegraph quickly set a new standard in long distance communication, and its use quickly spread. The telegraph and the growing dominance of the railroad for mass transportation and shipping are credited as important factors in the westward expansion of the United States (Dilts, 1996). During the American Civil War, the telegraph was used extensively to issue commands to troops on both sides of the conflict and to report troop movements. More importantly, it was also used to report casualty lists and to secure scarce medical supplies. Although the telegraph proved to be an important technological step in the communication of medical information, it is critical to note that Morse code has outlived the device. Since its invention, various militaries, first responders, and other civil service personnel continue to use the code to relay information in situations when other devices have failed.

Whereas Morse perfected wired communication, a relatively unknown inventor, Mahlon Loomis, experimented with what he called "wireless telegraphy." In 1866, Loomis demonstrated his invention between two mountain peaks in Virginia. Although mostly lost to history, Loomis' invention was a forerunner to modern-day radio transmissions, but it would take another three decades before the Italian inventor, Guglielmo Marconi, would be credited with its invention in 1895.

Dr. Alexander Graham Bell: The Telephone and the Photophone

In 1875, Dr. Alexander Graham Bell uttered the immortalized words, "Mr. Watson, come here, I want you!" into a rather crude transmitter after spilling acid on his leg. In the next room, Thomas A. Watson, a lab assistant, heard Dr. Bell's voice clearly through the receiver. In that moment, if this incident occurred, a new form of mass communication was born—the telephone. The acid incident could possibly have been the first documented example of someone seeking medical-specific intervention via "modern" technology (Carson, 2007).

Although Bell later understood the wider implications for his invention, his initial experiments focused on how to transmit speech across a wire. Bell, a noted elocutionist and teacher of the deaf, believed that children with even the most significant hearing loss could develop intelligible spoken language if given appropriate instruction. The telephone, therefore, was a product of his work with childhood hearing loss, the primary medical and educational interest of his life.

Although Bell became quite famous for the invention of the telephone, he believed that his photophone would be recognized as his greatest and most important invention. The photophone was designed to use a modulated light beam to transmit a person's voice over a distance. Both the transmitter and receiver consisted of a plane of mirrors and a selenium cell. The modulating light from the transmitter would be interpreted as a speech signal and would be reproduced in the receiver. Bell first transmitted a message through his photophone when he sent a message a distance of 700 feet between two rooftops in Washington, DC in April 1880.

Unfortunately, Bell's wish for the photophone to revolutionize telephone communication would not be immediately realized. Because the photophone depended on bright light for signal transmission, he could not overcome the effects of inclement weather. However, the basic concepts employed by the photophone became the precursors for modern fiberoptic communication, which uses light to transmit large amounts of information at extremely high speeds.

Early 20th Century: The Telephone Spreads and Radio Emerges

By the turn of the century, telephones were in use and physicians were among the first to utilize the technology in medical care. Gunsch (2011) observes that telemedicine began—on a limited basis—in the early 1900s when electrocardiograms, a graphic display of the electrical changes in the heart, were transmitted over telephone lines and physicians were able to read the results. Within the next decade, radio communication was in place. For convenience, physicians and other medical personnel used radio to provide a range of health consultations. Radio continued to be the primary long-distance communication technology used in times of military engagement (i.e., World War I and II, Korean, and Vietnam conflicts) and was often used to dispatch medical teams, communicate injury reports, and order helicopters or other transportation to evacuate the injured (Zundel, 1996).

Mid 20th Century: Television and Space Exploration

The 1950s ushered in widespread use of black and white televisions, which were quickly becoming one of the primary mediums of entertainment and communication for the masses. In terms of medical applications, the ability to visualize a patient's condition rather than rely on an audio description greatly enhanced diagnosis and the confidence of those engaged in treatment (House & Roberts, 1977). During this time, the Nebraska Psychiatric Institute, with funding from the National Institute for Mental Health, is credited with being one of the first facilities to use closed-circuit television for health care purposes (Wurm, Hofmann-Wellenhof, Wurm, & Soyer, 2008). An interactive, closed-circuit television system was established between two hospitals that were over 100 miles apart, and doctors were able to effectively conduct interviews with psychiatric patients.

By the early 1960s, the space race was in full gear as President John F. Kennedy pledged to go to the moon by the end of the decade. As a result, the National Aeronautics and Space Administration (NASA) collected physiologic measures of astronauts during spaceflight, which also led to wider use of satellite technology for telecommunications. Using telemetric data transmitted from the astronauts' spacesuits, medical personnel in ground control were able to continuously monitor heart rate, blood pressure, and electrocardiograms (Wurm et al., 2008). Through the 1990s, NASA continued to support a variety of early telemedicine research projects to determine preferred practices in the remote diagnosis and treatment of a range of medical conditions. (For more information on this history, see Allan, 2006; Welsh, 1999; and Wurm et al., 2008.)

Late 20th Century: Telecommunication Technology Established

In the early to mid-1970s, several projects around the country continued to perfect telemedicine and telepractice applications. One innovative project was led by Dr. Kenneth T. Bird of Massachusetts General Hospital in Boston who established an interactive system using direct microwave transmission from Logan Airport to the hospital to provide medical care for travelers (Thrall, 2007).

Another project, the Space Technology Applied to Rural Papago Advanced Health Care (STARPAHC), was developed by NASA and managed by the U.S. Indian Health Service. The project used advanced telecommunication technology to deliver medical services on the Papago Indian reservation (Freiburger, Holcomb, & Piper, 2007). The project was active from 1973 until 1977 and proved significant by demonstrating the effectiveness of telepractice applications, as summarized by Bashshur (1980):

- NASA and the Indian Health Services demonstrated the organizational and technological capacity to provide medical care to remote populations;
- The approach to the design and implementation of this mode of care delivery was effective and held promise for other situations;
- The project demonstrated the efficacy of remote telemetry and nonphysician personnel in the provision of health care services; and
- The cooperation and advance planning on the part of all participants in the project can serve as a model for others.

Although these projects demonstrated overall effectiveness of providing medical care over distance, the majority of these early experiments were not sustainable due to the high cost associated with the project. Additionally, the technology available at the time could not provide adequate quality, and the cost-to-benefit ratio led many of these efforts to be discontinued (Wurm et al., 2008). For much of the 1980s, the exploration of telemedicine applications declined. NASA, the Department of Veterans Affairs (VA), and branches of the military continued to support some projects, and other isolated programs labored on. However, in the early 1990s interest in telemedicine and telepractice began to grow again, spurred on by rapid advancements in information and telecommunications technology and digital data transmission, especially via the Internet (Wurm et al., 2005).

1990s Through Today: Internet Expands and Computers Increase Capacity

Recognizing the potential positive impact on health care, federal departments and agencies, the military, private industry, for-profit and nonprofit medical institutions, and universities increased the study of and support for telemedicine and telepractice models and their broad applications. This was made possible due in large part to the development of the Internet.

With the creation of computers in the 1950s came the need for a system that allowed for "connected" communication and information sharing. By the 1960s, the U.S. government provided research funding to design and build an interconnected network or "internet" that would allow computers around the globe to communicate seamlessly with each other using various protocols. Subsequent additional federal funding from the National Science Foundation in the 1980s as well as other nonfederal, commercial, and private funding continued to expand the Internet (Hafner, 1998).

Today, the World Wide Web is a collection of millions of web pages that can be viewed on a web browser from any computer, utilizing hypertext transfer protocol (HTTP). E-mail, another subnetwork of the Internet, utilizes simple mail transfer protocol (SMTP) and post office protocol (POP) to send text and picture messages from one private inbox to another or several others. Scientists continue to improve the quality of data transfer through these protocols over the Internet. Today, more than 66% of U.S. adults use high-speed, broadband Internet connections in their homes, up from only 55% in 2008 (Smith, 2010).

With the rapid proliferation of broadband Internet connections, the relatively inexpensive telecommunications and computing technology (e.g., laptops, desktop computers, smartphones), and the availability of online software and teleconferencing websites (e.g., Skype, ooVoo, Google Hangout, Facetime, etc.), telemedicine and telepractice service delivery models have become more widely available, reliable, and cost-efficient. Distance learning technology and telecommunications equipment are increasingly being adopted by physicians and other health care providers, hospitals, and medical centers to provide diagnostics and treatment in a variety of areas, resulting in a range of discipline-specific terminology such as telemental health, telenursing, telepharmacy, telecardiology, telepathology, teleradiology, telepsychology, telerehabilitation, teletherapy, teleintervention, and telepractice. Bashshur, Shannon, Krupinski, and Grigsby (2011) also address this challenge of the taxonomy of telemedicine, discussing the various working definitions with the intent of clarifying the proliferation of nomenclature in telemedicine but also providing a useful guide for research and policymaking. To this end, practitioners and some professional associations and organizations are adopting the term "telehealth" as the preferred term, regardless of discipline.

Innovation in Telemedicine and Telepractice: The Department of Veterans Affairs

The Department of Veterans Affairs (VA) began utilizing telemedicine in the 1970s and continues its use of these services today to reach veterans who may not have health care services in their community. With almost 39% of veterans residing in rural areas, access to a VA hospital or medical center is not always an option. To provide greater access to health care, the VA established community-based outpatient clinics (CBOC). However, due to the lack of trained staff and services offered at the CBOCs, the VA was determined to find a better way to reach the rural population of veterans (Dennis, Gladden, & Noe, 2012). With the establishment of the Office of Telehealth Services (OTS) in 2003, an array of health care services became available for veterans, regardless of their geographical location. Following the establishment of the OTS, telemental health was added later in 2003, telerehabilitation (including Speech-Language Pathology) and teleretinal imaging in 2005, and primary care telehealth in 2011 (Dennis et al., 2012).

Today, the VA focuses on three services provided via telepractice: clinical video telehealth (CVT), home telehealth (HT), and store and forward telehealth (SFT). Through clinical video telehealth, a remote patient can use real-time interactive videoconferencing to receive mental health services and specialty consultations. Home telehealth is a way for providers to monitor and manage patients with acute and chronic diseases while they are living at home. Home telehealth strives to improve clinical outcomes and reduce the need for further hospitalizations or complications. The store and forward telehealth program uses technology to obtain and transfer a patient's health care information between providers (Dennis et al., 2012; IOM, 2012). Each service area has its own national training center, operated by OTS, at various locations across the United States. As of 2012, almost 600,000 patients were receiving telemedicine services, making the VA a national leader in telehealth services (Dennis et al., 2012).

Telepractice and Speech-Language Pathology

As videoconferencing technology has become more widely available, the associated equipment costs have declined, and these services have become more cost-efficient. As a result, the use of web-based videoconferencing technology to provide health-related services has been used by a variety of medical and allied health disciplines, including speech-language pathology. However, whereas current technology capabilities have allowed for more rapid adoption of telepractice service delivery models, speech-language pathologists actually have used these models for nearly 40 years.

In the mid-1970s, one of the first pioneering applications of telepractice service delivery in speech-language pathology occurred at the Birmingham Veterans Administration (VA) Hospital in Alabama (Vaughn, 1976). Dr. Gwenyth Vaughn, Chief of Audiology and Speech Pathology Services, developed a "Tele-Communicology" project that would provide remote, supplementary treatment and evaluation for patients with speech, language, and hearing disorders—typically over the telephone. More specifically, Dr. Vaughn investigated methods to identify, modify, and design interventions that assisted clinicians when working with patients with neurological impairments and those with alaryngeal speech.

A decade later, Wertz et al. (1987) examined the reliability of diagnostic testing of adults by comparing three modes of assessment: traditional face-to-face (i.e., in-person), telepractice using a closed-circuit television, and telepractice using a video laser disc and telephone system. The closed-circuit television system was set up in two existing rooms at the therapy center. A video camera and monitor (television) were set up in both rooms so that real-time audio and video feeds could be transmitted between the rooms.

The clinician and patient could hear and see each other during the assessment process. For the laser disc method, testing material was recorded onto the laser disc and played for the client on a television that contained a touch screen in the patient's setting. The clinician was able to monitor responses to the touch screen at the same time the patient responded. A speaker phone was used to allow for audio communication during the session. As with the television method, the laser disc and telephone system was set up in two existing therapy rooms within one facility. With both methods, a volunteer was present in the room with the patient to assist with access to technology and ordering of testing materials (Wertz et al., 1987).

Thirty-six patients were tested using the three delivery methods, and data were analyzed to identify any variance in testing scores and diagnosis as a result of the system used. Assessments administered included The Western Aphasia Battery (Kertesz, 1982), Porch Index of Communicative Ability (Porch, 1967), sections from the Mayo Clinic Procedures for Language Evaluation (unpublished), and the Reading Comprehension Battery for Aphasia (LaPointe & Horner, 1979). The study found a 93% overall agreement between assessments conducted face-to-face and via closed-circuit television, and a 91% overall agreement between assessments conducted face-to-face and via computer-controlled video laser disc. In addition, there was a 91% overall agreement between the two modes of telepractice (Wertz et al., 1987).

Similarly, the Mayo Clinic began using telepractice to diagnose speech and language disorders a program known as Telemedicine Consultants (TMCs) (Duffy, Werven, & Aronson, 1997) in 1987. Technology involved with this project allowed the clinician to control the video and audio transmitted from the patient in order to change camera angles for a desired view or to adjust sound levels to comfort. The program assessed patients with suspected neurogenic motor speech disorders and other conditions. The project reported successful administration of oral mechanism exams with the use of an assistant at the location of the client. The clinician used a "close-up view" to observe physical characteristics of the patient's oral structures and function. The assistant was used to probe reflexes and other hands-on testing. Motor speech exams were conducted by asking the client to repeat desired phonemes, words, phrases, and paragraphs. Language testing was also conducted, which included both expressive and receptive tasks. A writing sample was sometimes generated and transmitted over the system for the clinician to review. The administration of these types of testing was well within the limits of the technology available (Duffy et al., 1997).

Although telepractice in speech-language pathology dates back almost four decades, the past decade has seen more rapid adoption of this service delivery model. Mashima and Doarn (2010) completed a recent review of the prevailing literature and described broad application of telepractice in the field, including treatment of neurogenic communication disorders, fluency disorders, voice disorders, dysphagia, and childhood speech and language disorders. Likewise, in a similar review of the literature, Theodoros (2011) found that roughly 25% of all studies investigated reported client and/or clinician satisfaction data, and the majority conveyed positive outcomes associated with telepractice service delivery. (See Chapter 2 for more information on the efficacy of telepractice applications in speech-language pathology.)

The American Speech-Language-Hearing Association and Telepractice

Since the late 1990s, the American Speech-Language-Hearing Association (ASHA) has studied the potential impacts and application of videoconferencing and distance learning technology within telepractice service delivery models. In 1998, ASHA published the Telehealth Issues Brief (ASHA, 1998), which described to date various telepractice applications in the field. To further inform its members, ASHA incorporated telepractice into its 2001–2003 Focused Initiative on Technology, an association effort to increase members' knowledge and access to ASHA products, information, and activities related to the use of telepractice in the delivery of clinical services in audiology and speech-language pathology (ASHA, 2005).

In 2002, to gather additional data about telepractice applications in the field, ASHA conducted a telephone survey (ASHA, 2002) of members, receiving responses from 1,667 participants regarding their experiences and knowledge of telepractice. They found that 11% delivered services via telepractice. Of those members who were providing telepractice services, the data also revealed that:

- 93% reported that they delivered telepractice via the telephone;
- 74% reported utilizing e-mail;
- 40% reported using Web-based information/resources;
- 13% used Web-based conferencing; and
- 8% utilized video teleconferencing.

The most common use of telepractice was for consultation with other professionals (42%). Direct patient care came in second at 38%, followed by education (15%) and supervision (6%). Of the patient care services, 76% were follow-up, 66% counseling, 37% treatment, and 16% equipment check (ASHA, 2002).

ASHA has worked to educate members on the area of telepractice. Between 2001 and 2003, ASHA collaborated with the National Rehabilitation Hospital's Rehabilitation Engineering Research Center on Telerehabilitation to create presentations for ASHA members to present at various meetings to inform other members about telepractice (ASHA, 2005f). In 2003, ASHA provided $4,000 grants to three programs to develop materials that would inform members about their telepractice activities (ASHA, 2005f).

ASHA Policy Documents

With the increase in the use of telepractice in both speech-language pathology and audiology, ASHA has developed policy positions and documents to guide practitioners in development and implementation of telepractice programs. In 2003, the Telepractice Working Group was formed and subsequently developed a position statement, technical reports, and knowledge and skills documents for each profession (Brown, 2011). Those documents, listed in the following, have created a foundation of practice on which current telepractice has been built.

- Telepractices and ASHA: Report of the Telepractices Team (ASHA, 2001)
- Audiologists Providing Clinical Services via Telepractice: Position Statement (ASHA, 2005a)
- Audiologists Providing Clinical Services via Telepractice: Technical Report (ASHA, 2005b)
- Knowledge and Skills Needed by Audiologists Providing Clinical Services via Telepractice (ASHA, 2005c)
- Knowledge and Skills Needed by Speech-Language Pathologists Providing Clinical Services via Telepractice (ASHA, 2005d)
- Speech-Language Pathologists Providing Clinical Services via Telepractice: Position Statement (ASHA, 2005e)
- Speech-Language Pathologists Providing Clinical Services via Telepractice: Technical Report (ASHA, 2005f).

As Brown (2011, pp. 4–5) states, "the enduring contribution of these documents for the past decade has been to establish the use of the term telepractice and to provide guidance about how to evaluate the quality of a service without specifying the type of technology, thus allow for continued growth in the rapidly expanding areas of connectivity and equipment."

ASHA's position statement defines telepractice as "the application of telecommunications technology to deliver professional services at a distance by linking clinician to client, or clinician to clinician for assessment, intervention, and/or consultation" (ASHA, 2005e, 2005f). Furthermore, as Brown (2011) notes, ASHA's position statement supports telepractice as "an appropriate model of service delivery" and the same Code of Ethics and Scope of Practice as well as applicable state and federal laws also apply to every practitioner (ASHA, 2005e, 2005f). As well, the position statement establishes that "the quality of services delivered via telepractice must be consistent with the quality of services delivered face-to-face (e.g., in person; ASHA, 2005e, 2005f; Brown, 2011). Thus, the practitioner must ensure that telepractice is an appropriate service delivery model that can meet the specific diagnostic and/or treatment needs of the patient being served.

To accommodate changes in technology and practice, ASHA updated its earlier report and appointed an Ad Hoc Committee on

Telepractice in Speech-Language Pathology in 2008. The committee, comprised of four speech-language pathologists and a rehabilitation engineer, developed the document, Professional Issues in Telepractice for Speech-Language Pathologists (ASHA, 2010). The document expanded on the previous 2005 reports to include updated terminology and addressed components of quality of service delivery in telepractice, such as technology, clinician competency, reliance on available evidence, and the use of outcome measures (Brown, 2011).

And finally, to provide more focused attention to telepractice applications in both speech-language pathology and audiology, ASHA established the Telepractice Special Interest Group (SIG 18) in 2010. Through this newly formed SIG and its publication, *Perspectives*, members can share information, promote efficacious practices, and work collaboratively to address many of the prevailing professional issues that face both practitioners and consumers of the services.

Professional Issues in Telepractice

ASHA (2010) continues to detail a range of professional issues that have the potential to impact clinicians providing services through telepractice (ASHA, 2010). Three of the most important professional issues include privacy regulations, licensure, and reimbursement for services.

Privacy

In some settings, telepractice may not be allowed for fear of violating the Health Insurance Portability and Accountability Act of 1996 (HIPAA). HIPAA addresses a patient's protected health information and requires that telepractice sessions be protected from unauthorized access. When utilizing VoIP software, such as Skype, consistent protection from third parties is not guaranteed. In addition, many of these companies are based in countries outside of the United States where data would not be protected under federal privacy laws (Cohn & Watzlaf, 2011). In order to stay within HIPAA compliance guidelines and the ASHA code of ethics, it is best to choose a secure software program that can provide necessary data transfer protection and in turn guarantee the security of clients' personal information.

Although HIPAA is in place to protect health information, the legislation does not specify the method of protection when conducting telepractice. Some facilities have made reasonable accommodations by carefully selecting software and hardware that offer protection from unwanted access through effective encryption and network security. For example, the Internet connection between the provider and the patient can be secured by establishing virtual private networks (VPNs), using enhanced firewall software on the provider's and patient's computers, and password protection when logging into secure websites or videoconferencing services.

Licensure

Licensure remains a challenge for telepractice providers in most states. According to ASHA (2010), only a small number of state licensure boards have addressed telepractice in their legislation or regulatory language, but this situation is slowly changing. Considerable variability exists among states in terminology and the specificity of existing regulations. Providing telepractice services across state lines requires securing and maintaining licensure in both states. This requirement is often cost prohibitive and requires considerable administrative support and oversight. For these reasons, providers usually limit their services to their home state. Currently, several organizations (e.g., the Federation of State Medical Boards, American Telemedicine Association) are exploring and advocating systems of licensure portability that remove barriers and improve access to interstate telepractice services. Similarly, credentialing and privileging by proxy, when allowed by the originating site where the patient is located, is based on reciprocity by the consultants' primary organization. This type of reciprocity facilitates the provision of telepractice services while ensuring that the provider is appropriately qualified to deliver the service. The Centers for Medicare and Medicaid Services (CMS) has adopted this option, which, it so happens, had already been implemented by the Joint Commission, the national organization tasked to approve and monitor the accreditation of hospitals throughout the United States.

Reimbursement for Telepractice Services

Reimbursement for services continues to be a challenge for providers who are utilizing telepractice models. Romanow and Brannon (2010) describe some of these challenges and the fact that as telepractice in health care continues to grow, CMS, Medicare, and Medicaid either do not allow telepractice or restrict reimbursement for audiological and speech-language services provided through a telepractice model. Although this is disheartening, some states have modified their state regulations regarding Medicaid or have passed legislation that defines how reimbursement can occur. Although not perfect, practitioners should investigate if and how these services have been addressed in their state as well as nationally, such as via CMS and other payers. Changes in health care funding paradigms beyond the traditional fee-for-service model should also allow coverage for audiology and speech-language services. In 2010, the Patient Protection and Access to Care Act (PPACA) was passed, which has created new opportunities to explore innovative service delivery models that improve access to health care and have the potential for lowering associated costs. These efforts will hopefully lead to recognition by CMS and more widespread reimbursement for telepractice services (Brown, 2011).

Conclusion

The need to communicate health-related information quickly and efficiently has often been a driving force behind new technological advancements especially over the past 2 centuries. Today, modern technology allows constant connectivity from a range of devices and the ability to see and hear others in real time, whether they are just down the street or thousands of miles away. Inevitably, the widespread availability of this technology—used in combination with the Internet—has allowed professionals to provide a range of speech and language services through telepractice. The growth of telepractice service delivery models is a means of improving access to critical diagnostic and treatment services, improving patient outcomes, and reducing overall costs. Although challenges remain, resolutions for some of the issues are forthcoming as multiple disciplines embrace the large-scale implementation of telehealth and telepractice as standards of care for the patients they serve. If history is our teacher, the next decade will assuredly see even more improvement in technology and service delivery models that will only enhance telepractice, and, in turn, foster better outcomes for those receiving these services.

References

Allan, R. (2006). *A brief history of telemedicine.* Penton Media. Available from http://electronicdesign.com/print/components/a-brief-history-of-telemedicine

American Speech-Language-Hearing Association. (1998). *Telehealth issues brief.* Rockville, MD: Author.

American Speech-Language-Hearing Association. (2001). *Telepractices and ASHA: Report of the telepractices team.* Rockville, MD: Author.

American Speech-Language-Hearing Association. (2002). *Survey report on telepractice use among audiologists and speech-language pathologists.* Rockville, MD: Author.

American Speech-Language-Hearing Association. (2005a). *Audiologists providing clinical services via telepractice: Position statement* [Position Statement]. Available from http://www.asha.org/policy

American Speech-Language-Hearing Association. (2005b). *Audiologists providing clinical services via telepractice: Technical report* [Technical Report]. Available from http://www.asha.org/policy

American Speech-Language-Hearing Association. (2005c). *Knowledge and skills needed by audiologists providing clinical services via telepractice* [Knowledge and skills]. Available from http://www.asha.org/telepractice.htm

American Speech-Language-Hearing Association (2005d). *Knowledge and skills needed by speech-language pathologists providing clinical ser-*

vices via telepractice [Knowledge and skills]. Available from http://www.asha.org/telepractice.htm

American Speech-Language-Hearing Association. (2005e). *Speech-language pathologists providing clinical services via telepractice: Position statement* [Position Statement]. Available from http://www.asha.org/telepractice

American Speech-Language-Hearing Association. (2005f). *Speech-language pathologists providing clinical services via telepractice: Technical report* [Technical report]. Available from http://www.asha.org/policy

American Speech-Language-Hearing Association. (2010). *Professional issues in telepractice/telespeech for speech-language pathologists.* Available from http://www.asha.org/telepractice.htm

Bashshur, R. L. (1980). *Technology serves the people: The story of a co-operative telemedicine project by NASA, the Indian Health Service and the Papago people.* Tucson, AZ: Indian Health Service, Office of Research and Development, pp.107–109.

Bashshur, R. L., & Shannon, G. W. (2009). *History of telemedicine: Evolution, context, and transformaton.* New Rochelle, NY: Mary Ann Liebert, Inc.

Bashshur, R. L., Shannon, G. W., Krupinski, E., & Grigsby, J. (2011). The taxonomy of telemedicine. *Telemedicine and e-Health, 17*, 484–494.

Brown, J. (2011). Asha and the evolution of telepractice. *Perspectives on Telepractice, 1*(1), 4–9. doi: 10.1044/tele1.1.4

Carson, M. K. (2007). *Alexander Graham Bell: Giving voice to the world.* New York, NY: Sterling Publishing Company.

Darkins, A., & Cary, M. (2000). *Telemedicine and telehealth: Principles, policies, performance and pitfalls.* New York, NY: Springer Publishing Company, Inc.

Dennis, K. C., Gladden, C. F., & Noe, C. M. (2012). *Telepractice in the Department of Veterans Affairs. Hearing review, 19*(10), 44–50. Retrieved from http://www.hearingreview.com/practice-management/17321-telepractice-in-the-department-of-veterans-affairs

Dilts, J. D. (1996). *The Great Road: The building of the Baltimore and Ohio, the nation's first railroad, 1828–1853.* Palo Alto, CA: Stanford University Press.

Duffy, J. R., Werven, G. W., & Aronson, A. E. (1997). Telemedicine and the diagnosis of speech and language disorders. *Mayo Clinic Proceedings*, *72*(12), 1116–1122. Retrieved from http://www.mayoclinicproceedings.org/article/PIIS0025619611636732/fulltext

Freiburger, G., Holcomb, M., & Piper, D. (2007). The STARPAHC collection:

Part of an archive of the history of telemedicine. *Journal of Telemedicine and Telecare*, *13*, 221–223.

Gunsch, J. (2011). *What is telemedicine? Conjecture corporation.* Available from http://www.wisegeek.com/what-is-telemedicine.htm

Hafner, K. (1998). *Where wizards stay up late: The origins of the Internet.* New York, NY: Simon & Schuster.

House, A. M., & Roberts, J. M. (1977). Telemedicine in Canada. *Canadian Medical Association Journal, 117*(4), 386–388.

IOM (Institute of Medicine). 2012. *The role of telehealth in an evolving health care environment: Workshop summary*. Washington, D.C.: National Academies Press.

Kertesz, A. (1982). *Western aphasia battery.* New York, NY: Grune and Stratton.

LaPointe, L. L., & Horner, J. (1979). *Reading comprehension battery for aphasia.* Tigard, OR: C. C. Publications, Inc.

Mashima, P. A., & Doarn, C. R. (2008). Overview of telehealth activities in speech-language pathology. *Telemedicine and e-Health*, *14*(10), 1101–1117. Retrieved from http://www.americantelemed.org/files/public/membergroups/PICATA/tmj_2008_0080.pdf

Mayo Clinic Procedures for Language Evaluation. (Unpublished).

Porch, B. E. (1967). *Porch index of communication ability.* Palo Alto, CA: Consulting Psychology Press.

Romanow, K., & Brannon, J. A. (2010, November 2). Telepractice reimbursement is still limited. *The ASHA Leader.*

Thrall, J. H. (2007). Teleradiology: Part 1. History and clinical applications. *Radiology*, *243*, 613–617.

Welsh, T. S. (1999). *Telemedicine. Telemedicine Network.* Available from http://ocean.st.usm.edu/~w146169/teleweb/telemed.htm

Wertz, R. T., Dronkers, N. F., Berstein-Ellis, E., Shubitowski, Y., Elman, R., Shenaut, G. K., Deal, J. L. (1987). Appraisal and diagnosis of neurogenic communication disorders in remote settings. *Clinical Aphasiology*, *17*, 117–123. Retrieved from http://aphasiology.pitt.edu/archive/00000925/01/17-12.pdf

Wurm, E. M. T., Hofmann-Wellenhof, R., Wurm, R., & Soyer, H. P. (2008). Telemedicine and teledermatology: Past, present and future. *Journal of the German Society of Dermatology*, *6*, 106–112.

Zundel, K. M. (1996). Telemedicine: History, applications, and impact on librarianship. *Bulletin of Medical Librarian Association*, *84*(1), 71–79.

2

Efficacy of Telepractice in Speech-Language Pathology

Arlene Stredler-Brown

Introduction

Telepractice is gaining global acceptance as evidence of its benefits emerge. Telepractice has been utilized in the diagnosis and treatment of children and adults in the fields of medicine, rehabilitation (e.g., psychology, speech-language pathology, audiology), and early intervention. According to the Agency for Healthcare Research and Quality (AHRQ), telepractice is described as the use of telecommunication technologies to deliver health-related services and information that support patient care, administrative activities, and health education (Dixon, Hook, & McGowan, 2008). In practical terms, telepractice is a service that is provided at a distance to a patient or client.

Many terms have been introduced to describe this service delivery model. Telemedicine provides medical services, delivered by a physician or at a hospital, from a distance (Darkins & Cary, 2000; Fong, Fong, & Li, 2011). Terms such as telecardiology, telepathology, teleradiology, and teledermatology have been used to describe services delivered remotely by medical subspecialties. Other professional disciplines have created their own terminology to describe these remote services. Psychologists use the term telemental health or telepsychology (Koocher, 2007; Nelson & Bui, 2010; Nelson, Bui, & Velasquez, 2011; Rabinowitz, Brennan, Chumbler, Kobb, & Yellowlees, 2008; Richardson et al., 2009). Telerehabilitation is a broad term that typically encompasses diagnosis and treatment provided by allied health professions (e.g., speech-language pathology, audiology, occupational therapy, physical therapy) (Brennan et al., 2010; Cason, 2009, 2011; Waite, 2010; Watzlaf, Moeini, Matusow, & Firouzan, 2011). To further refine the term "telerehabilitation," disciplines within the field of rehabilitation use terms such as tele-audiology (Hayes, Eclavea, Dreith, & Habte, 2012), tele-speech (Brennan et al., 2010), teletherapy (Brennan et al., 2010; Cason, 2009; Koocher, 2007; McCullough, 2001; Waite, 2010), and telepractice (ASHA, 2005a, 2005b, 2010). For infants and toddlers, early intervention programs have coined the term tele-intervention (Behl, Houston, & Stredler-Brown, 2012). In the field of education, tele-school has been used (McCarthy, 2012).

As Baker and Bufka (2011) stated, "terms are frequently used interchangeably as there is yet no universal definition or term used by legislators, policymakers, government agencies, and payers" (p. 405). Until stakeholders create standard terminology to avoid confusion and to provide consistency for readability, the term telepractice will be the predominant term used in this review of the literature. The term telepractice was selected, in part, because the American Speech-Language-Hearing Association (ASHA) defines service delivery at a distance as "telepractice" for practitioners in audiology and speech-language pathology (ASHA, 2005a, 2005b, 2010).

The use of telepractice started with a need to assist those living in remote or rural areas to access services. Almost 15 years ago, Pickering et al. (1998) reviewed the difficulty some clients had accessing speech-language services in rural, outback, and bush communities in six different countries: Australia, Canada, Hong Kong, South Africa, the United Kingdom, and the United States. Pickering et al. (1998) reported that access to services was challenging for a variety of reasons: (a) people living in remote communities may not have a speech-language pathologist (SLP) practicing there; (b) unique linguistic characteristics of some people living in less populated areas made it difficult to access services in the client's native language; and (c) it was difficult to identify providers who were aware of and respectful of the client's unique cultural identity.

With the expansive growth in the field of technology, telepractice has become ever more available and viable. Cason (2011) reported that telepractice supported these performance indicators: (1) timely receipt of services, (2) more consistent services due, in part, to fewer cancellations, and (3) delivery of services in a natural environment such as the home. Telepractice has been shown to mitigate provider shortages (Cason, 2011; Mashima & Doarn, 2008; McCarthy, Munoz, & White, 2010). More recently, programs in urban areas have engaged in telepractice (McConnochie et al., 2005; Shaikh, Cole, Marcin, & Nesbitt, 2008).

This review of the literature follows the emergence of telepractice in the medical field, its uptake in the field of psychology, past and current interest in the field of speech-language pathology, and nascent efforts in early intervention. The focus is on studies that deliver treatment rather than assessment.

Telepractice in the Medical Field

The medical profession was an early adopter of telepractice (i.e., telemedicine) service delivery models, which have been used to distribute limited resources, increase access to services, and close gaps in health disparities (Hailey, Roine, & Ohinmaa, 2002). Telepractice has been associated with decreased costs for services and improved health and wellness for recipients of care (Harper, 2006; Marcin et al., 2004). Five specialty areas from the health care profession were selected to demonstrate the effective use of telepractice in the medical field: absence from child care due to illness, dermatology, childhood obesity, psychiatry, and services delivered to children with special health care needs (CSHCN). These disciplines were selected for several reasons. Absence from child care due to illness has had health, education, and economic ramifications for families in urban areas (McConnochie et al., 2005). The application of telepractice in the field of dermatology had longitudinal studies of care (Bowns, Collins, Walters, & McDonagh, 2006; Loane et al., 2001). Studies on childhood obesity were selected, because the study designs included measures of client outcomes, which were considered more informative than measurements of client satisfaction (Mulgrew, Ulfat, & Nettiksimmons, 2011; Shaikh et al., 2008). A study from psychiatry was of interest because it addressed the ability to establish meaningful adult-to-adult relationships remotely (Hilty, Nesbitt, Kuenneth, Cruz, & Hales, 2007). And, research conducted with the CSHCN population had implications for several rehabilitation disciplines (i.e., occupational therapy, physical therapy, speech-language pathology) (Harper, 2006).

Absence from Child Care Due to Illness

McConnochie et al. (2005) investigated the impact of telepractice on children's absence from child care due to illness (ADI). This study, conducted in New York, engaged five child care centers from impoverished inner-city neighborhoods. The intent was to learn if attendance in child care would be affected with the adoption of telepractice. The investigators collected baseline attendance data for 18 weeks before initiating telepractice. After telepractice was implemented, there was a 63% reduction in children's absence from child care due to illness. Telepractice (i.e., telemedicine) was able to address health-related issues quickly and effectively without requiring parents to leave their own workplace and take their children home. It was notable that the medical professionals providing services were available promptly—within an average of 30 minutes from the time the service was requested. This speed of response was deemed beneficial to all parties—daycare providers, parents, and children.

Dermatology

The United Kingdom's Multicentre Teledermatology Trial was one of the world's largest telepractice research trials (Loane et al., 2001). First, Loane et al. (2001) established the clinical effectiveness and cost-effectiveness of using telepractice conducted in real time (RT) versus store-and-forward (S&F) mechanisms. In this study, a general practitioner saw each patient in the office while the patient received a consultation with a dermatologist located at a remote site. The study used a repeated measures design; all patients were seen in both telepractice conditions—RT and S&F. The results of this study demonstrated that telepractice conducted in RT was more efficient.

Having committed to RT telepractice, Loane et al. (2001) conducted another study that demonstrated the cost effectiveness of RT dermatology delivered through telepractice compared to conventional face-to-face (f2f) care. The results pointed out the cost benefit of telepractice; clinical outcomes demonstrated that dermatologists who saw patients in the telepractice condition recommended a further f2f hospital appointment less often. Fifty-six percent of the patients in the telepractice group were referred for a subsequent appointment, whereas 70% were referred from traditional f2f visits. Of note, the realized cost benefit was for patients living in rural areas; these patients benefited more than the providers.

Another group of researchers in the United Kingdom (Bowns et al., 2006) investigated diagnosis and treatment of dermatological disorders in both f2f and telepractice conditions. Based on the Patient Satisfaction Questionnaire (PSQ) (Ware, Snyder, Wright, & Davies, 1983), there was no statistical difference between the two groups. Only 38% of the patients preferred to discuss their condition in person, whereas 76% of the patients preferred to receive services remotely rather than wait for an f2f appointment.

Childhood Obesity

Articles on childhood obesity were selected because the study designs included measures both of satisfaction and, more importantly, client outcomes. Shaikh et al. (2008) conducted a survey in California that focused on patient outcomes as a result of telepractice consultations. The outcomes included: (a) improvements in patient nutrition, (b) increased activity levels, and/or (c) changes in weight. Results of this study showed that 80.6% of the patients receiving telepractice improved their diet; 69.4% demonstrated increased activity levels; 21% exhibited a slower rate of weight gain or weight maintenance; and 22.6% exhibited weight reduction.

Mulgrew et al. (2011) conducted a recent study of patient satisfaction as an indicator of the effectiveness of telepractice. In this study, the parents of children diagnosed as obese were exposed to both forms of health care delivery: f2f and telepractice. Mulgrew et al. (2011) noted no difference in overall parent satisfaction between the two groups. Parents reported that the provider using telepractice gave easy-to-understand directions. As well, parents were comfortable discussing their children's health problems. That said, parents rated telepractice visits slightly lower than f2f visits when asked if the provider explained things about the child's health in a way that was easy to understand. The authors suggested this concern might be due to the lack of access to visual support materials. If this were true, the criticism would be easy to ameliorate. Studies have shown that visual support materials can be made available by using a document reader, mailing printed materials, and making materials available on a website (Wade, Wolfe, Brown, & Pestian, 2005; Wilson & Wells, 2009).

Psychiatry

Hilty and colleagues (2007) studied the impact of psychiatry, delivered through telepractice, with a cohort of patients in California. The impact of treatment was measured using reports of participant satisfaction. The opinions of all participants were solicited including: patients, primary care providers (PCP), and participating psychiatrists. Reported on a 5-point Likert scale, all participant groups' mean scores indicated satisfaction with the telepractice model. The patient mean on the topic of being able to talk freely was 4.49. The patient mean on the topic of having needs met was 4.28. PCPs rated the quality of consultations at a mean of 4.83. It was also noted by the researchers that satisfaction with telepractice may have reflected the existing shortage of psychiatric providers in rural areas; hence, those living in geographically challenged areas were more inclined to be satisfied with any service versus no service at all (Hilty et al., 2007). Access was a motivation for accepting telepractice; satisfaction was statistically higher for those living in rural areas than for patients living in suburban areas.

Children with Special Health Care Needs (CSHCN)

To study whether services delivered through telepractice were as good as those delivered in the f2f condition, an interdisciplinary telemedicine team conducted evaluations of children on the CSHCN registry in Iowa (Harper, 2006). Professionals participating in this study worked in general practice (e.g., physicians, nurses), rehabilitation (e.g., social workers, psychologists, speech-language pathologists), and education. Groups of clients were matched for age, gender, socio-economic status (SES), and type of disability. A 55-item satisfaction survey, completed by parents and professionals, was conducted by phone. Parents in the telemedicine group viewed the consultations as at least as effective as direct onsite evaluations. A subgroup of parents experienced both f2f and telepractice conditions; they reported no significant differences in their ratings of the two experiences according to these indices: (a) quality of care, (b) allocation of physician and professional time, (c) ease of appointment making, and (d) quality of physician and professional care. Many professionals who participated in the telemedicine study were positive in their evaluations as well. Those providers who reported telemedicine as more favorable reported that it provided access to higher quality care, generated positive feedback from patients, had higher participation rates, and was a productive use of their professional time.

Marcin et al. (2004) investigated access to subspecialty consultations by children on the CSHCN registry in California. The satisfaction with telepractice, delivered by specialty consultants, was determined by using a 5-point Likert scale to measure satisfaction. Surveys were distributed to the primary care providers (PCPs and physician assistants) and to parents. Parents were asked five questions about: (1) training of staff, (2) ability to talk freely, (3) having needs met, (4) understanding the consultant, and (5) overall satisfaction. PCPs and physician assistants (PAs) were asked to address these topics: (1) quality of the video, (2) quality of the audio,

(3) confidence performing the examination, (4) understanding the consultant providing the service, and (5) overall satisfaction. Parents rated all questions in the 4 to 5 range and 98% wanted to continue receiving consultations through telepractice. Likewise, the PCPs and the PAs also scored all questions in the 4 to 5 range; scores for providers were even higher than those for parents.

The use of telepractice in the medical field (i.e., telemedicine) as it related to the fields of dermatology, childhood obesity, psychiatry, and children with special health care needs suggested telepractice was an effective service delivery platform that was also convenient, timely, and cost effective. Most importantly, patients were generally satisfied (Bowns et al., 2006; Hilty et al., 2007; Mulgrew et al., 2011).

Telepractice in Rehabilitation Fields

Subsequent to the implementation of telemedicine programs, practitioners in several rehabilitation disciplines have initiated trials with telepractice. Practitioners in psychology were pioneers. Some of the issues that propelled the development of telepractice in the field of psychology, such as the lack of psychologists in rural and remote areas (Rabinowitz et al., 2008), were deemed applicable to other client populations. Use of telepractice emerged in the fields of speech-language pathology and audiology. The adoption of telepractice models by early interventionists, serving children birth to 3 years of age, has been even more recent.

Psychology

Telepsychology has been defined as the use of real-time videoconferencing for the interaction of client and practitioner in the provision of psychology services that were usually delivered in person (Nelson & Bui, 2010). The American Counseling Association and the National Association of Social Workers endorsed the delivery of psychological services through telepractice (Epstein, 2011). The National Board of Certified Counselors also supported telepractice

(Gournaris, 2009). Short of an endorsement, per se, the American Psychological Association (APA) mentioned e-therapy in the introduction to its code of ethics as one of several therapeutic modalities (Epstein, 2011).

Rabinowitz et al. (2008) reviewed 380 studies using telepractice. Of these, only 14 studies had sample sizes greater than 10 and incorporated objective assessments and/or satisfaction surveys. Rabinowitz et al. (2008) persistently stated the need for multisite investigations on diverse ethnic populations using outcome variables other than satisfaction.

Nelson, Barnard, and Cain (2006) evaluated cognitive-behavioral therapy (CBT) treatment for childhood depression using traditional f2f treatment and interactive televideo (ITV) (i.e., telepractice). There were two strengths to the design of this study. One was the random assignment of clients to either f2f or telepractice settings. The other was that both the f2f treatment and the telepractice treatment were implemented in the clinic. Therefore, clients needed to travel to receive services one way or the other. The results show that CBT treatment across both delivery methods was effective in decreasing depressive symptoms. A measure of success was that 23 out of the 28 clients no longer met depression criteria at the end of treatment.

Wade et al. (2005) examined the feasibility and efficacy of using a hybrid approach (Nelson et al., 2006) that included both telepractice sessions and the use of Web-based modules with children diagnosed with traumatic brain injury (TBI). Each child received weekly sessions with the therapist. In addition, families accessed 7 to 11 online self-guided sessions on the Internet. The results were based on satisfaction with services from different perspectives: the children, the parents, and siblings. Participants rated telepractice sessions as very to extremely helpful. The children with TBI did not rate the services quite as favorably as their parents or their siblings, but this distinction was not statistically significant. The parents of all but one child reported improvements in the behavior problems exhibited by their children.

Nelson and Bui (2010) conducted a case study of one child and her mother using telepractice. Eight sessions were delivered over the course of 4 months and then maintenance therapy was offered one time each month thereafter. The outcomes of the therapy were measured using the Behavior Assessment System for Children (Reynolds & Kamphaus, 1992). At the end of treatment, the child's performance fell in the nonclinical range in all areas. This improvement was paired with a report of more adaptive functioning at home. There were some surprising perceived advantages to telepractice. One was that the client was less self-conscious. Another was the decreased concern about confidentiality, because services were delivered outside of the client's community.

Some researchers investigated specific treatment effects. For instance, working alliance is a central component of successful psychotherapy (Cook & Doyle, 2002). Working alliance, in the field of psychology, is measured according to three subscales on the Working Alliance Inventory (WAI) (Horvath & Greenberg, 1989): task, bonds, and goals. The task subscale measured collaboration between therapeutic partners—therapist and client—on specific technical in-session behaviors. The subscale for goals measured the degree to which therapist and client agreed on the desired outcomes of therapy. The bonds subtest looked at the quality of the human relationship between therapist and client (i.e., trust, attachment). Working alliance is of interest in that the telepractice condition may be perceived by some to limit or alter the quality of a relationship. Cook and Doyle (2002) investigated the development of working alliance through telepractice with participants in the United States and Canada. Clients were adults and ranged in age from 19 to 80 years old. Both groups received individual counseling services for a variety of problems. The results showed no significant differences or trends on any of the subscales or the composite score of the WAI based on the type of presenting problem. And, most importantly, all subscales and the composite score were actually higher for the telepractice group. Clients and therapists reported a positive experience; the results suggested "an empathic relationship can be strongly established regardless of modality of communication" (Cook & Doyle, 2002, p. 102). An added interest was the outcome for those who used a hybrid approach (e.g., more than one modality such as therapy and phone or therapy and e-mail) to have even higher composite and subscale scores on the WAI.

Corroborating the findings by Cook and Doyle (2002), Preschl, Maercker, and Wagner (2011) compared working alliance with clients receiving CBT in the f2f condition and via telepractice. The strength of this study was its experimental design and the number of participants. The researchers randomized clients to f2f therapy ($n = 28$) or telepractice ($n = 25$). Results using the Beck Depression Inventory (BDI) (Beck, Steer, & Brown, 1996), which was completed posttreatment, and the German version of the Working Alliance Inventory (WAI), which was completed at the middle and end of intervention, demonstrated the two groups did not differ significantly in ratings of working alliance. The therapists actually rated the tasks subscale on the WAI significantly higher for the group receiving telepractice. The results were promising; they supported the effectiveness of telepractice, corroborated previous research, and used an experimental design.

Speech-Language Pathology

The position statement of the American Speech-Language-Hearing Association (ASHA) (2005a) supports emerging efforts in telepractice and states:

"Telepractice is an appropriate model of service delivery for the profession of speech-language pathology. Telepractice may be used to overcome barriers of access to services caused by distance, unavailability of specialists and/or subspecialists, and impaired mobility. Telepractice offers the potential to extend clinical services to remote, rural, and underserved populations and to culturally and linguistically diverse populations" (ASHA, 2005a, p. 1).

ASHA has also specified parameters for standards of practice that are consistent with its prevailing code of ethics (ASHA, 2010). Although not an endorsement, these documents support the advancement of telepractice.

Many investigators have studied the use of telepractice to deliver speech and language services. Of the published articles, many are simply descriptive in nature. Fewer studies are empirically based; among these, many different research methodologies are used. Some studies investigated assessment procedures whereas others focused on treatment. Some studies were conducted with adults and fewer with children. This review of the literature in the field of speech-language pathology describes, briefly, the proof of concept for telepractice (Mashima & Doarn, 2008; Theodoros, 2008, 2011). A short review of studies on adults, with varying types of disabilities, follows (Clark, Dawson, Scheideman-Miller, & Post, 2002; Constantinescu et al., 2011; Howell, Tripoliti, & Pring, 2009; Mashima et al., 2003; Theodoros et al., 2006). The focus shifts to the use of telepractice to treat pediatric clients with various speech and language disorders in the United States (Forducey, 2006; Grogan-Johnson, Alvares, Rowan, & Creaghead, 2010) and in other countries (McCullough, 2001; Rose et al., 2000; Sicotte, Lehoux, Fortier-Blanc, & Leblanc, 2003; Waite, Cahill, Theodoros, Busuttin, & Russell, 2006). Whenever possible, studies were selected that used empirical methods of research with controlled samples. It should be noted, however, that there was a persistent request by many of the researchers to conduct studies with more rigorous design methodologies as most studies to date do not meet a high level of evidence; they require larger sample sizes, statistical analyses, or randomization of participants to treatment groups (Reynolds, Vick, & Haak, 2009).

Proof of Concept

Theodoros (2008), a noted Australian researcher in telepractice, suggested practitioners and administrators look at telepractice and ". . . the importance of service delivery models that are flexible, responsive to individual needs and sustainable" (Theodoros, 2008, p. 222). An overview of the literature was conducted by Mashima and Doarn (2008), which resulted in an observation that still holds true today. Of the 40 articles reviewed by these authors, most were pilot studies and provided anecdotal accounts rather than reports on well-controlled, randomized, clinical trials.

More recently, Theodoros (2011) stated that there continued to be a persistent need for telepractice. In addition, Theodoros

(2011) presented some new and forward-thinking ideas. Although there was a dogged need for telepractice to provide access to those living in rural or remote geographic areas, new considerations support the use of telepractice in urban areas as well. Some of the factors found to limit access to speech-language services in urban areas included the disability itself, the client's mobility, financial issues (e.g., cost to travel to a center), restrictive work schedules, and family support needs.

Adults

Clark and colleagues (2002) followed one stroke patient who received speech-language treatment via 62 telepractice sessions. The client's performance was evaluated with the Functional Communication Measure (FCM) (ASHA, 2003) before and after therapy. The client demonstrated improvement in all areas of the FCM following treatment.

Four treatment studies investigated the feasibility and validity of providing the Lee Silverman Voice Treatment using telepractice with clients with Parkinson's disease (PD) (Constantinescu et al., 2011; Howell et al., 2009; Mashima et al., 2003; Theodoros et al., 2006). Clients in the Howell et al. study (2009) demonstrated significant progress in sustained phonation, reading, and conversational speech. In a similar study by Theodoros et al. (2006), all 10 clients with PD showed significant improvements for vowel prolongation, reading, and conversational monologue, and pitch range. More recently, Constantinescu et al. (2011) conducted a randomized controlled trial with 34 clients with PD and found there was no significant difference between participants randomly assigned to f2f and remote treatment conditions when tested for sustained vowel phonation, reading, and monologue. Mashima et al. (2003) compared the outcomes of 51 individuals who received voice treatment who were randomly assigned to either f2f ($n = 28$) or remote ($n = 23$) treatment conditions. Results of this study indicated that there was no significant difference between groups for voice quality perceptual measures, acoustic changes for jitter and shimmer, and laryngeal changes. Positive treatment effects for both jitter ($d = .29$) and shimmer ($d = .12$) were noted for pre/post comparisons.

Pediatrics

Forducey (2006) supported the use of telepractice as an effective and efficient means to provide services for school-age children. Other studies focused on experimental treatment (versus diagnosis) of a variety of disorders in the pediatric population in the United States (Grogan-Johnson et al., 2010; Jessiman, 2003), in Ireland (Rose et al., 2000), in the United Kingdom (McCullough, 2001), and in Canada (Sicotte et al., 2003).

Forducey (2006) reported on a model of telepractice used with school-age children with speech and hearing disorders in Oklahoma. The Speech TeleTherapy program utilized real-time, two-way interactive video-conferencing throughout the state. This program was recognized by the Oklahoma Department of Education as an alternative to on-site speech services for children in rural and remote areas. A total of 11,000 sessions were provided by five part-time SLPs to 99 students in seven school districts. Anecdotal reports from the SLPs reported that students actively participated and accomplished their speech and language goals. Administrators at the building and district levels supported the project stating that telepractice provided consistent services that had been previously inaccessible.

Fluency

Sicotte and colleagues (2003) followed students with a diagnosis of stuttering living in Montreal, Canada. Each student attended two 1-hour treatment sessions with a parent. An analysis of fluency was conducted by measuring, as a dependent variable, the percentage of syllables stuttered (PSS). Videotapes were made of therapy sessions to gather this information. A videotape of each student was made two times before the therapy started, two times after the therapy ended, and three times during maintenance after treatment was terminated. Anything less than 50% PSS was considered an acceptable goal. Before treatment, the students demonstrated PSS rates ranging from 13% to 36%. After treatment, fluency rates were 2% to 26%. At the end of maintenance, students demonstrated rates ranging from 4% to 32%. Overall, there was a 52% decrease in stuttering for these students. This was especially laudable given the short duration of therapy compared to studies conducted in the f2f condition. The researchers stated that, ". . . this type of intervention is more demanding for the clinician, particularly when it comes to dealing with young children, and for parents, who must take an active role during treatment" (Sicotte et al., 2003, p. 57).

Articulation and Language

Four studies examined the treatment of a variety of communication disorders among preschool and school-aged children (Grogan-Johnson et al., 2010; Jessiman, 2003; McCullough, 2001; Rose et al., 2000). All had favorable outcomes for services delivered using telepractice.

An early effort in the United Kingdom studied preschool-aged children (Rose et al., 2000). This 3-year research project investigated quality of therapy and clinical effectiveness of treatment. The evaluation considered two models of therapy—telepractice and traditional f2f therapy. Parents reported overall satisfaction with minimal reservations about telepractice. Unfortunately, at the time of publication, no firm conclusions could be made based on clinical assessments.

McCullough (2001) provided services to five preschool-age children in Belfast, Ireland. The Attract Project explored the benefits of telepractice to child, caregiver, and clinician. This nonrandomized feasibility study was conducted with four clients with Down's syndrome ($n = 3$) and Cornelia de Lange syndrome ($n = 1$) and used surveys to measure caregiver satisfaction. The total response rate was 89%. Responses to the survey were measured on a 5-point Likert scale or by answering yes/no questions. In response to questions about their children's improvement, the mean parent score was 4.7. In response to the query, "Was the system useful in developing your skills with your child?" parents answered that the program was *very useful* (score of 5/5). When asked if the system enabled the parents to feel a part of the therapy program, parents also answered that it was *very useful* (score of 5/5). Parents reported that their knowledge of their children's language development improved (4/5). And, they answered resoundingly that they would miss the opportunity to receive services through telepractice when the project ended. The therapist also reported substantial improvements in the children's receptive and expressive vocabulary and vocal imitation skills according to informal records. One limitation to this study, so prevalent in the literature, is the absence of quantifiable or statistically measured outcomes.

An investigation by Jessiman (2003) included the treatment of two children using telepractice. The children, aged 7 years, and 5 years, 4 months, received biweekly therapy sessions for a 2-month period. Several articulation and language goals were targeted. Although there was no control group for comparison, Jessiman (2003) reported that both children made promising gains in their speech and language skills. Jessiman (2003) concluded that this improvement was at least partly due to the intervention, as no improvement was observed for three months between the initial assessment and the start of therapy. Questionnaires revealed that parents were satisfied with the improvements made during treatment using telepractice.

Of most interest was the recent study conducted by Grogan-Johnson et al. (2010) in Ohio. This study compared f2f therapy with telepractice using random assignment to one of the two treatment groups. Furthermore, each child in the study experienced both treatment conditions. Each student experienced one treatment condition for 4 months before switching to the other treatment mode. The dependent variable was the score on the Goldman-Fristoe Test of Articulation–2 (GFTA-2) (Goldman & Fristoe, 2002), which was administered at 4-month intervals. The results suggested that student performance in the telepractice condition was similar to student performance in the conventional f2f treatment condition. There was no significant difference between the two groups at the start of treatment (p = .16). There was no significant difference after the first 4 weeks in the initial treatment condition (p = .06). And, there was no significant difference after the second 4 weeks that were experienced in the alternative treatment condition (p = .21). The researchers also collected qualitative information from the participating SLPs. Perceived disadvantages of telepractice were that it was harder to collaborate with the classroom teachers and, subsequently, to relate the therapy to the classroom curriculum. On the other hand, there were perceived advantages. The SLPs thought IEP goals were accomplished, that a free and appropriate public education (FAPE) was provided, and that telepractice was easy to do. The study by Grogan-Johnson et al. (2010) had two limitations. The treatment in the two groups differed; the therapy in the f2f condition was group therapy whereas the therapy in the telepractice condition was individualized. A second limitation was that the SLPs for any one student were often different in the two treatment conditions.

Family-Centered Early Intervention (FCEI)

Family-centered early intervention (FCEI) has many unique characteristics. For instance, FCEI actively engages the parents of infants and toddlers by incorporating coaching techniques wherein the provider teaches the parents specific skills to practice with their children (Espe-Sherwindt, 2008; Fleming, Sawyer, & Campbell, 2011; Rush, Shelden, & Hanft, 2003; Woods, Wilcox, Friedman, & Murch, 2011). The use of coaching techniques has been supported by professional organizations working with infants and toddlers with disabilities (American Speech Language Hearing Association, 2008a, 2008b, 2008c; JCIH, 2007; Sandall, Hemmeter, Smith, & McLean, 2005). It is interesting to note that in spite of early support for the use of a coaching model (Rush et al., 2003), 10 years later, practitioners and administrators are still discussing ways to encourage its use. It seems fair to say that uptake has been difficult for most practitioners. Even when intervention sessions occur in the home, sessions tend to be predominantly child-focused rather than supporting interactions between parent and child (Campbell & Sawyer, 2007; Hebbeler, Spiker, Morrison, & Mallik, 2008; Peterson, Luzc, Eshbaugh, Jeon, & Kantz, 2007). After years of discussion, it is still unknown what might motivate practitioners to learn and use participatory practices such as coaching. It is possible, indeed likely, that telepractice will encourage this practice as infants and toddlers cannot be expected to actively engage with an interventionist remotely. Although the major incentive to adopt telepractice has been access to high-quality services for children living in remote and rural areas, telepractice may incidentally facilitate the use of coaching strategies by providers. Fortunately, the ability to form relationships between provider and adult client remotely has been affirmed in studies from the field of psychology (Cook & Doyle, 2002; Preschl et al., 2011).

The need for infants and toddlers with disabilities to access family-centered early intervention impacts many professional disciplines (e.g., speech-language pathology, occupational therapy, physical therapy) (Baharav & Reiser, 2010; Cason, 2009; Heimerl & Rasch, 2009; Kelso, Fiechtl, Olsen, & Rule, 2009). In general, results from studies on this population corroborated one another and produced a common recommendation for future investigations to compare outcome measurements in f2f and telepractice conditions. This type of experiment goes well beyond more common measurements of satisfaction.

A study by Baharav and Reiser (2010) used a quantitative research methodology and a research design that included client outcome data. These researchers investigated the use of telepractice to coach parents of two children with autism. The researchers hypothesized that there would be no difference in outcomes between f2f and telepractice models. A repeated-measures, single-subject design was conducted. The study enrolled each family in f2f therapy, two times each week, for 6 weeks. Then, for the following 6 weeks, each family received one session in the f2f condition and one session in the telepractice condition. Two assessment measures were used to measure child outcomes: (1) the Words and Gestures Subtest of the MacArthur Communicative Development Inventory (Fenson et al., 1993); and (2) an analysis of 20-minute videotaped therapy segments. In light of the small sample, the results were encouraging. Based on videotape analyses, one child used a similar number of communicative initiations (e.g., gestures, picture-pointing, verbalizations) per session at the end of treatment while the other child increased the number of communicative initiations relative to the f2f clinical sessions. When evaluating communicative responses (e.g., following directions), both children increased the percentage of their responses in the telepractice condition. And, both children increased the percentage of time spent in social interactions. These trends hold promise, especially considering the short length of treatment, 6 weeks only, using telepractice.

Kelso et al. (2009) set out to examine the satisfaction of parents and interventionists, parental knowledge of therapeutic outcomes, cost effectiveness, time effectiveness, and the use of coaching strategies via telepractice. Just four families, living in rural communities, participated in this study. The providers delivering the FCEI included two SLPs, one occupational therapist, and one physical therapist. Results were mixed. Parent satisfaction was higher than that of the providers. Parents also rated the telepractice platform as more usable than the providers. There were cost savings with telepractice; therapists who delivered f2f therapy were paid for their driving time, and this cost was eliminated. The increased use of coaching strategies in the study (Kelso et al., 2009) was encouraging. The therapists reported, and this is notable due to the documented challenges in using family-centered strategies, that they were less comfortable using coaching and modeling strategies than they were delivering traditional child-centered therapy in the f2f condition.

A study by Cason (2009) corroborated the findings of Kelso et al. (2009). Cason (2009) set out to determine if early intervention services could be delivered cost effectively by occupational therapists using telepractice in rural Kentucky. The providers engaged in the study provided early intervention to two families. The need in this community was dire; to this point, the families were receiving only one f2f treatment session each month. Both families received 12 weeks of intervention through telepractice. This qualitative study used interviews and journaling to collect the data. The data were analyzed using member checking and triangulation and identified three themes: (1) benefits and strengths of telepractice, (2) challenges and weaknesses, and (3) recommendations for program improvement. Results demonstrated telepractice had the potential to cost effectively provide the intervention.

A study by Heimerl and Rasch (2009), funded by the Office for the Advancement of Telehealth, explored the use of telepractice to deliver occupational therapy services in New Mexico. Children with developmental disabilities, all birth to 3 years of age, received home-based, f2f services from a developmental specialist as the primary provider while a second provider (i.e., SLP, occupational therapist, physical therapist, psychologist) offered consultation through telepractice. The results demonstrated that telepractice was a viable service delivery method that included some persistent barriers. For instance, in spite of the theoretical support for the use of coaching strategies, many providers, sometimes unwittingly, resorted to the use of familiar and traditional child-centered practices (Dunst, Boyd, Trivette, & Hamby, 2002). One major limitation of the study by Heimerl and Rasch (2009), as stated by the authors, was the lack of developmental assessments and, hence, the absence of child outcome data.

Olsen, Fiechtl, and Rule (2012) used telepractice in their Virtual Home Visit (VHV) Project to serve families living in three rural counties in northern Utah. The providers represented several professional disciplines including: physical therapy, occupational therapy, speech-language pathology, child development, and special education. Coaching strategies were assumed to be standard practice. VHV sessions were recorded for evaluation purposes. During the first year of the project, the six providers' mean ratings of satisfaction were: very satisfied at 32%, somewhat satisfied at 47%, somewhat dissatisfied at 10%, and very dissatisfied at 11%. During the second year, the providers' mean satisfaction ratings improved with 52% being very satisfied, 38% somewhat satisfied, 5% somewhat dissatisfied, and 5% very dissatisfied. Families also completed an online survey; this survey described parental experiences after each VHV. The percentage of parents rating virtual visits as better than face-to-face sessions ranged from 8% (one parent) to 39% (five parents) over the course of the 2-year project. The number of parents who rated VHVs as worse decreased over time. Olsen et al. (2012) included analyses of the recorded sessions conducted in both f2f and virtual conditions. Nine types of interactions were coded. No statistical significance was found for these three interaction types: (1) interactions of the parent with other people in the home, (2) interactions of the provider with others in the home, and (3) interactions in which the provider talked to the child as the parent engaged the child in an interaction to encourage a particular behavior. There were some statistically significant differences. Coaching strategies were used more often during VHVs than f2f visits and teaching and modeling techniques occurred more often during f2f visits.

Two studies investigated early intervention with infants and toddlers who were deaf and hard of hearing (DHH). The use of telepractice with this population has been in response to a unique combination of factors; families living in remote or rural communities, the low incidence of hearing loss, and the lack of qualified practitioners in the field (McCarthy, Duncan, & Leigh, 2012; Titus & Guthmann, 2010; Wilson & Wells, 2009).

The study by McCarthy et al. (2010), like so many others, did not look at child outcomes; it measured parent satisfaction. The program adhered to the principles of a family-centered approach and focused on coaching families to become the primary facilitators of their children's listening and spoken language development (Campbell, 2004; Campbell & Sawyer, 2007; Dunst et al., 2002; Marturana & Woods, 2012; Rush et al., 2003; Woods et al., 2011). The participants received services at the Royal Institute for Deaf and Blind Children (RIDBC) in Australia. A team of highly trained and experienced teachers of the deaf and speech-language pathologists implemented the project. The program adhered to the principles of a family-centered approach and focused on guiding and coaching families to become the primary facilitators of their children's listening and spoken language development (Campbell, 2004; Campbell & Sawyer, 2007; Dunst et al., 2002; Marturana & Woods, 2012; Rush et al., 2003; Woods et al., 2011). The parents and providers reported benefits from telepractice. First, parents seemed to acquire skills more rapidly than in a traditional f2f model. Furthermore, the role of the provider was defined, in part, by limited physical access to the child. This made it difficult, if not impossible, for the provider to engage in activities directly with the child. Rather, the provider had to ". . . regard the parents as the primary participants" (McCarthy et al., 2010, p. S56). So, it seemed that telepractice did, indeed, support the use of family-centered practices.

Behl, Houston, Guthrie, and Guthrie (2010) also reported on family satisfaction; reports by parents participating in the Sound Beginnings Program in Utah were collected through structured interviews. This program provided services to families who chose listening and spoken language as the desired outcome for their children. The typical session followed traditional participatory-based routines and procedures (Campbell, 2004; Campbell & Sawyer, 2007). The knowledge acquired and the skills used by the parents were monitored to determine if parents successfully used recommended language facilitation techniques with their children. The interview results indicated that the providers implemented coaching techniques. Subsequently, the parents reported that their children were more responsive, followed their directions better, and generally improved their interactions with them.

Summary

For decades, individuals have utilized communication technologies as a means to relay or transmit health-related information (Bashshur & Shannon, 2009). In the past, if the technology did not exist or if it failed to do an adequate job, users sought new technological advancements to develop or enhance services. This is exactly what seems to be happening with the adoption of telepractice. The intent for this body of information, from multiple disciplines, is to motivate readers to move forward with this initiative.

To date, many of the studies of telepractice have not focused on empirically based client or patient outcomes. Rather, the research more frequently reported on subjective and comparative studies. The need for empirical evidence using higher-level research strategies is lacking. As stated by McCarthy et al. (2010), "It is important to note that there is not enough systematic, rigorously collected evidence to demonstrate that such services would really be less costly or equally effective as the face-to-face services that are typically provided currently" (p. S54).

Yet, the implications are profound. There was a common theme that transcended each professional discipline—the incentive to harness current technology to provide high-quality treatment to more patients or clients. Where a client lives need not dictate access to services; nor must one's geographic location dictate the type of services. Through telepractice, patients have the potential opportunity to engage with professionals who practice at previously insurmountable distances. Telepractice can span time zones and continents. In the 21st century, technology is burgeoning while the need for high-quality medical and rehabilitation services persists. With additional research, added guidance, and needed regulations, advanced technology and the need for speech-language pathology services are bound to coalesce, and, in so doing, contribute to improved access and improved outcomes for clients with disabilities.

References

American Speech-Language-Hearing Association. (2003). *National Outcomes Measurement System (NOMS): Adult speech-language pathology user's guide.* Washington, DC: Author.

American Speech-Language-Hearing Association. (2005a). *Audiologists providing clinical services via telepractice: Position statement.* Available from http://www.asha.org/policy.

American Speech-Language-Hearing Association. (2005b). *Speech-language pathologists providing clinical services via telepractice: Position statement.* Available from http://www.asha.org/policy.

American Speech-Language-Hearing Association. (2008a). *Core knowledge and skills in early intervention speech-language pathology practice*. Available from http://www.asha.org/policy.

American Speech-Language-Hearing Association. (2008b). *Roles and responsibilities of speech-language pathologists in early intervention: Guidelines*. Available from http://www.asha.org/policy.

American Speech-Language-Hearing Association. (2008c). *Roles and responsibilities of speech-language pathologists in early intervention: Technical report*. Available from http://www.asha.org/policy.

American Speech-Language-Hearing Association. (2010). *Professional issues in telepractice for speech-language pathologists (professional issues statement).* Available from http://www.asha.org/policy.

Baharav, E., & Reiser, C. (2010). Using telepractice in parent training in early autism. *Telemedicine and e-Health, 16*(6), 727–731. doi: 10.1089/tmj.2010.0029.

Baker, D. C., & Bufka, L. F. (2011). Preparing for the telehealth world: Navigating legal, regulatory, reimbursement, and ethical issues in an electronic age. *Professional Psychology: Research and Practice*, *42*(6), 405–411.

Bashshur, R. L., & Shannon, G. W. (2009). *History of telemedicine: Evolution, context, and transformation*. New Rochelle, NY: Mary Ann Liebert, Inc.

Beck, A. T., Steer, R. A., & Brown, G. K. (1996). *Manual for the Beck Depression Inventory-II.* San Antonio, TX: Psychological Corporation.

Behl, D., Houston, K. T., Guthrie, W. S., & Guthrie, N. (2010). Tele-Intervention: The wave of the future fits families' lives today. *Exceptional Parent, 40*, 23–28.

Behl, D. D., Houston, K. T., & Stredler-Brown, A. (2012). The value of a learning community to support telepractice for infants and toddlers with hearing loss [Monograph]. *Volta Review, 112*(3), 313–327.

Bowns, I. R., Collins, K., Walters, S. J., & McDonagh, A. J. G. (2006). Telemedicine in dermatology: A randomized controlled trial. *Health Technology Assess, 10*(43), 1–63.

Brennan, D., Tindall, L., Theodoros, D., Brown, J., Campbell, M., Christiana, D., Lee, A. (2010). A blueprint for telerehabilitation guidelines. *International Journal for Telerehabilitation, 2*, 31–34.

Campbell, P. H. (2004). Participation-based services: Promoting children's participation in natural settings. *Young Exceptional Children, 8*, 20–29.

Campbell, P. H., & Sawyer, L. B. (2007). Supporting learning opportunities in natural settings through participation-based services. *Journal of Early Intervention, 29*(4), 287–305.

Cason, J. (2009). A pilot telerehabilitation program: Delivering early intervention services to rural families. *International Journal of Telerehabilitation, 1*, 29–37.

Cason, J. (2011). Telerehabilitation: An adjunct service delivery model for early intervention services. *International Journal of Telerehabilitation, 3*(1), 19–28.

Clark, P. G., Dawson, S. J., Scheideman-Miller, C., & Post, M. L. (2002). Telerehab: Stroke therapy and management using two-way interactive video. *Journal of Neurologic Physical Therapy, 26*(2), 87–93.

Constantinescu, G., Theodoros, D., Russell, T., Ward, E., Wilson, S., & Wootton, R. (2011). Treating disordered speech and voice in Parkinson's disease online: A randomized controlled non-inferiority trial. *International Journal of Language and Communication Disorders, 46*(1), 1–16.

Cook, J. E., & Doyle, C. (2002). Working alliance in online therapy as compared to face-to-face therapy: Preliminary results. *CyberPsychology and Behavior, 5*(2), 95–105.

Darkins, A., & Cary, M. (2000). *Telemedicine and telehealth: Principles, policies, performance and pitfalls.* New York, NY: Springer Publishing Company, Inc.

Dixon, B. E., Hook, J. M., & McGowan, J. J. (2008). *Using telehealth to improve quality and safety: Finding from the AHRQ Portfolio (Prepared by the AHRQ National Resource Center for Health IT under contract No. 290-04-0016).* AHRQ Publication No. 09-00120EF. Rockville, MD: Agency for Healthcare Research and Quality.

Dunst, C. J., Boyd, K., Trivette, C. M., & Hamby, D. W. (2002). Family-oriented program models and professional helpgiving practices. *Family Relations, 51*(3), 221-229.

Epstein, R. (2011). Distance therapy comes of age. *Scientific American Mind, 22*(2), 60-63.

Espe-Sherwindt, M. (2008). Family-centered practice: Collaboration, competency and evidence. *Support for Learning, 23*(3), 136-143.

Fenson, L., Dale, P. S., Reznick, J. S., Thai, D., Bates, E., Hartung, J. P., Reilly, J. (1993). *MacArthur communicative development inventories.* San Diego, CA: Singular Publishing Group, Inc.

Fleming, J. L., Sawyer, L. B., & Campbell, P. H. (2011). Early intervention providers' perspectives about implementing participation-based practices. *Topics in Early Childhood Special Education, 30*(4), 233-244. doi: 10.1177/0271121410371986.

Fong, B., Fong, A. C. M., & Li, C. K. (2011). *Telemedicine technologies: Information technologies in medicine and telehealth.* West Sussex, United Kingdom: John Wiley & Sons.

Forducey, P. G. (2006, August 15). Speech telepractice program expands options for rural Oklahoma schools. *ASHA Leader.*

Goldman, R., & Fristoe, M. (2002). *Goldman-Fristoe Test of Articulation-2.* Circle Pines, MN: American Guidance Service, Inc.

Gournaris, J. J. (2009). Preparation for the delivery of telemental health services with individuals who are deaf: Informed consent and provider procedure guidelines. *Journal of the American Deafness and Rehabilitation Association, 43*(1), 34-51.

Grogan-Johnson, S., Alvares, R., Rowan, L., & Creaghead, N. (2010). A pilot study comparing the effectiveness of speech language therapy provided by telemedicine with conventional on-site therapy. *Journal of Telemedicine and Telecare, 16,* 134-139. doi: 10.1258/jtt.2009.090608.

Hailey, D., Roine, R., & Ohinmaa, A. (2002). Systematic review of evidence for the benefits of telemedicine. *Journal of Telemedicine and Telecare, 8*(Suppl. 1), 1-7.

Harper, D. (2006). Telemedicine for children with disabilities. *Children's Health Care, 35*(1), 11-27.

Hayes, D., Eclavea, E., Dreith, S., & Habte, B. (2012). From Colorado to Guam: Infant diagnostic audiological evaluations by telepractice [Monograph]. *Volta Review, 112*(3), 243–253.

Hebbeler, K., Spiker, D., Morrison, K., & Mallik, S. (2008). A national look at the characteristics of Part C early intervention services. *Young Exceptional Children, Monograph Series No. 10: Early Intervention for Infants and Toddlers and Their Families: Practices and Outcomes*, pp. 2–18.

Heimerl, S., & Rasch, N. (2009). Delivering developmental occupational therapy consultation services through telehealth. *Developmental Disabilities Special Interest Section Quarterly, 32*(3), 1–4.

Hilty, D. M., Nesbitt, T. S., Kuenneth, C. A., Cruz, G. M., & Hales, R. E. (2007). Rural versus suburban primary care needs, utilization, and satisfaction with telepsychiatric consultation. *Journal of Rural Health, 23*(2), 163–165. doi: 10.1111/j.1748-0361.2007.00084.x.

Horvath, A. O., & Greenberg, L. S. (1989). Development and validation of the Working Alliance Inventory. *Journal of Counseling Psychology, 36*, 223–233.

Howell, S., Tripoliti, E., & Pring, T. (2009). Delivering Lee Silverman voice treatment (LSVT) by Web camera: A feasibility study. *International Journal of Language and Communication Disorders, 44,* 287–300.

Jessiman, S. M. (2003). Speech and language services using telehealth technology in remote and underserviced areas. *Journal of Speech-Language Pathology and Audiology, 27*, 45–51.

Joint Committee on Infant Hearing. (2007). Year 2007 position statement: Principles and guidelines for early hearing detection and intervention programs. *Pediatrics, 102*(4), 893–921.

Kelso, G., Fiechtl, B., Olsen, S., & Rule, S. (2009). The feasibility of virtual home visits to provide early intervention: A pilot study. *Infants and Young Children, 22*(4), 332–340. doi: 10.1097/IYC.0b013e3181b9873c.

Koocher, G. P. (2007). Twenty-first century ethical challenges for psychology. *American Psychologist, 62*(5), 375–384. doi: 10.1037/0003-066X .62.5.375.

Loane, M. A., Bloomer, S. E., Corbett, R., Eedy, D. J., Evans, C., Hicks, N., et al. (2001). A randomized controlled trial assessing the health economics of real-time tele-dermatology compared with conventional care: An urban versus rural perspective. *Journal of Telemedicine and Telecare, 7,* 108–118.

Marcin, J. P., Ellis, J., Mawis, R., Nagrampa, E., Nesbitt, T.S., & Dimand, R. J. (2004). Using telemedicine to provide pediatric subspecialty care to children with special health care needs in an underserved rural community. *Pediatrics, 113*(1), 1–6.

Marturana, E. R., & Woods, J. J. (2012). Technology-supported performance-based feedback for early intervention home visiting. *Topics in Early Childhood Special Education, 32*(1), 1-10,14-23.

Mashima, P., Birkmire-Peters, D., Syms, M., Holtel, M., Burgess, L., & Peters, L. (2003). Telepractice: Voice therapy using telecommunications technology. *American Journal of Speech-Language Pathology, 12*, 432-439.

Mashima, P. A., & Doarn, C. R. (2008). Overview of telehealth activities in speech-language pathology. *Telemedicine and e-Health, 14*(10), 1101-1117. doi: 10.1089/tmj.2008.0080.

McCarthy, M. (2012). RIDBC Teleschool: A hub of expertise [Monograph]. *Volta Review, 112*(3), 373-381.

McCarthy, M., Duncan, J., & Leigh, G. (2012). Telepractice: The Australian experience in an international context [Monograph]. *Volta Review, 112*(3), 297-312.

McCarthy, M., Munoz, K., & White, K. R. (2010). Teleintervention for infants and yong children who are deaf or hard-of-hearing. *Pediatrics, 126*, S52-S58. doi: 10.1542/peds.2010-0354J.

McConnochie, K. M., Wood, E., Kitzman, H. J., Herendeen, N. E., Roy, J., & Roghmann, K. J. (2005). Telemedicine reduces absence resulting from illness in urban child care: Evaluation of an innovation. *Pediatrics, 115*(5), 1273-1282.

McCullough, A. (2001). Viability and effectiveness of teletherapy for preschool children with special needs. *International Journal of Language and Communication Disorders, 36*(Suppl.), 321-326.

Mulgrew, K. W., Ulfat, S., & Nettiksimmons, J. (2011). Comparison of parent satisfaction with care for childhood obesity delivered face-to-face and by telemedicine. *Telemedicine and e-Health, 17*(5), 383-387. doi: 10.1089/tmj.2010.0153.

Nelson, E., Barnard, M., & Cain, S. (2006). Feasibility of telemedicine intervention for childhood depression. *Counselling and Psychotherapy Research, 6*(3), 191-195. doi: 10.1080/14733140600862303.

Nelson, E., & Bui, T. (2010). Rural telepsychology services for children and adolescents. *Journal of Clinical Psychology, 66*(5), 490-502. doi: 10.1002/jclp.20682.

Nelson, E., Bui, T. N., & Velasquez, S. E. (2011). Telepsychology: Research and practice overview. *Child and Adolescent Psychiatric Clinics of North America, 20*, 67-79. doi: 10.11016/j.chc.2010.08.005.

Olsen, S., Fiechtl, B., & Rule, S. (2012). An evaluation of virtual home visits in early intervention: Feasibility of "virtual intervention" [Monograph]. *Volta Review, 112*(3), 267-281.

Peterson, C. A., Luze, G. J., Eshbaugh, E. M., Jeon, H., & Kantz, K. (2007). Enhancing parent-child interactions through home visiting: Promising practice of unfulfilled promise? *Journal of Early Intervention, 29*(2), 119–140.

Pickering, M., McAllister, L., Hagler, P., Whitehill, T. L., Penn, C., Robertson, S. J., McCready, V. (1998). External factors influencing the profession in six societies. *American Journal of Speech-Language Pathology, 7*(4), 5–17.

Preschl, B., Maercker, A., & Wagner, B. (2011). The working alliance in a randomized controlled trial comparing online with face-to-face cognitive-behavioral therapy for depression. *BMC Psychiatry, 11*, 189–198.

Rabinowitz, T., Brennan, D. M., Chumbler, N. R., Kobb, R., & Yellowlees, P. (2008). New directions for telemental health research. *Telemedicine and e-Health, 14*(9), 972–976. doi: 10.1089/tmj.2008.01.

Reynolds, A. L., Vick, J. L., & Haak, N. J. (2009). Telehealth applications in speech-language pathology: A modified narrative review. *Journal of Telemedicine and Telecare, 15*, 310–316. doi: 10.1258/jtt.2009.081215.

Reynolds, C. R., & Kamphaus, R. W. (1992). *Behavior Assessment System for Children: Manual*. Circle Pines, MN: American Guidance.

Richardson, L. K., Frueh, B. C., Grubaugh, A. L., Egede, L., Elhai, J. D. (2009). Current directions in videoconferencing tele-mental health research. *Clinical Psychology: Science and Practice, 16*(3), 323–338.

Rose, D. A. D., Furner, S., Hall, A., Montgomery, K., Katsavras, E., & Clarke, P. (2000). Videoconferencing for speech and language therapy in schools. *British Telecom Technology Journal, 18*(1), 101–104.

Rush, D. D., Shelden, M. L., & Hanft, B. E. (2003). Coaching families and colleagues: A process for collaboration in natural settings. *Infants Young Children, 16*(1), 33–47.

Sandall, S., Hemmeter, M. L., Smith, B. J., & McLean, M. E. (Eds.) (2005). *DEC recommended practices: A recommended guide for practical application in early intervention/early childhood special education.* Longmont, CO: Sopris West.

Shaikh, U., Cole, S. L., Marcin, J. P., & Nesbitt, T. S. (2008). Clinical management and patient outcomes among children and adolescents receiving telemedicine consultations for obesity. *Telemedicine Journal and e-Health, 14*, 434–440. doi: 10.1089/tmj.2007.0075.

Sicotte, C., Lehoux, P., Fortier-Blanc, J., & Leblanc, Y. (2003). Feasibility and outcome evaluation of a telemedicine application in speech-language pathology. *Journal of Telemedicine and Telecare, 9*, 253–258.

Theodoros, D. (2008). Telerehabilitation for service delivery in speech-language pathology. *Journal of Telemedicine and Telecare, 14*, 221–224. doi: 10.1258/jtt.2007.007044.

Theodoros, D. (2011, September). Telepractice in speech-language pathology: The evidence, the challenges, and the future. *Perspectives on Telepractice, 1,* 10–21. doi: 10.1044/tele1.1.10.

Theodoros, D. G., Constantinescu, G., Russell, T., Ward, E. C., Wilson, S. J., & Wootton, R. (2006). Treating the speech disorder in Parkinson's disease online. *Journal of Telemedicine and Telecare, 12,* 88–91.

Titus, J. C., & Guthmann, D. (2010). Addressing the black hole in substance abuse treatment for deaf and hard of hearing individuals: Technology to the rescue. *Journal of the American Deafness and Rehabilitation Association, 43*(2), 92–100.

Wade, S. L., Wolfe, C. R., Brown, T. M., & Pestian, J. P. (2005). Can a Web-based family problem-solving intervention work for children with traumatic brain injury? *Rehabilitation Psychology, 50*(4), 337–345. doi: 10.1037/0090-5550.50.4337.

Waite, M. (2010). *Online assessment and treatment of childhood speech, language, and literacy disorders* (Unpublished doctoral dissertation). University of Queensland, Australia.

Waite, M., Cahill, L., Theodoros, D., Busuttin, S., & Russell, T. (2006). A pilot study of online assessment of childhood speech disorders. *Journal of Telemedicine and Telecare, 12*, 92–94.

Ware, J. E., Snyder, M. K., Wright, R., Davies, A. R. (1983). Defining and measuring patient satisfaction with medical care. *Evaluation and Program Planning, 6*, 247–263.

Watzlaf, V., Moeini, S., Matusow, L., & Firouzan, P. (2011). VoIP for telerehabilitation: A risk analysis for privacy, security, and HIPAA compliance, Part II. *International Journal of Telerehabilitation, 3*(1), 3–10. doi: 10.5195/ijt.2011.6070.

Wilson, J. A. B., & Wells, M. G. (2009). Telehealth and the deaf: A comparison study. *Journal of Deaf Studies and Deaf Education, 14*(3), 386–402. doi: 10.1093/deafed/enp008.

Woods, J. J., Wilcox, M. J., Friedman, M., & Murch, T. (2011). Collaborative consultation in natural environments: Strategies to enhance family-centered supports and services. *Language, Speech, and Hearing Services in Schools, 42*, 379–392. doi: 10.1044/0161-1461(2011/10-0016).

3

Getting Started: Building a Successful Telepractice Program

Sena Crutchley, Robin L. Alvares, and Michael F. Campbell

Introduction

Creating and establishing a telepractice program in speech-language pathology is a way to provide speech-language pathology services to those who otherwise might not have access. Building a telepractice program that is successful requires a thoughtful approach, careful planning, and a commitment to ensuring its sustainability. Without such dedicated efforts, a program is likely to struggle and may ultimately fail. Although there is some overlap across the stages of developing and implementing a successful telepractice program, it is recommended that professionals seeking to establish telepractice services follow these basic steps: define, research, plan, promote, implement, and evaluate and adjust. This chapter provides an overview of this process.

Define

To Telepractice or Not to Telepractice: That Is the Question!

The first question a practitioner must ask is, "Why telepractice?" Telepractice is a service delivery model—not an approach to therapy. The primary rationale for providing services via telepractice is to overcome geographic or mobility limitations ***on the part of the client***, and the quality of telepractice services must be commensurate with those available when the client and clinician are in the same location. This service delivery model is most appropriate for those clients who may have difficulty accessing qualified personnel, difficulty accessing center-based services, and/or who prefer not to travel. Some patients who have access to center-based services may appreciate the convenience of receiving services in their home rather than travel even short distances. Rural school districts and health care facilities may have difficulty recruiting and retaining qualified personnel even if there is a sufficient client base to sustain center-based services. The telepractice service-delivery model also may be attractive to clients who want specialty consultation. For example, a school district may establish a telepractice program to allow specialized providers (e.g., bilingual speech-language pathologists) to deliver services throughout the district from one location. The practitioner needs to keep in mind that telepractice should not be used simply because it is more convenient for the practitioner. Although there may be less travel involved, telepractice requires not only the knowledge and skills practitioners already possess but additional knowledge and skills, many of which are described in this chapter.

There are a number of venues in which telepractice may be incorporated. Each will have its advantages and disadvantages for clients and clinicians, and each model will have different challenges to service delivery. The primary ways that telepractice have been used are center-to-center, practitioner home to remote center, center-based to client home, or practitioner home to client home.

There are numerous applications of this service delivery model that maintain the goal of increasing the clients' access to quality services. Telepractice may be used as the exclusive service delivery model, as an extension of a center-based model (e.g., to do a "virtual" home visit or to meet with a group of family members), as an adjunct to on-site speech-language services, for follow-up after an intensive or residential program (e.g., speech camp, rehabilitation services), or for a single session of specialty consultation.

A speech-language pathologist (SLP) should also consider the extent to which one may engage in telepractice. If a clinician wishes to add additional clients to an existing caseload through telepractice, it might be advantageous to consider the option of engaging with an established telepractice provider. These established providers who use the telepractice delivery model exclusively have already navigated many of the issues that will be discussed in this chapter, such as billing, licensing, technology, and insurance. They may have their own software platforms and resources, such as assessment materials, that will decrease the need for start-up funds. An established telepractice may also allow the clinician to be part of a practice community that provides support and problem solving. The clinician may be able to make a more informed decision as to whether this model provides the desired job satisfaction. Based on one of the authors' experiences, clinicians accustomed to collaboration who also choose to engage exclusively in telepractice as sole practitioners or independent contractors may experience professional isolation, which may decrease the attractiveness of the model.

When planning to start telepractice either as an independent contractor or as part of an existing practice, it is of primary importance to determine who is to be served and what kind of services are to be offered. Will the program serve adults or children? Are there specific disorders that the organization is interested in addressing through telepractice? Some telepractice programs provide services to a broad spectrum of clients, such as children in the public schools. Others are more specialized, such as serving individuals with hearing loss or fluency disorders or those needing augmentative-alternative communication. Will services be provided to individuals, families, or groups? Although it is important to decide what population or populations will be served, such decisions are sometimes dictated by the population already served by one's facility.

A clinician also needs to determine the potential benefits of telepractice to the practitioner or facility. Without a clear benefit, there would be no value in investing time and resources to develop a telepractice program. Telepractice may provide an additional revenue stream or reduce travel time for clinicians. Staff with physical disabilities or other health conditions might benefit from working from home or from one office. Will the implementation of telepractice allow graduate students access to a greater variety of clinical experiences? Services could be provided to incarcerated individuals in jails, prisons, and juvenile detention facilities without risk to the speech-language pathologist's physical safety. A clinician may also want to branch outside the state, or choose to deliver SLP services internationally. Ultimately, one must decide which benefits are relevant to one's practice and whether the benefits justify implementing a telepractice program.

One final area to define is that of potential barriers to a successful telepractice program. The barriers will vary somewhat according to the features of the service delivery model that have been described so far. However, it is imperative that one carefully ascertain any potential barriers. The likelihood of any unanticipated challenges can be minimized with careful planning. These challenges may be fiscal, technological, perceptual, or regulatory. Each of these will be addressed in more detail in subsequent chapters.

- Is there enough capital available, or can enough be generated to furnish and maintain the needed equipment and personnel?
- Is there an income source (e.g., third-party payer, school contract) to pay for one's services? Telepractice is not covered by Medicare and is only covered by Medicaid in 12 states at the time of this writing. Some third-party insurers reimburse for services delivered via telepractice. In those states where telepractice is not covered by third-party payers, the provider may be able to deliver services through a fee-for-service model as it would when providing in-person services (ASHA, 2010).
- Will there be adequate connectivity at the provider's and client's sites to allow for a strong and reliable signal?

- Is there stakeholder buy-in? A thriving telepractice program will have support from the SLPs, administration, information technology (IT) staff (sometimes referred to as information systems [IS]), support staff, family, and community.
- Is there adequate training and support for primary and support personnel?
- Can telepractice be done within the regulatory constraints of the provider's state of residency and to the remote site of the client? Lack of support from one's licensure board or the inability to deliver services across state lines without an additional license can negatively impact one's telepractice program (American Speech-Language-Hearing Association, 2010). One would need to identify any other barriers that are relevant to the unique circumstances of your proposed project.

Once these key aspects of service delivery have been clearly defined, the specifics of a telepractice program may be researched more in depth. Considering the previous factors may determine whether a clinician or practice proceeds with implementing a telepractice service delivery model.

Research

Telepractice in speech-language pathology is an evolving service delivery model that has a small but growing body of literature. It is vital that those beginning a telepractice program be familiar with the existing evidence base. There may not be data supporting the use of telepractice with certain populations or using some technologies. To engage in telepractice where there is limited data or even contraindications could conceivably put clients as risk as well as create liability issues for the practitioner.

Awareness of the existing literature is also important to assist in stakeholder buy-in. While some stakeholders readily embrace this service delivery model, others may be skeptical as to its efficacy. Knowledge of current efficacy research and professional guidelines will assist practitioners with obtaining third-party reimbursement.

Even with efficacy data, some clients have chosen not to participate in services via telepractice.

Most of the existing studies have focused on specific aspects of service delivery (e.g., validity and reliability of administration of specific standardized assessments) or efficacy with specific populations/disorders (e.g., fluency) (Grogan-Johnson, Gabel, Taylor, Rowan & Alvares, 2011; Mashima et al., 2003; Sicotte, Lehoux, Fortier-Blanc, & Leblanc, 2003; Waite, Theodoros, Russell, & Cahill, 2010; Wilson, Onslow, & Lincoln, 2004). A few studies have looked at the viability of providing speech and language services to more heterogeneous populations (Grogan-Johnson, Alvares, Rowan, & Creaghead, 2010). Others have addressed the issue of stakeholder and SLP satisfaction (Crutchley & Campbell, 2010; Grogan-Johnson et al., 2010; Tucker, 2012). Many of the studies are described and/or cited in Chapter 2.

The American Speech-Language-Hearing Association (ASHA) has established a Special Interest Group (SIG 18) devoted to issues related to telepractice. Special Interest Group 18 provides practitioners with a number of resources, including access to an online community. Like other ASHA SIGs, SIG 18 publishes *Perspectives*, which is a biannual electronic peer-reviewed journal. Some state professional associations, such as the Ohio Speech-Language-Hearing Association, have published journals on the topic of telepractice. There are several journals within the discipline of speech-language pathology that have published data on telepractice, including *The American Journal of Speech-Language Pathology* and *Communication Disorders Quarterly*. In addition, there are journals of telemedicine and telerehabilitation (e.g., *International Journal of Telerehabilitation*, *Journal of Telehealth and Telecare*) that have published articles specific to speech-language pathology.

In addition to resources based in the United States, other countries offer resources that relate to telepractice. For example, the Canadian Association of Speech-Language Pathologists and Audiologists (CASLPA) has published a position paper on telepractice for SLPs and audiologists (CASLPA, 2006). For those outside the United States, it is recommended that one check with national or state organizations about the use of telepractice, recognizing that "telepractice" may not be the term used in that area. ASHA provides an online list of associations outside the United States (ASHA, n.d.).

Training

As of April 2013, The American Speech-Language Hearing Association (ASHA) is in the process of developing a practice portal for telepractice. This portal will be an online resource to allow clinicians to access preliminary information on telepractice (see Appendix B). With respect to acquiring the knowledge and skills necessary for telepractice, it is important to consult the Knowledge and Skills Document from ASHA (ASHA, 2005). The authors also recommend learning about doing telepractice by observing an experienced practitioner who will be using the service delivery model that would seem to best fit the needs of the client population that is being considered. In addition, there are an increasing number of venues to become trained in telepractice. The aforementioned SIG 18 provides a number of training opportunities, including sessions at professional conventions, online chats, and online seminars. There are training programs certified by the American Telemedicine Association that are available throughout the country. A few universities, such as Kent State University and The University of Akron, offer opportunities for students to engage in telepractice as part of their clinical practicum. In Figure 3-1, services at Kent State University are delivered through a telepractice model.

Regulatory Issues

State Licensure Requirements in the United States

Speech-language pathologists may only engage in telepractice in states in which they hold a professional license. Therefore, if the clinician and client reside in different states, the clinician MUST hold licensure in both states. If services are being provided to school-based clients, the state may require additional department of education certification.

Not only must the clinician meet credentialing requirements if he or she is telepracticing to a state different from their state of residence, the SLP must honor the licensure laws in each state in which he or she holds licensure and/or credentials. These laws may vary from state to state. For example, in Texas, an in-person contact

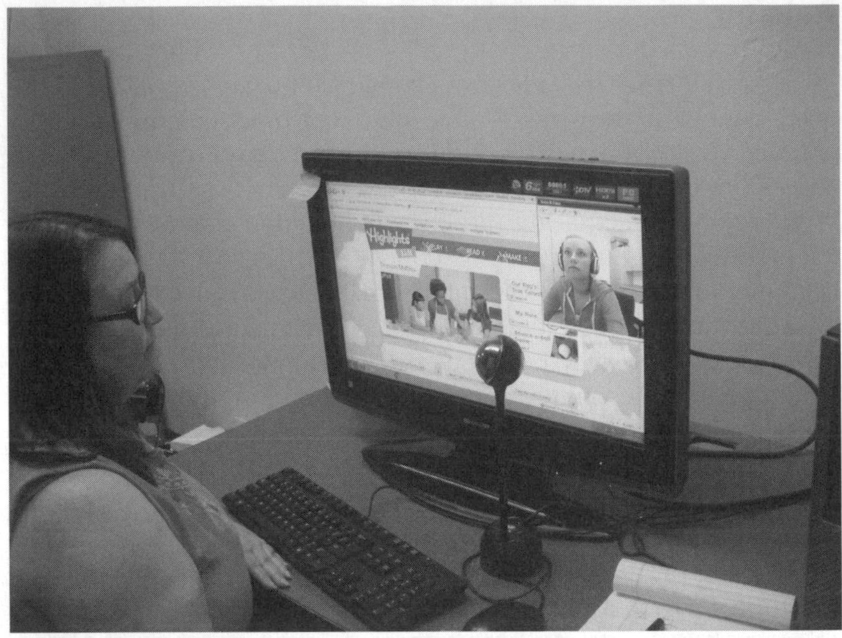

Figure 3–1. Telepractice from a hub site to a brick-and-mortar school using application sharing.

must be made prior to beginning telepractice services. Services may not be provided by telepractice in Delaware as of this writing. Practitioners will want to consult with state licensing boards and possibly state speech-language hearing associations prior to attempting telepractice within a state or across state lines.

It may be expensive and time-consuming to provide services in multiple states, so the costs and benefits must be weighed. This is an issue that is not exclusive to speech-language pathology and audiology, and the American Telemedicine Association (ATA) Telerehabilitation SIG is currently attempting to address this issue and raise awareness of the need for licensure portability in speech-language pathology, audiology, and other rehabilitation disciplines.

During presentations and online events, the authors have noted that one topic that seems to be receiving increasing interest is continuation of services when a clinician or client is on vacation and outside of the state in which the SLP is licensed. Because this issue has not been litigated, it would probably be unwise to engage in this practice until there is clear legal guidance.

International Telepractice

The authors have also noted during presentations and through the SIG 18 online community that there is considerable interest in the international use of telepractice. Issues related to regulation and client privacy vary considerably, but the clinician should follow the laws of the country to which he or she is telepracticing. Shprintzen & Golding-Kushner (2012) provide an excellent discussion on the delivery of telepractice services internationally. One suggestion is that international services be done on a consultative basis rather than as direct services.

Liability/Malpractice Laws

Individuals providing telepractice in speech-language pathology should have liability insurance that covers them both in their home state and in any state to which they may telepractice. Clinicians should consult their insurance carriers prior to engaging in telepractice to determine (1) if their services will be covered, and (2) if services will be covered across state lines. In addition, some carriers will provide coverage for the practitioner's state of residence and adjacent states only. Maheu, McMenamin, and Pulier (in press) advise that clinicians must inform their insurance carrier of the nature of their telepractice activities and "obtain its written agreement to cover you in those activities."

Malpractice in speech-language pathology and audiology telepractice remains a relatively unexplored area and relevant issues may not be clarified until there is significant litigation (Denton, 2003). It is best that those beginning telepractice are experienced clinicians who stay within their scope of expertise, are well versed in the technology they use to telepractice, are intimately familiar with local laws and regulations, and are capable of evaluating the suitability of telepractice services for each client. It is also recommended that SLPs considering telepractice consult an attorney prior to engaging in this modality.

Technology

Convenient access to teleconferencing from a variety of devices at first glance makes telepractice appear to be a relatively easy and efficient way to provide services. However, the services provided by telepractice must be of equal quality as those provided in person. Easily accessible means of teleconferencing platforms do not necessarily allow the clinician to provide optimal input or elicit optimal responses from clients. Many social telecommunication platforms (e.g., Skype, ooVoo, Google Hangout) are designed for social purposes rather than teleconferencing. It is recommended that clinicians consider platforms and equipment that are designed for business communications or distance learning purposes, because these configurations are designed not only for face-to-face interactions and incorporate the sharing of documents, whiteboards, document cameras, other software applications. These configurations vary widely in cost, but basic setups can be inexpensive while allowing the telepractitioner to provide a range of services.

The equipment configurations and teleconferencing platforms (software) described in this chapter are by no means exhaustive or comprehensive, but they will give readers a general sense of what has been used. The rapid advancement of technology provides a positive outlook for the future of telepractice services. Chapter 12 discusses future directions related to telepractice technology.

Researching available technologies may be conducted in a number of ways. Practices that already provide telepractice or telemedicine services may be consulted to ascertain what equipment is used and how it is configured. Professional conferences, webinar sessions, listservs, and professional publications also may allow SLPs to evaluate a variety of equipment configurations or teleconferencing platforms. Professional conferences (e.g., ASHA, ATA) also may provide access to vendors demonstrating products that may be used for telepractice. Seeing a variety of equipment configurations and teleconferencing platforms will allow the clinician to find the optimal system to provide quality services within specified budget guidelines.

Infrastructure

Technology and connectivity can certainly be a major challenge for any telepractice program. Many areas in which there is the greatest need (e.g., rural or other geographically remote areas) have limited infrastructure for Internet accessibility. Telepractice requires the transmission of a continuous video signal requiring considerable bandwidth for quality real-time, face-to-face interactions.

Before equipment and platforms are considered, it is crucial to identify the available infrastructure at the hub (the SLP's site) and the remote site (the client's site). If there is insufficient bandwidth to use teleconferencing software, the quality of the signal—and the quality of services—will be compromised. Local Internet service providers at both the hub and remote sites may be consulted. In the case of center-based services at either the hub or remote site, information technology (IT) professionals should be consulted in all aspects of choosing equipment and teleconferencing platforms. In fact, they must be consulted regularly to ensure a sustainable telepractice program. In addition, in the United States (U.S.), the National Telecommunications and Information Administration maintains a website (http://www.broadbandmap.gov/) that provides information about available broadband access across the United States.

If the hub is in an institutional setting (e.g., hospital, university, health clinic), it is advisable to meet with the IT department to determine available bandwidth. Telepractice often involves real-time video streaming and uses substantial bandwidth. At a larger institution, there may be competition for bandwidth that could potentially slow services, distort the signal, or make it difficult to use various teleconferencing features. It is possible to split bandwidth or give a signal priority; however, this is often an additional expense and has budgetary implications.

Telepracticing from a residence depends on the bandwidth available through one's Internet service provider. It is recommended that a clinician subscribe to the maximal bandwidth available using cable-based or digital subscriber line (DSL) Internet. Some wireless devices may not support the bandwidth necessary to support some videoconferencing platforms.

Equipment

Selecting the type of technology that will be used is one of the most important aspects of the planning phase. The technology selected will depend on the needs of the practitioners and clients, the physical spaces involved, and the available capital. Key components of any telepractice system include a computer (at a minimum a notebook or laptop), video monitor, videoconferencing software, a high-definition camera, and high-quality speakers and microphone at the hub and remote site.

Dedicated Teleconferencing System. There are dedicated systems that include a codec (a device that compresses and decompresses audio-video signals allowing for their efficient transmission and receipt), which essentially the videoconferencing device, and any other above mentioned components. These systems may allow for a videoconferencing connection between two sites or between multiple sites. These types of devices are best used when the hub and remote site are institutional sites. These systems currently tend to be expensive and may be cost prohibitive for a residence-based hub or remote site. Systems have a number of features that may or may not be useful, including zooming and panning of the camera, and attached peripherals such as a document camera and ability to engage in application sharing. Monitors at the remote site may be portable or stationary (wall mounted) or integrated into a desktop computer system. There is also the option of using a telepresence format in which the monitors are set up to simulate an in-person meeting. Additional components may be needed to make the system functional. For example, devices may be needed to traverse firewalls. With dedicated systems, it is recommended that several vendors and manufacturers be consulted in order to determine what system will work best for service delivery and budget. A detailed description of plans and available resources should be developed prior to approaching vendors or manufacturers.

Using Personal Computers. For those who wish to utilize readily available software for videoconferencing over the Internet via Voice over the Internet Protocol (VoIP) systems, there are several providers, some of which were mentioned earlier, and off-the-shelf devices available. A minimum of a laptop or notebook computer is necessary to run business and educational teleconferencing software. As with the dedicated systems, one would need to choose a monitor, a microphone, and a camera.

Monitor. Many teleconferencing platforms have features (e.g., whiteboards) that require multiple windows to be open simultaneously, and clinicians may find the screen size of most laptops or notebooks inadequate. A larger monitor may easily be added as a peripheral.

Video Camera. Laptop and notebook computers generally have built-in cameras; however, they limit the field of vision. In these cases, a webcam may be easily added as a peripheral. If telepracticing to a center where services might be provided to groups, a camera with wide-angle capabilities might be needed. A wide-angle camera may also be used to provide services to classrooms if there is a smart board upon which to display the SLP image. A wide-angle camera attached to a PC or Mac would allow the SLP to view the students.

As mentioned, dedicated systems typically include a camera that may allow the clinician the ability to zoom in and out on the patient. The ability to pan the room at the remote site may be a helpful feature during meetings to help the SLP see everyone who is present. Panning a room to determine who is present is also frequently used to ensure privacy before a telepractice session.

Microphones and External Speakers. In addition to built-in cameras, most laptops and notebook computers have built-in microphones. Peripheral webcams may also have microphones built in. These microphones may vary with respect to signal clarity. Information technology (IT) professionals may be consulted to determine which equipment configuration will be optimal. When the hub and/or remote site is in a residence, noise canceling headphones with a lavaliere microphone may be used to enhance signal clarity.

As with the cameras, dedicated systems typically include microphones. It would be beneficial to ensure that the microphones offer high fidelity sound. Speakers may be included in the system, or they may need to be added as peripherals.

Peripherals. Document cameras may be useful for presenting information, particularly worksheets, books, stimulus cards, and other similar material used in a therapy session. Although materials are increasingly available in digital format or online, the document camera may save money by allowing an SLP to use existing resources without having to purchase new material or scan the "oldies but goodies." It is highly recommended by the authors that the hub and remote site have access to a fax machine, a printer, and a document scanner. Often these are incorporated into one machine, and these machines are becoming increasingly affordable.

Teleconferencing Platforms

Dedicated systems, such as those manufactured by Polycom, Tandberg, and other companies, include their own videoconferencing software. These systems are typically point-to-point, meaning that both the hub and remote site need to have the software, and the initial costs to install the teleconferencing software at both sites may be expensive and may require periodic renewal of the site license. They may also offer multipoint software, in which the hub can connect to more than one remote site at a time, allowing for real-time meetings or treatment groups across several locations. These types of systems tend to be cost prohibitive with residential remote sites. It should also be noted that there are companies that engage exclusively in telepractice that have developed teleconferencing platforms specific to speech-language pathology.

There are a number of server-based teleconferencing platforms available. For these platforms, the hub subscribes to a service that provides a "room" for the origination site to which clients/patients are "invited." The cost of the subscription is often covered by the hub and generally does not result in additional cost to the client, though the client will need to download the software to be able to use the platform. This is often free for clients. Institutions (e.g., hospitals or universities) may have site licenses that are available at a reduced cost. An advantage to a group site license is that a reservoir of shared materials (e.g., therapy materials, assessments) may be developed and made available to practitioners in a group. It is beyond the scope of this chapter to review available platforms, but some sharing features (interactive features used by both the clinician and the client) are described in the following.

Whiteboard. With systems that do not include a document camera, at a minimum, the authors recommend that the teleconferencing system have a whiteboard. Presenting therapy materials by holding them up to a camera is inefficient and does not provide optimal input for the client. There are problems with relying exclusively on a whiteboard; the main limitation being the need for the client to use a keyboard. Young children or clients with limited manual dexterity may have difficulty using this feature. A mouse may be used to "write" on the whiteboard; however, the authors have found that using a mouse to write or draw is very difficult for many clients. Equipment may be available (e.g., touch screens) but often at increased cost to the client. Some teleconferencing platforms have enhanced whiteboards with features that can be used therapeutically (e.g., visual reinforcers) and can be easily accessed. These features are generally not available through free social conferencing software (e.g., Skype, ooVoo, Google Hangout).

Application Sharing. One of the most important features for increasing the flexibility of teleconferencing software is application sharing. Application sharing allows for the clinician and the client to access materials simultaneously. Application sharing may be used for any operation on the SLP's computer, such as therapy software programs, scanned materials, and video recordings. Joint access to the Internet provides SLPs with infinite therapy resources for stimulus materials (e.g., online books), therapy activities (e.g., Quia is a shared site with SLP therapy activities), and reinforcement sites (e.g., Discovery Kids *Build a Coaster* where the students can place a piece on a roller coaster after producing a sound). Incorporating the Internet is a vast topic and is not exclusive to telepractice; however, application sharing does require that multiple windows are open, and, as was mentioned previously, screens on notebook or laptop computers or tablet devices would not be practical. As of this writing, iPads do not allow for application sharing, but this feature could be added in future generations of this device. Application sharing can have its limitations; for example, many application sharing programs share only video and not audio to a remote site.

Regardless of the teleconferencing platform chosen, the practitioner must have ready access to IT support. If the SLP chooses to purchase a dedicated system from a vendor or service provider, it is highly recommended that the clinician inquire about technical support options. Such on-site support must also be available at the remote site, whether that is another center, a "brick and mortar" school, or a client's home.

Privacy and Security

Protecting the privacy of clients' records and personal health information is mandated in the United States by federal law (Health Insurance Portability and Accountability Act [HIPAA] and Family Educational Rights and Privacy Act [FERPA]), the ASHA Code of Ethics, and often state licensure laws. Telepractice services are being conducted through VoIP systems, such as Microsoft Office Live Meeting, Adobe Connect Now, ooVoo, LINC, and iChat (Watzlaf, Moeini, Matusow, & Firouzan, 2011; Watzlaf, Moeini, Firouzan, 2010). Many of these systems are server-based in which the meeting (or therapy session) participants are routed through a central server. (Because platforms are continually being created and updated, it is recommended that practitioners consult the American Telemedicine Association website for the most current platforms.) Some of these systems are automatically encrypted, which means the signal is encoded to prevent hacking and to ensure confidentiality. Some VoIPs require an additional fee for encryption. In addition to investigating the type of encryption used by providers, one also should ascertain how the service provider handles the data that passes through its system. Does it store the data, or is it simply a portal? Clinicians who do not use adequate encryption for the provision of telepractice services may be in violation of HIPAA and FERPA and subject to fines and other legal actions.

Planning

Having successfully navigated through the research process, the feasibility of being able to provide telepractice to a target population or region should be more apparent. Having an understanding of the regulatory issues and potential hurdles, available technology and infrastructure, and a familiarity with best practices for providing telepractice services will provide a clearer picture of how to approach the next phase of establishing a successful telepractice—planning.

The next step would be to determine if there is a need for one's services. This is accomplished by completing a needs assessment.

Needs Assessment

A needs assessment is a critical part of the planning process. If there is no need for telepractice services, it is unlikely that a telepractice project would be successful. At this stage, the SLP has an idea of to whom one would like to deliver services and where there is a potential need for services.

A needs assessment will be created as a guide to help a clinician determine if there would be a need for telepractice and the extent of that need. There may be a shortage of SLPs in a geographic region or with expertise in a particular area of practice. Depending on the initial perceived need, the SLP should contact the appropriate administrative staff to do a needs assessment. For schools, a clinician may contact the director of special education or the superintendent. For adult clients, a clinician may send a needs assessment survey to a director of rehabilitation at a hospital or skilled nursing facility. The needs assessment survey will determine if patients/students have no or limited access to qualified SLPs and the barriers to receiving services. If a need is not identified, a change in population focus or a change in location may be necessary.

Business Plan

A business plan is invaluable to any new venture. According to the U.S. Small Business Administration (SBA), "A business plan is an essential roadmap for business success. This living document generally projects 3 to 5 years ahead and outlines the route a company intends to take to grow revenues" U.S. Small Business Administration. (n.d.).

It is beyond the scope of this chapter to detail how to develop a business plan, although there are typical key components that will be highlighted. Much of the information necessary (e.g., market analysis) may have been gathered during the research process and needs assessment stages of investigation. The business plan is a place to clearly describe one's telepractice program, outline the structure of the organization and management, define how the program will be marketed and funded, and make financial projections. The above-mentioned SBA reference provides an excellent resource to help create a carefully designed business plan.

Physical Space

There are several components to consider when planning a physical telepractice space. These considerations must not be taken lightly as a poor location or a poorly designed room can negatively impact the outcome of a program. If the remote site is center-based, ideally the equipment, if not the space, will be dedicated to telepractice. In addition to a nondedicated space potentially compromising patient/client confidentiality, multiple users may inadvertently change settings, readjust cameras or microphones, or delete materials.

Location is an important factor (Crutchley, Campbell, & Christiana, 2012; Major, 2005). The telepractice rooms at the hub and the remote site should be located away from significant noise as would be preferable for on-site services. For example, at a school site, the telepractice room should be situated away from the cafeteria and gymnasium. If intermittent noise is an issue, noise canceling headphones may be used to minimize distraction. In addition, the telepractice rooms should be easily accessible to those who will be using them. They are more likely to be used if they are in accessible locations. For school programs, the shorter amount of distance the facilitator has to walk between classrooms and the telepractice room, the more productive the SLP can be. Additionally in the schools, if the telepractice room is readily accessible, teachers and administrators are more likely to visit the room to consult with the SLP.

If services are provided to a client at home, the clinician needs to work with the client and the client's family to ensure that conditions are optimal for the duration of telepractice sessions. The client should be in a place where noise and distractions can be minimized. In this situation, noise canceling headphones may be used to decrease exposure to ambient noise. These same factors should be considered if the site of origin is in the clinician's residence. These guidelines will vary based on the needs of the client. For example, a clinician providing services to a family may prefer to have those in the remote site in a more typical situation, for example, at the kitchen table for a family meal. In some cases, telepractice will allow the clinician to observe functional activities in real time in a client's home or vocational environment.

One also needs to ensure that the location ensures the privacy and security of the patients/students (ASHA, 2010). In addition to the room not being in a noisy location, the room should have enough soundproofing that those outside the room will not be able to hear sessions. Unauthorized people should not be able to look in the room to watch a session, so one may need to cover windows or position the telepractice equipment in such a way as to discourage such observation. The rooms should be of sufficient size to allow for any needed activities (Crutchley et al., 2012; Major, 2005). For example, if the room at a medical remote site is being used for consultation, it may need to be large enough to hold the patient, caregiver, and in-person SLP. The room should also be large enough for the patient/student to engage in gross motor activities. At a school site, ideally the room should be large enough to hold the entire Individualized Education Program (IEP) team (e.g., teacher, administrator, and parents).

Another option for meeting would be the use of a laptop or notebook. ETR (Evaluation Team Report)/IEP meetings could be done with hard copies of IEPs and/or ETRs without requiring the opening of multiple windows.

Of course, as was mentioned earlier, one also needs to consider the size of the room relative to the size of the equipment and any materials that would need to be stored in the room. With a large monitor, whether wall mounted or on a cart, the room would need to be large enough to allow for comfortable viewing. Consider whether or not hands-on materials would be more readily accessible if stored in the therapy room. If so, the room would need adequate storage space depending on the amount and size of the materials.

Another critical component of room planning is lighting (Major, 2005). Just as lighting is an important aspect of television show production, it is an important factor in videoconferencing. Without adequate lighting, it may be difficult for those involved in speech therapy/evaluation sessions to see each other clearly. Conversely, having light behind the clinician (e.g., a window), may create glare at the remote site, compromising vision. Depending on skin tone, poor lighting could result in the SLP and/or patient/student not being able to see the other's facial features. Clearly, that could have a negative impact on the quality of a speech services. Besides having ceiling-mounted lighting, having a light source in front of those involved in telepractice sessions may improve visual clarity and comfort on the eyes.

Also related to visual comfort, the color and décor of a telepractice room are important (Chan, Ho, Jarvis-Selinger, Payne, & Plohman, 2008; Major, 2005). Soft, muted colors are typically easier on the eye than bold, bright colors. Light blue is sometimes recommended as the ideal wall color. Regarding décor, minimal distractions typically allow for improved focus for the people involved. At the telepractice hub, a clinician might wish to display the name of the organization behind the clinician. If the clinician is telepracticing from his/her residence, care should be taken to minimize the personalization of the space. Again, these guidelines vary on a case-by-case basis.

In addition to visual clarity, sound clarity can also be addressed. Good acoustics depends on having some surfaces covered in sound-absorbing material (Major, 2005). Carpeted floors and/or acoustic tiles may be chosen to dampen excess noise in the room.

Human Resources

It has been the authors' experience that one of the most important people to identify during the development phase of a telepractice program is someone at the remote site who will champion the program. A telepractice champion is typically someone who understands your vision of how telepractice can help their facility meet the needs of their students and patients. They are also usually someone who values technology and sees its potential applications in improving student and patient care.

Stakeholders

All of the above-mentioned stakeholders will need to be trained in how the program works, what will be needed of them, and what to expect from the rest of the team (Crutchley et al., 2012). The training should be ongoing, as the program will likely be modified over time and the stakeholders may need an occasional review of what they learned during the initial training. In addition, the training should be tailored to the person's role in the program. It is important that everyone knows each other's role and responsibilities and who to approach with information, questions, and requests. For example, it seems obvious that the facilitator should be trained in his/her responsibilities as compared to those of the SLP. However, with a school-based program, it is also vital that the administrators understand each person's role. Otherwise, a school principal may approach the facilitator with questions that require the clinical judgment of the SLP. In the authors' experience implementing telepractice programs at nine school sites over the past 8 years, the most important school-based "champions" are the superintendent and/or principal, the director of special education, and the school psychologist. If one can have a good working relationship with them, one will typically be successful in that school district.

But this is only for school-based services to a "brick and mortar" school. In a hospital, the champion would likely be the information technology (IT) director, the hospital president or director, and/or the director of rehabilitation (J. Crutchley, personal communication, January 23, 2013). Essentially, an effective champion for any organization would be someone with influence who has the authority to make key decisions related to services and the funding of programs.

Because the people associated with telepractice are critical to the success of any telepractice program, it is important to maintain support for all involved (Crutchley et al., 2012). Some of the key players to plan for are the speech-language pathologists, facilitators, information technology staff, caregivers and/or significant others, and telepractice champions. Others (e.g., school principals, hospital administrators) may be key players depending on the type of setting one plans to pursue.

Telepractice SLP

Plans must be in place for the telepractice SLP, but considerations may also be made if there is an SLP at the remote site. The telepractice SLP is, ideally, creative, comfortable with technology, resourceful, and able to problem solve quickly on demand. These skills allow the SLP to adapt lessons to the telepractice modality, and they facilitate troubleshooting when technology-related issues arise. It is the opinion of the authors that the telepractice SLP also needs to be comfortable being physically alone in a space for long periods of time. Perhaps planning for occasional on-site interactions would prevent any sense of isolation. When providing services to a client's home, relationships are typically limited to the client and some or all of the family members. In an institutional setting, such as a school or hospital, each client has a variety of team members with whom the SLP needs to establish a professional relationship. For example, in a skilled nursing facility, and SLP will need to establish relationships with administrative personnel, nursing staff, and social workers. A school-based program requires interaction with team members including administrators, general education teachers, intervention specialists, school psychologists, and many others. This becomes a challenge when the types of interactions that take place tend to occur in the workroom or in the hall and are no longer available. SLPs telepracticing to institutional settings will have to develop strategies to become part of the school culture.

Another reason for visiting an institutional site or the community in which the client lives, if it is significantly remote from the SLP, is to better understand the community in which the client resides. This is not always possible if the client site is sufficiently remote, but when possible, it helps establish a stronger relationship between the telepractice SLP and patient. For example, clients or students may refer to landmarks in the community or local events that are important to the client that the clinician may be able to incorporate into a therapeutic activity. If the clinician does visit a remote site, the cost of transportation and lodging should be factored into the budget.

Facilitators

If a program will be providing telepractice services to children or to adults who will need some onsite support, facilitators or caregivers will be needed to fill that role (ASHA, 2010; Crutchley et al., 2012). Remuneration for facilitators must be included in the budget, as the use of volunteers is not advised. In an institutional setting, the facilitator is the face of the program. He or she will have a range of responsibilities outlined in the following, and it is important that they present a professional face and that there are clear guidelines for supervision. The use of volunteer facilitators may also present privacy and confidentiality issues. A detailed description of the responsibilities, knowledge, and skills for this person will need to be developed. In a center-based program, this position could be filled by an aide or paraprofessional. The roles and responsibilities of the paraprofessional need to be clearly defined. The primary responsibility of the paraprofessional will be to deal with technical issues that arise. The paraprofessional needs to make sure the equipment is in working order and should be able to troubleshoot when technical issues arise. Depending on the setting, the facilitator may have the responsibility of escorting students to and from classes, monitoring students' behavior, distributing reinforcers, and helping to manage materials. Facilitators must also be willing to "fade into the background" by not prompting the student or providing the student with reinforcement for communication behaviors.

The use of facilitators in a home-based environment needs to be considered on a case-by-case basis. Some clients may not require facilitators, but others, depending on age and/or disability, may require assistance in using the equipment and navigating the software. A home facilitator will also need to commit to being available to assist the client during the scheduled session. As with center-based facilitators, home-based facilitators will need to be trained, and the telepractice SLP will want to develop a training program that will help facilitators understand their role.

Technological Support Staff

Consideration of the information technology (IT) staff at the remote site and hub is undoubtedly an important part of the planning phase. It is critical that a telepractice program secures IT staff that is knowledgeable about and competent at working with videoconferencing systems. IT persons with limited knowledge of telepractice may require additional time and funds to train. In addition, when problems arise, it is probable that troubleshooting will take longer, resulting in missed telepractice sessions and possibly lost revenue. Such issues could occur with ill-prepared IT staff at either site. Even highly competent IT support would need to be made aware of your program's needs and resources. Thus, one should carefully plan for what information to share with the IT personnel.

Performance Monitoring

One remaining and very important item to address during the planning of a telepractice program is a means of monitoring the performance of the program. Because the quality of services delivered by telepractice must be comparable to those delivered in person, continuous quality monitoring must be built into the plan. There are a number of resources for quality monitoring in health care that a practitioner may consult, although there are few specific to telemedicine and telerehabilitation.

The planning stage of a telepractice program may be time-consuming and challenging; however, it is in this stage where you build the foundation to a successful program. Once the clinician has thoroughly planned the telepractice program, promoting the venture is the next step.

Promote

It is extremely important to collect the full support of the key team telepractice players. Most successful telepractice programs also have, as was mentioned earlier, a "telepractice champion" who advocates within the organization and the community. A telepractice champion who promotes the services can develop excitement and pass along program successes not only in his or her organization and community, but also to others who might benefit. These folks can help develop an extremely successful program and can also help to problem solve when issues arise.

When marketing telepractice to an existing speech-language pathology program, such as in a school district, it is best to demonstrate "that integrating technology services into a speech therapy program is not compromising in-person sessions but is expanding access to services while reducing travel and related expenses such as time" (ASHA, 2010; Crutchley et al., 2012, p. 32). Because it is difficult for many to visualize how telepractice works, it may be beneficial to provide demonstrations to administration, board of directors, as well as potential customers and community members. There must be an ongoing effort to educate and market the services to reduce the impression that the quality of service is less than in-person. Marketing should focus on addressing the needs of those who have limited to no access to a qualified speech-language pathologist. Telepractitioners should engage in ethical practices to acquire and retain clients as well as contracts.

Implement

Once a program has been carefully developed and designed, it can begin to be implemented. Although the specifics of the program will vary depending on the exact services one will be providing, there are certain commonalities to implementing any telepractice program. It is important to generate a prioritized task list that will be followed as the program is being established (Grogan-Johnson, 2012). Examples of items for that task list include: finalizing any contracts and billing services, hiring needed personnel, acquiring telepractice equipment and materials, conducting videoconference trials with the remote site(s), training relevant personnel, and sending notifications or acquiring informed consent.

Billing will vary depending on the type of services one will be providing. For example, if a clinician will be providing services in a school, a contractual arrangement may be needed. If a clinician intends to provide services through a hospital or skilled nursing facility, an understanding of coding and billing for telepractice, and what third-party payers reimburse for telepractice services, is needed.

When it is confirmed that one's program will have a reliable source of revenue, it will be time to acquire telepractice equipment and materials. The hardware and software will be acquired from a vendor that understands one's needs and wishes. The equipment will either be installed by the vendor or local IT personnel. Once it is installed, a connection will be established that allows for access and the use of any needed applications yet ensures privacy and security (ASHA, 2010).

Whether or not telepractice personnel are newly hired or recruited from existing staff, they will need to be explicitly trained in their roles and responsibilities, how to use the equipment, and how to troubleshoot any technological issues. As was mentioned earlier, tailored training will also need to be provided to other key personnel (e.g., administration). If home health services are to be provided, one will need a plan for installing equipment and/or software into patients' homes.

Documentation guidelines developed during the planning stage should include a means to notify patients or acquire informed consent (Dudding, Crutchley, Grogan-Johnson, & Alvares, 2012). If providing school-based services, one will complete this process at the beginning of program implementation. As new students enter the program, this process will need to be repeated on an individual basis. If providing services through a medical facility, one can acquire informed consent following facility guidelines.

Evaluate and Adjust

There are a number of components that may be considered when looking at evaluation and quality improvement. As mentioned earlier, there are existing resources for continuous quality monitoring in health care, but few are specific to telepractice. The principles, however, remain the same. The most important consideration is client or patient outcomes. There are multiple means of assessing client outcomes qualitatively and quantitatively. Measuring these outcomes is an integral part of clinical practice, and the types of quantitative and qualitative measures that are used in telepractice are no different than those used in on-site therapy. There may be challenges to completing certain types of outcome measures; as it may not be possible to observe classroom performance directly, for example. These challenges may be overcome if the telepracticing SLP is willing to think outside of the box. In the case of classroom observation, the student's performance may be audio or video recorded, as long as all privacy guidelines are followed. It is important that the telepracticing SLP assess the factors contributing to the client's success and identify any barriers to progress. If there are barriers, one needs to determine if they are due to telepractice or other factors.

The service delivery model itself should also be evaluated. Quantitative data, such as the number of sessions held, clinician productivity, and the number of clients/patients served, can be calculated and compared to similar data for on-site services. Qualitative data in the form of stakeholder interviews and surveys can determine the level of satisfaction with services and identify any problems that should be addressed. Studies of stakeholder satisfaction have recorded high degrees of satisfaction with telepractice (Crutchley & Campbell, 2010; Grogan-Johnson et al., 2010; Tucker, 2012).

It was stated earlier that quality monitoring should be continuous, though identifying specific timelines for reporting results is recommended. Any evaluation plan should include regular meetings with stakeholders to resolve any problems that arise. These meetings should be relatively frequent at the initiation of a telepractice program. Establishing a climate and a process for dealing with problems when they arise will go far in ensuring the success and sustainability of the program.

In addition to measures of client outcomes and stakeholder satisfaction, it is imperative to have a plan for analyzing ongoing program costs after the program has been initially piloted. A brief description of cost analysis will be provided here. For more detail, see chapter 8.

Essentially, one needs to calculate the program's expenses, including those that are fixed (e.g., space, equipment) and those that are variable and may also be considered an investment (e.g., marketing materials), and the realistic potential for revenue (e.g., third-party payers, school contracts) generated by the program (D. Christiana, personal communication, February 6, 2013). This cost analysis helps to determine if a program has the potential to be self-sustaining and if there needs to be a change in course. If the expenses outweigh the revenue, questions can be raised as to the long-term sustainability of the program. Cost analysis provides an objective measurement of a program's viability.

Conclusion

This chapter has presented considerations and guidelines for the implementation of a successful telepractice program. The first step is to determine if the telepractice service delivery model best meets the needs of a client population. The clinician considering telepractice needs to be aware of the regulatory issues specific to telepractice. Hardware, software, and infrastructure considerations were described. Guidelines for developing a business plan, suggestions for implementation of a telepractice program, and means by which the success of a telepractice program may be measured were also presented. We, as authors, have found our respective journeys full of challenges and frustrations yet still stimulating, invigorating, and just plain fun. We have worked with dedicated colleagues to establish a practice community committed to providing quality speech and language services to individuals who might not otherwise receive services, and this has been most satisfying. We hope that after reading this chapter, future telepractice SLPs will join us to further develop this service delivery model to help enhance the quality of life for our clients/patients and their families.

Acknowledgment

We wish to thank Diana Christiana of Clinical Communications for generously giving of her time and knowledge, Susan Grogan-Johnson of Kent State University for her support and assistance, Michael Towey of the Voice and Swallowing Center of Maine for his contribution, and K. Todd Houston of The University of Akron for his support and patience. We would also like to thank Sena Crutchley's husband, Jonathan Crutchley, for his contribution related to hospital-based telemedicine.

References

American Speech-Language-Hearing Association. (n.d.). *Audiology and speech-language pathology associations outside of the United States.* Retrieved February 2, 2013, from http://www.asha.org/members/international/intl_assoc.htm.

ASHA. (2005). *Knowledge and skills needed by audiologists providing clinical services via telepractice.* Available from http://www.asha.org/policy.

ASHA. (2010). *Professional issues in telepractice for speech-language pathologists* [Professional issues statement]. Available from http://www.asha.org/policy.

Canada Association of Speech-Language Pathologists and Audiologists. (2006). *Position paper on the use of telepractice for CASLPA S-LPs and auds.* Retrieved February 2, 2013, from http://www.caslpa.ca/PDF/position%20papers/telepractice.pdf.

Chan, E., Ho, K., Jarvis-Sclinger, S., Payne, R., & Plohman, K. (2008). Clinical telehealth across the disciplines: Lessons learned. *Telemedicine and e-Health, 14*(7), 720.

Crutchley, S., & Campbell, M. (2010). TeleSpeech Therapy pilot project: Stakeholder satisfaction. *International Journal of Telerehabilitation, 2*(1), 23–30.

Crutchley, S., Campbell, M., & Christiana, D. (2012). Implementing a school-based telepractice program. *Perspectives on Telepractice, 2*(1), 31–41.

Denton, D. (2003). Ethical and legal issues related to telepractice. *Seminars in Speech and Language, 24*(4), 313–322.

Dudding, C., Crutchley, S., Grogan-Johnson, S., & Alvares, R. (2012, November). *Telepractice: Meeting Needs in the Public Schools.* Presentation at Annual Convention of the American-Speech-Language-Hearing Association, Atlanta.

Grogan-Johnson, S. (2012). Providing school-based speech-language therapy services by telepractice: A brief tutorial. *Perspectives on Telepractice, 2*(1), 42–48.

Grogan-Johnson, S., Alvares, R., Rowan, L., & Creaghead, N. (2010). A pilot study comparing the effectiveness of speech language therapy provided by telemedicine with conventional on-site therapy. *Journal of Telemedicine and Telecare, 16*(3), 134–139.

Grogan-Johnson, S., Gabel, R., Taylor, J., Rowan, L., & Alvares, R. (2011). A pilot exploration of speech sound disorder intervention delivered by telehealth to school-age children. *International Journal of Telerehabilitation, 3*(1), 31–41.

Maheu, M., McMenamin, J., & Pulier, M. (in press). Optimizing the use of technology in psychology with best practice principles. In G. Koocher, J. Norcross, & B. Greene (Eds.), *Psychologist's desk reference* (3rd ed.). New York, NY: Oxford University Press.

Major, J. (2005). Telemedicine room design. *Journal of Telemedicine and Telecare, 11*, 10–14.

Mashima, P., Birkmire-Peters, D., Syms, M., Holtel, M., Burgess, L., Peters, L. (2003). Telehealth: Voice therapy using telecommunications technology. *American Journal of Speech-Language Pathology, 12*(4), 432–439.

Shprintzen, R. J., & Golding-Kushner, K. J. (2012). International use of telepractice. *Perspectives on Telepractice, 2*(1), 16–25.

Sicotte, C., Lehoux, P., Fortier-Blanc, J., & Leblanc, Y. (2003). Feasibility and outcome evaluation of a telemedicine application in speech-language pathology. *Journal of Telemedicine and Telecare, 9*, 253–258.

Tucker, J. (2012). Perspectives of speech-language pathologists on the use of telepractice in schools: The qualitative view. *International Journal of Telepractice, 4*(2), 61–72.

United States Small Business Administration. (n.d.). *Create your business plan.* Retrieved February 3, 2013, from http://www.sba.gov/category/navigation-structure/starting-managing-business/starting-business/how-write-business-plan.

U.S. Small Business Administration. (n.d.). *How to write a business plan.* Retrieved February 2, 2013, from http://www.sba.gov/content/how-write-business-plan-1.

Waite, M., Theodoros, D., Russell, T., & Cahill, L. (2010). Internet based telehealth assessment of language using the CELF-4. *Language, Speech, and Hearing Services in Schools, 41*, 445–458.

Watzlaf, V., Moeini, S., & Firouzan, P. (2010). VOIP for telerehabilitation: A risk analysis for privacy, security and HIPAA compliance. *International Journal of Telerehabilitation, 2*(2), 3–14.

Watzlaf, V., Moeini, S., Matusow, L., & Firouzan, P. (2011). VOIP for telerehabilitation: A risk analysis for privacy, security and HIPAA compliance: Part II. *International Journal of Telerehabilitation, 3*(1), 3–10.

Wilson, L., Onslow, M., & Lincoln, M. (2004). Telehealth adaptation of the Lidcombe Program of Early Stuttering Intervention: Five case studies. *American Journal of Speech-Language Pathology, 13*, 81–93.

4

Family-Centered Early Intervention for Children with Disabilities Provided through Telepractice

K. Todd Houston, Kami Zeckzer Walters, and Arlene Stredler-Brown

Introduction

Children with special needs and their families need access to appropriate family-centered early intervention services that are delivered by professionals who are well trained and experienced in the use of current evidence-based practices. Unfortunately, a lack of qualified practitioners, especially in remote and rural communities, in addition to limited funding, can affect the quality of services that some children receive. However, advancements in telecommunication and distance learning technology have led to models of telepractice, such as teleintervention, that can provide access to appropriate services and reduce overall costs.

The program outlined in Part C of the Individuals with Disabilities Education Act (IDEA) of 1997 (PL 105-17) requires the implementation of family-centered intervention in a natural learning environment (Rush & Shelden, 2011). Family-centered early intervention is a service delivery model that is critical for infants and toddlers who have developmental and communication delays and is at the core of teleintervention. Through a teleintervention model, parents are the primary consumers of the service. That is, through regular videoconferencing sessions, appropriate strategies are modeled for the parents, and the parents are the ones who must carry out the activity with their child. Because the practitioner is not in the home, the model is heavily focused on parent coaching, an essential element of efficacious early intervention (Hamern & Quigley, 2012). Since parent coaching is an integral part of this service delivery model, professionals must expand their knowledge of coaching strategies, which includes an appreciation of the unique characteristics of adult learners.

Although more efficacy research is needed, preliminary findings support the delivery of family-centered early intervention services through telepractice (Behl, Houston, Guthrie, & Guthrie, 2010; Cason, 2009; Cohn & Cason, 2012; Hamern & Quigley, 2012; Houston, 2011; Kelso, Fiechtl, Olsen, & Rule, 2009; Olsen, Fiechtl, & Rule, 2012). Professionals who embrace models of telepractice can help to ensure that more children with special needs and their families receive the intervention to which they are entitled.

The Role of Part C and Early Intervention Applications

Children with special needs and their families should have access to appropriate early intervention services that are delivered by professionals who are well-trained and experienced in current evidence-based practices. Currently, all U.S. states, the District of Columbia, and five U.S. territories (i.e., American Samoa, Guam, Northern Mariana Islands, Palau, and Republic of the Marshall Islands) provide early intervention (EI) to children who have been identified as having a developmental delay or disability from birth through 3-years of age as mandated by Part C of the Individuals with Disabilities Education Act (IDEA) of 1997 (PL 105-17) (Cohn & Cason, 2012). For children and their families who qualify under this legislation, EI services are designed to enhance the quality of their lives by facilitating the parent's capacity to promote the development of skills in infants and toddlers (Cason, 2011).

Family-Centered Intervention in Natural Environments

The program outlined in Part C requires the implementation of family-centered intervention in a natural learning environment (Rush & Shelden, 2011). Natural environments are defined as "settings that are natural or normal for the child's same age peers who have no disabilities" (IDEA, 2004). A child's learning is most functional and socially adaptive when it transpires during natural activities occurring within the context of their everyday settings (Dunst, 2006). By recognizing and incorporating the interests of children within these settings (e.g., eating a meal, taking a bath, etc.), the parent capitalizes on numerous learning opportunities and teachable moments (Dunst, Bruder, Trivette, & Hamby, 2006; McWilliam, 2010; Rush & Shelden, 2011).

The requirement to provide services in the child's natural learning environment has created a shift from intervention programs that are child-centered, with intervention strategies implemented by professionals, to include interventions that are family-centered, with interventions implemented by the parent who is supported by the professional. During family-centered intervention, the professional focuses on enhancing the parent's ability, through coaching, to promote the growth and development of the infant or toddler during everyday learning opportunitics (Campbell & Sawyer, 2007; McWilliam, 2010; Rush & Shelden, 2011; Spagnola & Fiese, 2007; Trivette, Dunst, & Hamby, 2004). When parents follow their children's lead by supporting their interests and participation, there is a positive effect on the child's development and learning (Dunst et al., 2006).

Supporting Family-Centered Early Intervention: Contextually Mediated Practices

Contextually mediated practices (CMP) adhere to many of the tenets outlined in Part C and may be integrated into the telepractice service delivery model to provide high-quality, evidence-based early intervention. The four principles of CMP are as follows (McWilliam, 2010):

- Principle 1: The most meaningful learning opportunities increase the child's participation in family and community life. Therefore, the context for mastering functionally and socially adaptive behavioral competencies should be embedded in the culturally meaningful learning opportunities that exist in the child's everyday experiences.
- Principle 2: The child's ability to self-initiate and direct learning, which develops functional behavioral competencies, should be cultivated through his or her experiences. There is a fundamental difference between experiences that produce a child-desired consequence (e.g., pointing as a gesture to obtain a desired object) and those that elicit a child's behavior (e.g., labeling objects presented by an adult).
- Principle 3: Effective parent-mediated child learning strengthens the parent's confidence and competence. When adults recognize the importance of their influence on the development of their children, they will continue to provide them with the experiences necessary to maximize their child's development.
- Principle 4: The professional must use evidence-based practices to support and strengthen the parent's capacity to provide his or her child with quality experiences and opportunities, thereby strengthening the competence and confidence of the child and the parent (Dunst et al., 2006).

Parent Responsiveness

Another important dynamic that encourages a child's engagement and success in daily learning opportunities is the responsiveness of the parent. The quality, timing, appropriateness, and effect of the parent's responses are all factors that contribute to variations in the child's behavioral and developmental outcomes (Dunst, 2007). Therefore, it is important for the professional to focus on the parent's acquisition and implementation of effective responsive strategies. Responsive strategies may include turning daily routines into games, imitating the child, following the child's lead, and building on the child's interests. It is important to note that daily routines are activities that exist within the pattern of the child's family and school life; they are not lessons or activities to be imposed on the family or child. Incorporating interventions into the child's everyday routines for a large portion of the child's waking hours builds family involvement, maximizes learning opportunities, and normalizes learning (McWilliam, 2010). This type of interaction, which is a basis for successful intervention, promotes child development by supporting the parent as the primary interventionist, increasing responsive parent-child interactions, and occurs during real-life activities (Dunst, 2006; Mahoney, Boyce, Fewell, Spiker, & Wheeden, 1998; Rush & Shelden, 2011).

Collaboration and Accountability

Part C also requires interagency collaboration, and more recently, it mandates state accountability (IDEA, 2004; U.S. Department of Education, 2011). Through collaboration (e.g., collaboration between family members, early interventionists, other professionals), intervention services for each eligible child and family are planned, implemented, and evaluated through the development of an individualized family service plan (IFSP) (McWilliam, 2010). The objective of the IFSP is to ensure that the children served through Part C will have the outcomes and services necessary to establish a strong foundation, which is crucial for their success in preschool and kindergarten (U.S. Department of Education, n.d.). Despite legislation aimed at providing quality services to children with developmental delays or disabilities, statewide birth-to-three programs often struggle to provide appropriate early intervention services to these children and their families. A primary issue is the lack of qualified practitioners. Therefore, administrators and program directors are increasingly utilizing telepractice service delivery models to connect families of children with disabilities to fully qualified service providers. These models of telepractice are associated with positive outcomes (Cason, 2011; Houston, 2011; McCarthy, Munoz, & White, 2010; Olsen, Fiechtl, & Rule, 2012).

Family-Centered Early Intervention + Telepractice = Teleintervention

The rapid increase in the number of services delivered through two-way videoconferencing has led to the creation of a number of terms for this service delivery model. For example, the American Speech-Language-Hearing Association (ASHA) defines this service delivery as "telepractice" for speech-language pathologists and audiologists (ASHA, 2005a, 2005b, 2010). The American Telemedicine Association (ATA), however, refers to these services as telerehabilitation; this term is applied to practitioners in several disciplines (e.g., physical therapists, speech-language pathologists, occupational therapists, audiologists, rehabilitation physicians and nurses, rehabilitation engineers, assistive technologists, teachers, psychologists, and dietitians) (Brennan et al., 2010). More recently, professional associations and other organizations have endorsed the more general term "telehealth" to encompass all medical, intervention, or rehabilitative services in an effort to cause less confusion among consumers and to promote improved insurance reimbursement and licensure portability among practitioners.

In the fall of 2008, researchers at Utah State University initiated a project designed to evaluate the overall feasibility of delivering early intervention services through a telepractice model. Soon afterward, the faculty and staff involved in the project coined the term "teleintervention" to describe the early intervention services provided through distance technology. Teleintervention, a model of early intervention provided through distance technology, provides family-centered services to infants, toddlers, and young children with disabilities. This service delivery allows the provider to model strategies and coach parents in the use of language facilitation techniques (Houston & Behl, 2012). As one parent explained: "We had to drive two hours each way to get these services. We couldn't find an early interventionist in our area who had the experience and training to work with us. Teleintervention has been a lifesaver for our family. Our overall quality of life has improved, and I see tremendous improvement in her language already" (Houston & Behl, 2012).

As telepractice, telerehabilitation, and teleintervention services become more common and are integrated into existing standards of care, early intervention administrators will, no doubt, continue to embrace these models. In so doing, programs will eliminate barriers to services. However, providers must develop the knowledge and skills to effectively deliver these services.

Advantages of Teleintervention Within the Family

Although teleintervention is still a relatively new service delivery model for young children with special needs and their families, there are definite advantages and very few disadvantages. Even families who may live in a community where specialists are available find that receiving services via teleintervention can be very beneficial. For example, some families may live only a short distance from the center or program but may have other young children in the home. The process of packing up all of the children as well as the child with a disability and then traveling to the center is no small undertaking. Teleintervention allows the family to stay at home with less disruption to the family routine. In Figure 4-1, a mother, Nancy Guthrie, is enjoying a book with her son, Alex, during a teleintervention session in their home in Provo, Utah.

In addition, since the technology is available to record and store the sessions, all of the members of a family, as well as other professionals on the early intervention team, can benefit from the strategies offered through teleintervention. The option to record the session allows for it to be viewed at a later date, allowing those—either other professionals or family members—who did not attend the session to benefit. Benefits include opportunities to learn the strategies used in the session and to observe the child's progress from week to week (NCHAM, 2010).

For other families, the shortage of early interventionists who are highly skilled to meet the specific developmental or communication needs of the child and family may propel them toward a model of telepractice. Through teleintervention, parents may have greater access to professionals who could meet the communication needs

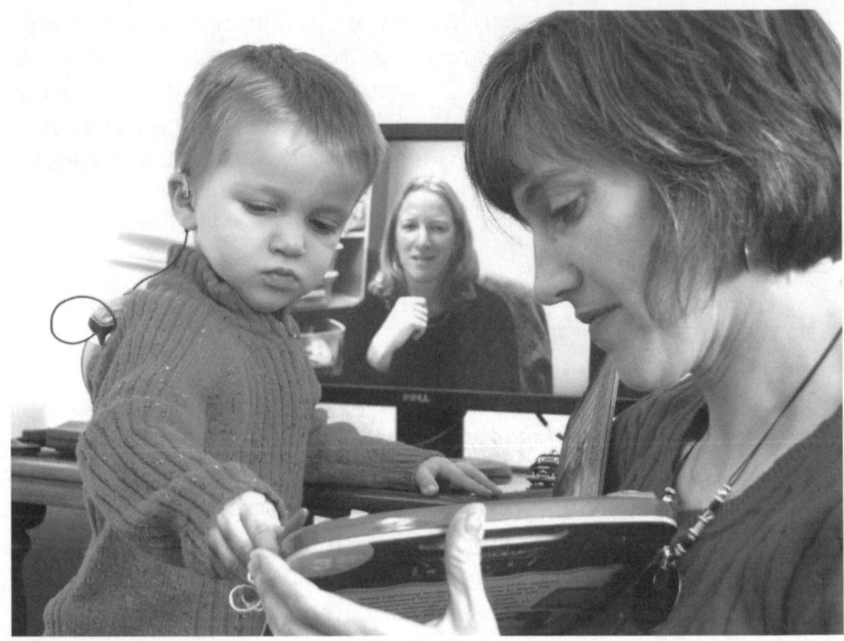

Figure 4–1. Nancy Guthrie describes a favorite book to her son, Alex, while speech-language pathologist Marge Edwards coaches through a teleintervention model.

of their child. And, because the telepractice platform necessitates the use of a coaching partnership, the interaction may be different than that of traditional in-person home visits. For example, when working with the young child, stranger anxiety may surface when the professional visits the home. Since the interventionist is able to coach the parent from a remote location when using a telepractice platform, the child's anxious reaction to the interventionist is circumvented (Hamren & Quigley, 2012). Furthermore, as a result of active engagement between parent and child during teleintervention sessions, parents are better equipped to integrate speech and language goals into the child's typical routines. Thus, in many situations, parents may actually prefer a model of teleintervention rather than pursue more traditional service delivery models.

Given the importance of intensive early intervention, teleintervention may prove to be a more efficient way to ensure consistency of services. With traditional home visits, a family may need to cancel a session if their child or someone else in the family has even a minor illness. However, with teleintervention, cancellations can be kept to a minimum. Even though the child or parent may not be feeling well, the session can proceed in most cases. For children who are medically fragile and/or may have a compromised immune system, this is an added comfort for parents. As a result of fewer cancellations, children receive more frequent services and, consequently, are more likely to obtain the goals outlined in the IFSP.

Telepractice and the Young Child

Cason (2011) addressed the use of telerehabilitation (i.e., telepractice or teleintervention) with young children, birth through age 2, with a disability or developmental delay and ways in which telerehabilitation can improve the annual performance of state Part C programs. Each state's Part C Program is required to report to the Office of Special Education Programs (OSEP) of the U.S. Department of Education annually. This report measures how the Part C program performs on 14 established indicators. Cason's work addresses 8 of these performance indicators and how telerehabilitation could impact the delivery of services.

- Timely Receipt of Services: OSEP requires reporting of the percentage of infants and toddlers with Individualized Family Service Plans (IFSPs) who receive the early intervention services listed on their IFSPs in a timely manner. Telerehabilitation can improve timely delivery of services by increasing access to providers anywhere in the state (or the region) when they are not available in the local community. Through telerehabilitation, children can receive more consistent services due, in part, to fewer cancellations. With traditional home visits, a family may need to cancel a session if their child or someone else in the family has even a minor illness. With teleintervention, cancellations can be kept to a minimum. For children who are medically fragile, teleintervention can be an added comfort for parents.

- Settings: OSEP requires reporting of the percentage of infants and toddlers with IFSPs who receive early intervention services primarily in the home or in community-based settings. Telerehabilitation maintains provision of services within the home or community-based setting though the use of technology. The provider, though at a distance, is actually conducting face-to-face intervention "virtually" (Olsen et al., 2012). The provider implements the same strategies and recommendations that would be provided in a traditional face-to-face setting.
- Infant and Toddler Outcomes: OSEP requires reporting of the percentage of infants and toddlers with IFSPs who demonstrate: improved social-emotional skills, acquisition and use of new skills (e.g., early language, communication), and use of appropriate behaviors to meet their needs. Telerehabilitation has the same potential to augment outcomes for infants and toddlers. Parents and caregivers are taught to enhance their child's skills during naturally occurring routines. Incidentally, telerehabilitation can also be used to conduct professional development activities including training to teach providers to collect and report child outcomes.
- Family Outcomes: OSEP requires reporting of the percentage of families participating in Part C who state that early intervention services have helped their families. This is measured by assuring families know their rights under the law, effectively communicate their children's needs, and help their children develop and learn. Telerehabilitation can be used to conduct ongoing provider training about the use of effective coaching strategies so that families' experiences in early intervention lead to the desired outcomes.
- Indicators #5 and #6—Child Find: OSEP requires each state to report the percentage of infants and toddlers, birth to 1, with IFSPs as compared to national data and the percentage of infants and toddlers, birth to 3, with IFSPs as compared to national data. Telerehabilitation promotes Child Find efforts by facilitating the development and implementation of public awareness activities and materials, engaging in

outreach activities with physicians and referring agencies, connecting experts with one another so they may explore best practices related to evaluation and assessment of children birth to 3, and providing immediate access to interpreters when families do not speak English.

- Forty-five Day Time Line: OSEP requires the reporting of the percentage of eligible infants and toddlers with IFSPs for whom an evaluation and an initial IFSP meeting were conducted within Part C's 45-day timeline. Telerehabilitation can improve this timely delivery of services by improving access to providers and services that are not available in a local community. In this way, telerehabilitation addresses existing personnel shortages.
- Transition: OSEP requires the reporting of the percentage of all children exiting Part C who received timely planning to support the child's transition to preschool and other community services. Telerehabilitation addresses this issue; professionals (e.g., service coordinator, early interventionist, preschool teacher) and multiple family members can call in to a transition conference by using distance technology.

The indicators described here relate specifically to the delivery of early intervention services by providing families in remote and rural areas with access to qualified personnel. Telerehabilitation may improve a state's performance on these, and other, early intervention indicators.

Virtual Home Visits

The Virtual Home Visit Project (VHV), a 2-year study by Olsen et al. (2012), investigated the delivery of early intervention services using videoconferencing to conduct home visits with parents and their children under 3 years of age. During this project, it was observed that coaching (i.e., discussing strategies with parents, listening to parent's opinions, providing feedback) occurred significantly more often during VHVs than in traditional face-to-face visits in the home.

In addition, the study demonstrated that VHVs supported learning within the child's natural environment and encouraged family members to use daily activities and routines to provide intervention for their child with disabilities. VHVs lessen the barriers of time, travel, availability of qualified personnel, and inequity of available services in rural areas. The study also showed that VHVs delivered effective early intervention, were cost-effective, time efficient, and may be a viable approach to strengthen the Part C system in delivering services to families with young children (Olsen et al., 2012).

The use of teleintervention adheres to the major tenets of early intervention services as required by Part C of IDEA. Specifically, services can be delivered in the child's natural environment or in community settings where typical developing peers are found; services can be family-centered and include parent coaching; services can be direct or consultative; and services can support a range of teaming models—multidisciplinary, interdisciplinary, or transdisciplinary. (For a more thorough discussion of possible early intervention services delivered through telerehabilitation, see Cason, 2011.)

Family-Oriented Program Models and Terminology

The foundation of early intervention services is established in a family-centered context that fosters the child's participation in typical family and community activities (Sandall, McLean, Santos, & Smith, 2005). In essence, the target of services is designed for the family and child collectively (Fleming, Sawyer, & Campbell, 2011). Mahoney et al. (1999) define family-centered therapy as a commitment to help families learn new information, receive emotional support, and learn specific communication strategies to augment their child's language development. Others endorse the need for the early interventionist to facilitate the child's development by teaching parents to embed specific strategies into their interactions with their children in naturally occurring activities and routines (Dunst, 1999; Fleming et al., 2011; Hanft, 2004; Klass, 2003; Muma, 1998; Rush & Shelden, 2011; Wasik & Bryant, 2001). Stredler-Brown (2005, 2011) specifically notes this paradigm adjustment for children who are deaf or hard of hearing. Family-centered intervention maximizes already existing learning opportunities while creating individualized learning opportunities for the child, which if indicated, may also include the use of adaptations and assistive technology (Fleming et al., 2011).

Within this context, there is a continuum of four family-oriented program models: professionally centered, family-allied, family-focused, and family-centered. Based on distinctive assumptions about families, each model emphasizes a different approach to involving families; and thereby, influences the roles the professional and family members assume in the intervention process (Dunst, Boyd, Trivette, & Hamby, 2002). In other words, the type of model that is adopted indicates the way the family and professional will assess help-giving practices, whether implicitly or explicitly (Trivette, Dunst, & Hamby, 1996).

In the professionally centered model, professionals are viewed as the experts. As a result, the professional determines the needs of the household, the desired outcomes for the family, and the best way to obtain those outcomes. Decisions are deferred to the professional, and minimal credence is given to the family's opinions (Dunst et al., 2002; Trivette et al., 1996). Additionally, in the professionally centered approach, the child's learning typically occurs using specialized materials during provider-designed activities. Generally, the caregiver is either not present during the session or observes as the professional interacts with the child (Fleming et al., 2011).

Proponents of the family-allied model regard family members as the agents of the professional, who is considered the expert. In this model, the family is recruited to implement the interventions that the professional deems necessary to improve the function of the child and family (Trivette et al., 1996). Families are considered capable of following professional recommendations, but they are viewed as requiring professional assistance to acquire the strategies and skills necessary to effectively influence their family's behavior and development (Dunst et al., 2002). In the early childhood education field, family-allied models are described as family-guided models (Slentz & Bricker, 1992), and in the help-giving field, they are referred to as direct-guidance models (Michlitsch & Frankel, 1989).

Supporters of the family-focused or consumer-directed model view the family as a consumer of professional services capable of making decisions from options recommended by the professional. In this model, after the family makes their decisions, the professional is responsible for providing the necessary assistance (Dunst et al., 2002).

Advocates of family-centered models follow participation-based practices (Fleming et al., 2011), which consider the professional an instrument of the family, and expect the professional to support the family in ways that are individualized, flexible, and responsive. Families are viewed as having existing capabilities, the ability to make informed decisions, the power to act on their decisions to strengthen family competence and improve family functioning, and the capacity to become increasingly competent (Trivette et al., 1996). As the families' existing capabilities are strengthened, functioning is improved, and the family becomes more competent, there is a shift from the family-professional relationships toward interfamily relationships (Dunst et al., 2002).

The Family-Centered Model and the Influence of the Parent

The focus on family-centered, participation-based practice has encouraged a shift from providing developmental services directly to the child, as in professionally centered models, to providing supports to the people in the child's life, their family (McWilliam, 2010). When delivering family-centered early intervention to the young child, professionals must continue to recognize the vital role of the parent and the sheer magnitude of the daily opportunities that the parent has to influence the developmental intervention of the child. For example, during the course of a typical week, a teacher allotting an average of 33 minutes per week to work one-to-one with a child will spend 990 minutes annually with that child. Similarly, a therapist meeting with a child for 30 minutes weekly will work one-to-one with the child for 25 minutes weekly or 750 minutes annually. In contrast, a parent or primary caregiver, who devotes 1 hour daily in activities such as holding, comforting, feeding, playing, and communicating with the child, will spend 420 minutes weekly or 22,000 minutes annually interacting with their child (Mahoney & McDonald, 2004).

Dunst (2006) expands on this concept by reporting that 20 everyday activities provide approximately 40,000 learning opportunities for a child in his or her first year of life. Likewise, research indicates that preschoolers average 50 different everyday activities (Dunst, Buder, Trivette, Raab, & McLean, 1998), which translates into 100,000 learning opportunities for each year of a child's life. This does not account for the multiple learning opportunities that are afforded within a single activity. Even if only five learning opportunities are provided by an activity, a child has 500,000 opportunities to practice an existing skill or learn a new one. Truly, parents have the greatest number of opportunities to influence their child, and therefore, the greatest direct effect on their child's development.

Because parents have the greatest potential for impact and studies demonstrate the effectiveness of parental engagement on the communication outcomes of their children (DesJardin & Eisenberg, 2007; McWilliam, 2010; Moeller, 2000; Zaidman-Zait & Young, 2007), it is essential for professionals to thoroughly understand and apply family-centered, participation-based (Fleming et al., 2011) practices as a key component of early childhood interventions (Rush & Shelden, 2011).

Participation-Based Practices and the Provider

Family-centered, participation-based services align with the Division of Early Childhood's early intervention recommended practices (Fleming et al., 2011; Sandall et al., 2005), as the provider directly teaches the parents to interact with their child through the use of strategies that promote their child's learning in naturally occurring activities and routines (Fleming et al., 2011). However, in contrast to this recommendation, research has indicated that many providers are not using participation-based practices in their daily interactions with children and their families (Campbell & Sawyer, 2007, 2009; Colyvas, Sawyer, & Campbell, 2010; Fleming et al., 2011; Peterson, Luze, Eshbaugh, Jeon, & Kantz, 2007; Wilcox & Lamorey, 2004), as they often do not have the necessary background and training to provide such services. This is regrettable because the skills of the provider are, at the very least, as important as the approach implemented by the parents (Miller & Rollnick, 2002).

This lack of training may, in turn, cause the professional to be apprehensive when working with parents and generate some reluctance to engage parents in the role of their child's primary language facilitator (Fleming et al., 2011; Houston & Bradham, 2011). When such is the case during traditional in-person therapy, providers may unwittingly revert to child-centered practices, because it allows them, as well as the parent, to remain in their comfort zones (Reiss, 2007). This is not a desired outcome as numerous studies demonstrate that effective parent engagement leads to improved communication outcomes in children with special needs (DesJardin & Eisenberg, 2007; McWilliam, 2010; Moeller, 2000; Zaidman-Zait & Young, 2007). However, through a telepractice model, parents must be engaged and professionals, because they are not physically in same room, cannot revert to child-centered practices.

In a study by Fleming and colleagues (2011), providers overwhelmingly identified the critical factors that hindered optimal service to be related to the family. In other words, "ideal" services tended to be implemented more frequently when the provider perceived the caregivers as attentive, involved during the visits, and willing to follow through on their suggestions. Similarly, when parental involvement was perceived to be limited and follow through was lacking, providers reported delivering a lower percentage of "ideal" visits. In the same study (Fleming et al., 2011), the researchers concluded that to consistently provide "ideal" services to families, the providers must have a broader understanding of participation-based practices, initiate strategies within the family's day-to-day lives regardless of the family's characteristics, and use effective modeling and other techniques to teach caregivers.

Coaching: Fostering Increased Parent Engagement

Coaching, a participation-based practice, is intended to develop the parent's ability to facilitate his or her children's participation and learning beyond what is expected to be naturally acquired in day-to-day life (Rush & Shelden, 2011). Parent coaching is a central component of teleintervention, as the very format of this service delivery necessitates the active participation of the parent. Because the professional is not in the room with the child during the teleintervention session, and therefore cannot take direct control of a situation, it is virtually impossible for the parent to passively observe while the professional interacts with the child (Hamren & Quigley, 2012). Teleintervention makes it necessary for the professional to move into the role of coach to educate the parent in appropriate, participation-based, family-centered intervention strategies. As a result, the parent must learn to become the primary facilitator of the child's communication, language, and behavior; take control of interactions with the child; and practice the new skills they have learned.

This process may remove some parents from their comfort zone; however, the benefits outweigh any temporary discomfort as the parent experiences the positive outcomes of coaching. Session by session, the parents, supported by training and feedback from the coach, become more proficient as language facilitators. Eventually, the parents feel more confident in their newly acquired skills (Reiss, 2007). Through this process, the professional develops a partnership with the parent, and the coaching relationship emerges. At the basis of this relationship is the recognition of the parent as the one who has the greatest knowledge of his or her child's interests and temperament (Peterson et al., 2007). When parents move to the place where accomplishments are recognized, goals have been met, and a sense of achievement has been attained, they have moved from the discomfort zone to the "anything's possible" zone (Reiss, 2007).

Coaching: A Family-Centered Strategy in Telepractice

Coaching is a successful strategy that has been used to support parents with the intervention provided to their children (Hendrickson,

Gardner, Kaiser, & Riley, 1993; Marchant & Young, 2001; Peterson et al., 2007; Shanley & Niec, 2010). As part of the coaching relationship, the professional develops the parents' proficiency using specific strategies and increases the parent's confidence in the use of these techniques in each telepractice session. Through this process, parents learn to reinforce appropriate speech, language, listening, and/or communication targets during structured activities in natural everyday settings.

When assuming the role of the coach, the professional is in the position to collaborate with the parent (i.e., coachee) to create an opportunity during the telepractice session where current practices may be jointly examined. To encourage the development of new skills and competencies, feedback is given to the parent, problem-solving strategies are discussed, and mutually agreed-upon strategies are implemented. Effective coaching encourages lifelong learning (Rush & Shelden, 2011) and sustains the performance of the coachee through self-reflection, self-correction, and the generalization of the learned skills (Flaherty, 1999; Kinlaw, 1999).

The quality of the adult's (i.e., parent's) interactions with the child is the most important part of instruction and shows the greatest correlation to a child's development (Justice & Vukelich, 2008). Through the coaching relationship, the professional works to increase the parent's confidence and interaction skills by reinforcing appropriate speech, language, and listening targets during play activities in each telepractice session. As a result of this active engagement, parents are better equipped to integrate communication and language goals into their typical routines.

The Key Components of Coaching

There are five key components of the coaching process (Mc William, 2010; Rush & Shelden, 2011). The first component involves joint planning where the coach and parents cooperatively develop a plan that includes a purpose and an outcome. The importance of parental involvement is threefold. First, research indicates a strong relationship between child benefit and incorporating a child's likes and preferences, as identified by the parents, to learning opportunities (Raab & Dunst, 2006). Secondly, when parents are involved in joint planning, they are more inclined to apply their newly acquired knowledge and skills between coaching sessions, thereby increasing the child's learning opportunities. Finally, a meaningful and relevant plan must consider the family's ecology. The ecology of a family includes: the individuals that make up the family; the supports and resources available to the family; and the activities that fill their day, whether academic, professional, or recreational. For a developmental strategy to be successful, it must promote the competence of a child's skill within the context of the family's unique situation while taking into consideration the family's priorities (McWilliam, 2010).

Next, during the observation step, which does not generally occur during each session, an opportunity is provided for either the professional to observe the parent or for the parent to observe the coach (i.e., the professional) modeling a strategy. When the coach selects a strategy for the parent, it involves a three-step process, which includes: preparation, modeling, and reflection. To prepare, the coach discusses with the parents what is going to be demonstrated and asks them to make observations. The modeling period is a demonstration of strategies that builds upon what is already being implemented by the parent. Finally, there is to be prompt reflection by the parents to ascertain how the modeling reflected their intent.

The third phase is the action step, which allows for parents to demonstrate their new skills. This may occur whether or not the coach is present during a planned or spontaneous event. The goal of this phase is to provide an opportunity for the parent to practice the learned strategy, which is key to building the competence of the coachee. Research indicates that parenting competence is strengthened when children demonstrate positive functioning as a result of parents building child-learning opportunities into everyday activities (Dunst et al., 2006). It has also been proven effective for parents to incorporate interaction styles known to strengthen and promote child competence in addition to increasing their child's participation in these activities. In a study by Dunst et al. (2006) it took less than two weeks for parents to increase the number, frequency, and quality of everyday child learning opportunities.

The action step is followed by a time of reflection, as the coach encourages the parent to think about what happened during the session, what should have happened, and what changes could be made. This provides the parents with time to analyze the strategies, which is necessary for them to improve their skills. Two types of self reflection seem to influence parents' actions: the extent to which the learning opportunities have helped their child reach desired outcomes; and the extent to which the competence and confidence in their parenting capabilities has improved due to their decisions and actions (Dunst, 2006).

Finally, through evaluation and feedback, the coach creates the right environment for reflective learning (Cox, 2006). During this time the parent reflects, recaptures, discerns, and re-evaluates his or her decisions and actions. The coach responds by affirming the reflections, offering additional input, relating relative research, and sharing ideas. Through this process, together, the coach and parent strive to develop strategies to help the child succeed in reaching his or her goals while increasing the parent's competence (Dunst, 2006). Parent competence is measured in terms of child interest identification, selection of everyday activities resulting from the child's expression of interests, parenting efforts to increase child participation in the telepractice session and in everyday activities, and parents' roles in supporting child learning in these activities. Ultimately, this process leads to the parents' personal development (Cox, 2006) and directly contributes to their confidence and competence in their role as their child's primary interventionist. As a result, the experiences and benefits provided to their child are positively impacted (Dunst, 2006).

In addition, special attention is placed on self-efficacy beliefs, which are known to be mediators of these parenting behaviors. Cox (2006) describes self-efficacy as one's belief in his or her capacity to successfully accomplish tasks. It is rooted in the theory that individuals are proactive in their development; therefore, their actions influence outcomes (Bandura, 1994; Pajares, 2002). Self-efficacy is built on the mastery of experiences; enhanced through the sharing of experiences and modeling behavior; reinforced by positive physiologic states and attitudes; and heightened through positive, honest feedback. In family-centered practices, self-efficacy is measured in terms of parents' judgments about their abilities to plan and provide their children with interest-based everyday learning opportunities that lead to desired outcomes.

As the parent's confidence grows, the same speech, language, or communication strategies should be incorporated into the child's daily routines. For example, the parent may learn how to appropriately model and expand language during a cookie-baking activity. By reinforcing communication targets during these regularly occurring activities within the home, the parent's skills become more habitual and can easily transfer to other commonly occurring activities, such as bath time, getting dressed, or setting the table for dinner.

Coaching and the Adult Learner in Telepractice

When engaging in coaching practices, it is important to consider that the parent is an adult learner. Theories associated with adult learning have significant relevance to telepractice service delivery models, especially teleintervention. Many adult learners have grown up in the digital world, and as a result, they have acquired a new means of learning, processing, and understanding novel information. Consequently, a multifaceted approach that melds contemporary adult learning theories and the social learning theory with the digital world is emerging (Baird & Fisher, 2005). Cercone (2008) claims that professionals who design online environments for adults must understand adult learning theory, especially in terms of its relationship to distance or online learning. Today, telepractice provides a platform for integrating adult learning theories while making provisions for the demands of the adult's busy schedule to create an environment that best meets the needs of the child. This is significant for parents as adult learners generally have numerous responsibilities associated with their family, careers, and finances that often result in demanding personal schedules (U.S. Department of Education, 2005). Consequently, minimal time is usually available for the parent to pursue additional activities that occur outside of the home, such as center-based therapy for his or her child. In contrast, telepractice eases the demands on the family's time by providing therapy within the home environment.

The adult learner brings a wide range of abilities, personal experiences, and educational and cultural backgrounds to the learning experience. Therefore, the learner's background is an essential component of the andragogy theory (Baird & Fisher, 2005). In the andragogy theory, Malcom Knowles (1980) identifies the characteristics of the adult learner (Baird & Fisher, 2005; Cercone, 2008), and views the adult as a mature, self-motivated, equal participant who is engaged in a learning relationship with the teacher or coach. In this theory, the coach's primary role is to help the learner achieve his or her primary self-determination. Five assumptions about the adult learner are present in this theory (Baird & Fisher, 2005; Cox, 2006).

Adult learners:

1. are self-directed in their learning, goal-oriented, and seek relevant material;
2. bring an abundance of life experiences to their learning, which becomes an increasing resource for their learning;
3. require learning to be relevant, useful, and helpful in solving life dilemmas;
4. necessitate a practical application for the information they are learning;
5. and are intrinsically motivated.

Learning styles are also an important consideration when determining how individuals approach learning tasks (Baird & Fisher, 2005), as they affect the way learners receive and process information (Felder, 1996). According to Silver, Strong, and Perini (1997), learning styles are associated with the way people think, feel, and interact as they solve problems. If students are motivated to learn by understanding their learning style, they can heighten their lifelong learning (Coffield, Moseley, Hall, & Ecclestone, 2004).

Because adults must balance the demands of learning with the numerous responsibilities of their everyday lives, the best way to motivate them is to involve them in the development of a relevant plan that takes into consideration adult learning characteristics, emphasizes the importance of their role in their child's intervention, recognizes the unique contributions they have to offer, and decreases the barriers that keep them from assuming this new role. Research indicates that coaching practices are consistent with how people learn. Therefore, coaching is a viable way for parents to interact in their children's lives (Rush & Shelden, 2011).

A Model of Teleintervention for Children with Hearing Loss

There are challenges inherent to the provision of early intervention services to children with disabilities, including children with hearing loss and their families. Some of these challenges include limited communication options available within the family's community (Roush, 2011) and a lack of well-trained professionals with expertise in hearing loss, including educators of the deaf, speech-language pathologists, and audiologists (Houston, Munoz, & Bradham, 2011; Houston & Perigoe, 2010; JCIH, 2007), and a need for home-based intervention in addition to center-based intervention. The School of Speech-Language Pathology and Audiology at The University of Akron created a model of teleintervention for children with hearing loss through the Telepractice and eLearning Lab (TeLL) to overcome these challenges and to provide children with hearing loss and their families with high-quality family-centered early intervention services. Furthermore, the TeLL offers an enhanced learning experience for graduate students in speech-language pathology to develop their knowledge and skills in the provision of telepractice services to families of children with hearing loss.

The principal investigators for the Telepractice and eLearning Lab (TeLL) at the University of Akron (UA) seek to evaluate the outcomes of teleintervention. For this research, families have chosen listening and spoken language as the desired outcome for their children. The knowledge acquired and the skills used by the parents are carefully monitored to determine if they successfully employed recommended language facilitation techniques with their children.

Currently, the TeLL utilizes the distance learning software Collaborate, which is produced by Blackboard, to deliver telepractice services. Although other videoconferencing equipment and software were evaluated, Collaborate provided the flexibility that was required, and the University of Akron was able to provide technological support as needed. Because the software is designed for distance learning applications, it creates a "virtual classroom" whereby the "student" can enter and have access to complete audio and video of the "lecturer" in real time (i.e., synchronously). In the TeLL's telepractice sessions, parents can log into the virtual classroom using their laptop or desktop computer from their home. In a similar manner, the clinician can enter the classroom and can see and hear the parent clearly. The equipment requirements have remained minimal.

Through the TeLL, families receive weekly telepractice sessions that support listening and spoken language development in children with hearing loss. Prior to each weekly 60-minute session, each family receives via e-mail a lesson plan and materials that can be printed that were developed to meet the child's current goals in speech, language, and listening. Many of the materials, such as colorful scenes to foster language use, can be posted within the virtual classroom as a PowerPoint file. The parent and the child can see these materials as images on their computer screen. Each session begins with a discussion of the speech, language, and listening goals targeted during the prior session and about how previously demonstrated communication strategies had been integrated into the child's daily routines. The faculty member, graduate students, and parent discuss any new communication behaviors that might be relevant to the child's progress, such as new or emerging speech sounds, language targets, or listening behaviors that have been noticed. Once these updates have occurred, the faculty member and graduate students introduce the goals for that day's session, explaining the desired speech, language, listening, and interactive behaviors.

After discussing the materials and activities that would most engage the child, the SLP and graduate students demonstrate the activity before asking the parent to engage the child. The parent repeats the activity while the faculty member and graduate students observe. At this point in the session, the practitioner's role shifts to that of a coach. The faculty member and/or graduate student provides positive reinforcement and constructive feedback to the parent based on how the activity was implemented and how the communication strategies that promote listening and spoken language were applied. This same scenario is repeated as one activity ends and a new activity is initiated. Throughout the session, the parent, the faculty member, and graduate students closely monitor the child's attention level.

Following the session, the parent is given ample opportunity to discuss any concerns about the child's progress, to ask questions about and provide input in forming short- or long-term communication goals, or to seek input about troubleshooting the child's hearing technology (e.g., digital hearing aids, cochlear implants, and/or FM systems). The faculty member and graduate students summarize the goals and facilitation strategies that were modeled and practiced during the session. Based on the child's performance and developmental level, new or additional communication goals are discussed that will be targeted in the home the following week.

The TeLL telepractice program continues to demonstrate its effectiveness as a service delivery model, which is depicted in Figure 4–2. As one mother of a 4-year-old son with bilateral cochlear implants explained:

> *What I've found is that telepractice has benefitted him in many, many ways. First, we have the consistency of weekly therapy back in place. Second, my son is more comfortable with telepractice than he was going to see a therapist and having more traditional services sitting at a table in a therapy room. With telepractice, he's in his home, and I'm working with him. If he needs to get down and stretch his legs or grab a glass of water, he can. It is quite natural for him. Most importantly, because he feels more comfortable being at home, I see him talking more during the sessions. He doesn't "clam up" like he used to when we visited the therapist. Another benefit of telepractice is the coaching I receive as the parent, and that I receive weekly lesson plans and other materials that I can refer to after the session.*

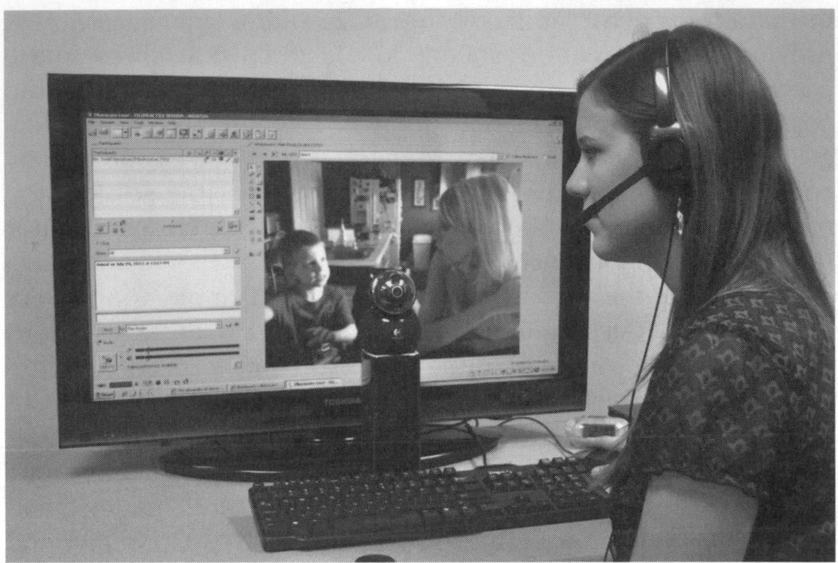

Figure 4–2. Kelly Brown, a graduate student in speech-language pathology at the University of Akron, provides auditory-verbal therapy to Tammy Kenny and her son, Aiden.

> *We'll continue to work on the goals and do the activities throughout the week. Telepractice has been great for my son and our family.* (personal communication, November, 2012)

Considerations Before Starting Teleintervention

Program or center administrators must carefully select the providers who will be delivering teleintervention services and the families who will receive them. Professionals may recognize that some parenting and other behavior management issues are better addressed through a traditional, in-person service delivery model. Likewise, some parents may not feel comfortable with teleintervention and may decide that they prefer a more traditional, in-home service delivery model. However, these families may consider starting services at a center or in the home and slowly move to a teleintervention model.

Some professionals and parents are "techno-phobes" and may feel intimidated by the technology. For providers who are reluctant to use technology in this manner, it may be helpful for them to observe practitioners who are currently providing teleintervention. It is important to recognize that once the equipment is in place and functioning well, the sessions focus less on the operation of the technology and more on the intervention. Most of the technology—from the more expensive videoconferencing equipment to the standard laptop and webcam—are relatively simple to use. Tutorials on setting up and using the technology are available online and offered by many manufacturers and service providers (i.e., SKYPE, ooVoo, etc.). Regardless of how efficient a provider becomes using the equipment, it is critical to have support from information technology (IT) specialists who are experts in telecommunication technology. These specialists inform providers about new trends and products that can enhance teleintervention and troubleshoot problems that may arise.

Another consideration is the type of Internet connection available in the remote community and at the professional's site. The speed of the Internet connection is a critical component for a successful interaction. It cannot be assumed that a family has access to a high-speed Internet connection. Even with access to a high-speed Internet connection, the volume of users on the network at any given time may cause the transmission time to slow. A busy clinic may need to evaluate and accommodate the Internet connection to allow for high-speed access.

Conclusion

Young children with special needs and their families require access to appropriate early intervention services delivered by well-trained professionals who implement evidence-based practices that are in compliance with Part C of IDEA. Family-centered interventions enhance the quality of the family's lives, occur in the child's natural learning environment, educate the parents in appropriate family-centered intervention strategies, and promote the development of the young child's skills. These principles are also supported by Contextually Mediated Practices, which provide a conceptual framework for effective family-centered practices. Through family-centered models, families are viewed as have existing capabilities, the ability to make informed decisions, the power to act on their decisions, and the capacity to become increasingly competent (Trivette et al., 1996).

Obstacles to providing family-centered intervention may occur when a professional lacks training and therefore becomes reluctant to engage parents in the role of their child's primary language facilitator (Fleming et al., 2011; Houston & Bradham, 2011). However, because numerous studies demonstrate that effective parent engagement leads to improved communication outcomes in children with special needs (DesJardin & Eisenberg, 2007; McWilliam, 2010; Moeller, 2000; Zaidman-Zait & Young, 2007), these obstacles must be overcome.

Teleintervention makes it necessary for the professional to assume the role of coach. The coaching process provides an effective way to develop the parent's ability to facilitate a child's participation and learning. As a result of the coaching process, the parent learns to take control of the interactions with the child to become the primary facilitator of the child's communication, language, and behavior. As the coach, the professional is in the position to collaborate with the parent to create an environment where current practices may be jointly examined; feedback may be used to encourage the development of new skills and competencies; and problem-solving strategies may be discussed and implemented. Effective coaching encourages lifelong learning (Rush & Shelden, 2011) and sustains the performance of the coachee through self-reflection, self-correction, and the generalization of the learned skills (Flaherty, 1999; Kinlaw, 1999).

When engaging in coaching practices, it is important for the professional to consider the parent as an adult learner. The adult learner brings a wide range of abilities, personal experiences, academic learning, and cultural background to the learning environment. Theories associated with adult learning have significant relevance to teleintervention. In addition, teleintervention provides a platform for integrating adult learning theories while making provisions for the demands of the adult's schedule to create an environment that best meets the needs of the child.

Advances in telecommunication and distance learning technology offer a new option for implementing family-centered early intervention services. Programs increasingly are utilizing models of telepractice or teleintervention to ensure access to appropriate services for the families they serve. Parents also are requesting and seeking these services, especially when highly skilled early interventionists or other practitioners are not available in their communities. Programs that embrace models of telepractice and teleintervention are in a better position to meet this growing demand.

The use of telerehabilitation adheres to the major tenets of early intervention services as required by Part C of IDEA (Cason, 2009). It is too soon to know if the term "teleintervention" will withstand the test of time. This terminology addresses family-centered early intervention for infants and toddlers under 36 months of age. What is known is that telepractice—and teleintervention—eliminate many of the barriers to services that continue to affect young children with special needs and their families.

References

American Speech-Language-Hearing Association. (2005a). *Audiologists providing clinical services via telepractice: Position statement.* Available from http://www.asha.org/policy.

American Speech-Language-Hearing Association. (2005b). *Speech-language pathologists providing clinical services via telepractice: Position statement.* Available from http://www.asha.org/policy.

American Speech-Language-Hearing Association. (2010). *Professional issues in telepractice for speech-language pathologists (professional issues statement).* Available from http://www.asha.org/policy.

Baird, D. E., & Fisher, M. (2005). Neomillennial user experience design strategies: Utilizing social networking media to support "always on" learning styles. *Journal of Educational Technology Systems, 34*(1), 5–32.

Bandura, A. (1994). Self-efficacy. In V. S. Ramachaudran (Ed.), *Encyclopedia of human behavior* (Vol. 4, pp. 71–81). New York, NY: Reprinted in H. Friedman (Ed.), *Encyclopedia of mental health.* San Diego, CA:

Academic Press, 1998. Retrieved April 5, 2013, at http://p20motivationlab.org/Bandura-Publications.

Behl, D., Houston, K. T., Guthrie, W. S., & Guthrie, N. (2010). Tele-Intervention: The wave of the future fits families' lives today. *Exceptional Parent*, *40*, 23–28.

Brennan, D., Tindall, L., Theodoros, D., Brown, J., Campbell, M., Christiana, D., Lee, A. (2010). A blueprint for telerehabilitation guidelines. *International Journal of Telerehabilitation*, *2*(2), 31–34.

Campbell, P. H., & Sawyer, L. B. (2007). Supporting learning opportunities in natural settings through participation-based services. *Journal of Early Intervention*, *29*(4), 287–305.

Campbell, P. H., & Sawyer, L. B. (2009). Changing early intervention providers' home visiting skills through participation in professional development. *Topics in Early Childhood Special Education, 28*, 219–234.

Cason, J. (2009). A pilot telerehabilitation program: Delivering early intervention services to rural families. *International Journal of Telerehabilitation*, *1*(1), 29–38.

Cason, J. (2011). Telerehabilitation: An adjunct service delivery model for early intervention services. *International Journal of Telerehabilitation*, *3*(1), 19–28.

Cercone, K. (2008). Characteristics of adult learners with implications for online learning design. *AACE Journal*, *16*(2), 137–159.

Coffield, F. J., Moseley, D. V., Hall, E., & Ecclestone, K. (2004). *Learning styles and pedagogy in post-16 learning: A systematic and critical review*. London, UK: Learning and Skills Research Centre.

Cohn, E., & Cason, J. (2012). Telepractice: A wide-angle view for persons with hearing loss. *Volta Review*, *112*(3), 207–226.

Colyvas, J. L., Sawyer, B. E., & Campbell, P. H. (2010). Identifying strategies early intervention occupational therapists use to teach caregivers. *American Journal of Occupational Therapy*, *64*, 776–785.

Cox, E. (2006). An adult learning approach to coaching. In D. R. Stober & A. M. Grant (Eds.), *Evidence-based coaching handbook* (pp. 193–217). Hoboken, NJ: Wiley & Sons.

DesJardin, J. L., & Eisenberg, L. S. (2007). Maternal contributions: Supporting language development in young children with cochlear implants. *Ear and Hearing*, *28*(4), 456–469.

Dunst, C. J. (1999). Placing parent education in conceptual and empirical context. *Topics in Early Childhood Special Education, 19*(3), 141–147.

Dunst, C. J. (2006). Parent-mediated everyday child learning opportunities: I. Foundations and operationalization. *CASEinPoint*, *2*(2), 1–10.

Dunst, C. J. (2007). Early intervention with infants and toddlers with developmental disabilities. In S. L. Odom, R. H. Horner, M. Snell, & J. Blacher (Eds.), *Handbook of developmental disabilities* (pp. 531-551). New York, NY: Guilford Press.

Dunst, C. J., Boyd, K., Trivette, C. M., & Hamby, D. W. (2002). Family-orientated program models and professional helpgiving practices. *Family Relations*, 51, 221-229.

Dunst, C. J., Bruder, M. B., Trivette, C. M., & Hamby, D. W. (2006). Everyday activity settings, natural learning environments, and early intervention practices. *Journal of Policy and Practice in Intellectual Disabilities*, 3, 3-10.

Dunst, C. J., Bruder, M. B., Trivette, C. M., Raab, M., & McLean, M. (1998). *Increasing children's learning opportunities through families and communities early childhood research institute: Year 2 progress report*. Asheville, NC: Orelena Hawks Puckett Institute.

Felder, R. M. (1996, December). *Matters of style.* Retrieved April 16, 2013, from http://www4.ncsu.edu/unity/lockers/users/f/felder/public/Papers/LS-Prism.htm.

Flaherty, J. (1999). *Coaching: Evoking excellence in others.* Boston, MA: Butterworth-Heinemann.

Fleming, J. L., Sawyer, B. L., & Campbell, P. H. (2011). Early intervention providers' perspectives about implementing participation-based practices. *Topics in Early Childhood Special Education*, *30*(4), 233-244.

Hamren, K., & Quigley, S. (2012). Implementing coaching in a natural environment through distance technologies. *Volta Review*, *112*(3), 403-407.

Hanft, B. E., Rush, D. D., & Shelden, M. L. (2004). *Coaching families and colleagues in early childhood*. Baltimore, MD: Brookes.

Houston, K. T. (2011). TeleIntervention: Improving service delivery to young children with hearing loss and their families through telepractice. *Perspectives on Hearing and Hearing Disorders in Childhood*, *21*(2), 66-72.

Houston, K. T., & Behl, D. (2012). Using telepractice to improve outcomes for children with hearing loss and their families. In Schmeltz, L. (Ed.), *EHDI E-Book*. Available at http://www.infanthearing.org/ehdi-ebook/index.html.

Houston, K. T., & Bradham, T. S. (2011). Parent engagement in audiologic habilitation: Increasing positive outcomes for children with hearing loss. *ASHA Leader*, *16*(8), 5-6.

Houston, K. T., Munoz, K. F., & Bradham, T. S. (2011). Professional development: Are we meeting the needs of state EHDI programs? *Volta Review*, *111*(2), 209-223.

Houston, K. T., & Perigoe, C. B. (Eds.). (2010). Professional preparation for listening and spoken language practitioners. *Volta Review, 110*(2), 86–354.

Individuals with Disabilities Education Improvement Act of 2004. (2004). *20 U.S.C. § 1400 et seq.*

Individuals with Disabilities Education Improvement Act of 2004, Pub. L. No. 108–446, 117 Stat. (2004). [Quotation is from Sec. 631 (a) (1), Findings and Policy.] Retrieved from http://nichcy.org/wp-content/uploads/dics/PL108-446.pdf.

Joint Committee on Infant Hearing. (2007). Year 2007 Position Statement: Principles and guidelines for early hearing detection and intervention programs. *Pediatrics, 120*(4), 898–921.

Justice, L., & Vukelich, C. (2008). *Achieving excellence in preschool literacy.* New York, NY: Guilford Press.

Kelso, G., Fiechtl, B., Olsen, S., & Rule, S. (2009). The feasibility of virtual home visits to provide early intervention: A pilot study. *Infants and Young Children, 22*(4), 332–340.

Kinlaw, D. C. (1999). *Coaching for commitment: Interpersonal strategies for obtaining superior performance from individuals and teams.* San Francisco, CA: Jossey-Bass.

Klass, C. S. (2003). *The home visitor's guidebook.* Baltimore, MD: Brookes.

Knowles, M. (1980). *The modern practice of adult education: From pedagogy to andragogy.* Englewood Cliffs, NJ: Prentice-Hall/Cambridge.

Mahoney, G., Boyce, G., Fewell, R., Spiker, D., & Wheeden, C. A. (1998). The relationship of parent-child interaction to the effectiveness of early intervention services for at-risk children and children with disabilities. *Topics in Early Childhood Special Education, 18*(1), 5–17.

Mahoney, G., Kaiser, A., Girolametto, L., MacDonald, J., Robinson, C., Safford, P., et al. (1999). Parent education in early intervention: A call for a renewed focus. *Topics in Early Childhood Special Education, 19*(3), 131–140.

Mahoney, G., & McDonald, J. (2004). *Responsive teaching: Parent-mediated developmental intervention.* Baltimore, MD: Paul H. Brookes.

Marchant, M., & Young, K. R. (2001). The effects of a parent coach on parent's acquisition and implementation of parenting skills. *Education and Treatment of Children, 24*(3), 351–373.

McCarthy, M., Munoz, K., & White, K. R. (2010). Teleintervention for infants and young children who are deaf or hard-of-hearing. *Pediatrics, 126*, S52–S58.

McWilliam, R. A. (2010). *Working with families of young children with special needs.* New York, NY: Guilford Press.

Michlitsch, J., & Frankel, S. (1989). Helping orientations: Four dimensions. *Perceptual and Motor Skills*, *69*, 1371–1378.

Miller, W. R., & Rollnick, S. (2002). *Motivational interviewing*. New York, NY: Guilford.

Moeller, M. P. (2000). Early intervention and language development in children who are deaf and hard of hearing. *Pediatrics*, *106*, 1–9.

Muma, J. (1998). *Effective speech-language pathology: A cognitive socialization approach*. Mahwah, NJ: Erlbaum.

National Center for Hearing Assessment and Management (NCHAM), (2010). *Telehealth survey of EHDI coordinators*. Retrieved from http://www.infanthearing.org/telehealth/index.html.

Olsen, S., Fiechtl, B., & Rule, S. (2012). An evaluation of virtual home visits in early intervention: Feasibility of "virtual intervention." *Volta Review, 112*(3).

Pajares, F. (2002). *Overview of social cognitive theory and of self-efficacy*. Retrieved April 5, 2013, from http://www.uky.edu/~eushe2/Pajares/eff.html

Peterson, C. A., Luze, G. J., Eshbaugh, E. M., Jeon, H. J., & Kantz, K. R. (2007). Enhancing parent-child interactions through home visiting: Promising practice or unfulfilled promise. *Journal of Early Intervention*, *29*, 119–140.

Raab, M., & Dunst, C. J. (2006). *Influence of child interests on variations in child behavior and functioning*. (Winterberry Research Syntheses Vol. 1, No. 21), Asheville, NC: Winterberry Press.

Reiss, Karla. (2007). *Leadership coaching for educators: Bringing out the best in school administrators*. Thousand Oaks, CA: Corwin Press.

Roush, J. (Ed.). (2011). A strategic analysis of state early hearing detection and intervention programs. *Volta Review, 111*(2), 83–293.

Rush, D., & Shelden, M. (2011). *The early childhood coaching handbook*. Baltimore, MD: Brookes.

Sandall, S., McLean, M. E., Santos, R. M., & Smith, B. J. (2005). DEC's recommended practices: The context for change. In: J. L. Fleming, L. B. Sawyer, & P. H. Campbell (Eds.), Early intervention providers' perspectives about implementing participation-based practices. *Topics in Early Childhood Special Education*, *30*(4), 233–244.

Shanley, J. R., & Niec, L. N. (2010). Coaching parents to change: The impact of in vivo feedback on parent's acquisition of skills. *Journal of Clinical Child and Adolescent Psychology, 39*(2), 282–287.

Silver, H., Strong, R., & Perini, M. (1997). Integrating learning styles and multiple intelligences. *Educational Leadership*, *55*(1), 22–27.

Slentz, K., & Bricker, D. (1992). Family guided assessment for IFSP development: Jumping off the family assessment bandwagon. *Journal of Early Intervention*, *16*, 11-19.

Spagnola, M., & Fiese, B. H. (2007). Family routines and rituals. A context for development in the lives of young children. *Infants and Young Children*, *20*(4), 284-299.

Stredler-Brown, A. (2005). Family-centered intervention: Proven strategies to assure positive outcomes. In R. Seewald & J. Bamford (Eds.), *A sound foundation through early amplification 2004: Proceedings of the Third International Conference* (pp. 185-195). Great Britain: Immediate Proceedings Limited.

Stredler-Brown, A. (2011). Early intervention: Serving infants and toddlers. In C. Deconde Johnson & J. Seaton (Eds.), *Educational audiology handbook* (pp. 445-465). Clifton Park, NY: Thomson Delmar Learning.

Trivette, C. M., Dunst, C. J., & Hamby, D. (1996). Characteristics and consequences of help-giving practices in contrasting human services programs. *American Journal of Community Psychology*, *24*(2), 273-293.

Trivette, C. M., Dunst, C. J., & Hamby, D. (2004). Sources of variation in and consequences of everyday activity settings on child and parenting functioning. *Perspectives in Education*, *22*(2), 17-35.

U.S. Department of Education. (n.d.). *IDEA 2004: Building the legacy.* Retrieved March 5, 2013, from http://idea.ed.gov/part-c/search/new.

U.S. Department of Education. (2005, May). *National Center for Education Statistics Brief: Reasons for adult's participation in work-related courses.* Retrieved from http://www.sreb.org/page/1397/who_is_th.

U.S. Department of Education. (2011). Early intervention program for infants and toddlers with disabilities. *Federal Register, 76*(60140-60309), 28.

Wasik, B. H., & Bryant, D. M. (2001). *Home visiting: Procedures for helping families* (2nd ed.). Thousand Oaks, CA: Sage.

Wilcox, M. J., & Lamorey, S. (2004, October). *Relationship-based practice in early intervention settings: The experimental investigation of impact and effectiveness: Final report* (Field-Initiated Research R305T00049). Washington, DC: U.S. Department of Education.

5

Teletherapy: Serving School-Age Children

Sue Grogan-Johnson

Introduction

This chapter focuses on implementing speech and language intervention telepractice services for school-age children. Based on the actual implementation of a telepractice service delivery model, this chapter includes: a procedure for developing and implementing a telepractice delivery model within a school setting; a needs assessment; and a description of the school-based telepractice project at Kent State University, Kent, Ohio.

In order for a school-based speech and language telepractice project to be successful, it must have a clearly defined scope and purpose. Then, it must be designed to accomplish that purpose. Throughout this chapter, focus questions are utilized to introduce each step in a five-step process for defining the scope and purpose and then implementing a school-based telepractice project.

Focus Question: How Do I Get Started?

The first step in implementing a school-based telepractice project is to review the rules and regulations related to the practice of speech-language pathology to ensure that telepractice is permitted in the state where the speech-language pathologist (SLP) resides and, if applicable, the state where services will be provided. The American Speech-Language Hearing Association (ASHA) maintains an updated list of telepractice requirements by state (http://www.asha.org/Practice/telepractice/StateProvisionsUpdate Telepractice/). Contact your state licensure board for the most current information.

Familiar adages such as "seeing is believing" and "a picture is worth a thousand words" are relevant during this first step as it is very helpful to observe a telepractice program in progress and/or consult with speech-language pathologists who are currently using the delivery model. Telepractioners may be found through the online community of ASHA Special Interest Group 18: Telepractice (http://www.asha.org/SIG/18), as well as through an Internet search for telepractice services. Actually viewing the service delivery model may help solidify a decision to try the service delivery model. Observing several different practitioners allows for comparison among different types of technology and videoconferencing options. Observation may also spark ideas for applying the service delivery model in your particular situation. Online communities also offer the opportunity to pose questions and ask advice of those who are currently providing telepractice services.

Additionally, Chapter 3 reviews essential documents and resources that outline the provision of effective and safe telepractice services based on currently available evidence and technology. In addition to these written materials, continuing education is becoming increasingly available with sessions targeted specifically to SLPs and audiologists. National organizations such as ASHA and the American Telemedicine Association (ATA) provide Webinars as well as in-person continuing education.

After researching state legal requirements, observing telepractice service delivery and reading relevant published materials related to the provision of speech-language telepractice, those choosing to move forward with telepractice must progress to defining the scope of the program and its essential elements.

The Kent State University (KSU) school-based telepractice project began in 2006. The acute shortage of SLPs had resulted in some school districts being unable to provide the services needed for students with communication impairments. In attempting to eliminate the shortage, the Ohio Department of Education (ODE) formed a task force with representatives from Ohio's universities, the Ohio Board of Speech-Language Pathology & Audiology (OBSLPA), Ohio Master's Network Initiatives in Education (OMNIE), and state professional associations. The group developed a program consisting of eight initiatives funded by ODE (Boswell, 2007). One of the initiatives, a pilot telepractice project, would provide speech-language therapy services to students in rural school districts using live interactive videoconferencing. The purpose of the pilot telepractice project was to collect data on students who received the services to determine if children make similar amounts of progress in speech-language therapy when they receive services via telepractice as compared to a traditional side-by-side service delivery model.

The KSU telepractice program began as a grassroots effort, without prior knowledge or experience in telepractice. After investigation of other programs delivering similar services, the KSU program was formulated, refined, and implemented with funding provided by the ODE. The program has grown and thrived. Now funded independently of the ODE, the program delivers speech-language intervention services to approximately 120 students in two rural school districts in Ohio.

How Do I Develop a Telepractice Program for the Public Schools?

An effective and systematic method for developing a telepractice program begins with the completion of a needs assessment. A needs assessment provides guiding questions designed to help the developer carefully consider the many variables inherent in developing a telepractice project. As with the KSU project, the development of a telepractice program is often motivated by a challenging situation or a gap that exists between available services and the need for services. Examples of such a gap in services include a school district that is unable to recruit an SLP to fill a vacancy or unable to obtain the services of an additional SLP to work part-time to assist with large caseloads. Other motivating needs include providing services to students who are home bound or in an alternate placement. Perhaps many hours of intervention time are lost weekly due to the travel requirements between buildings in a school district. Identifying the challenging situation/need is the first step in the needs assessment. The identified need(s) will help define the scope and initial focus of your telepractice project.

Consider the scenario of a small rural school district that employs only one SLP to provide services to children from preschool through high school. Increasing demands for student achievement and a growing population of children with disabilities has substantially increased her caseload. The SLP needs to provide effective services to the students on her caseload, but she would need "more hours in the day" to provide those services. The SLP analyzes her service delivery and identifies that she works collaboratively in the preschool through sixth grade classrooms so that a continued physical presence in the building is essential. The high school students on the caseload receive services through a coaching/mentoring model. By transitioning to a telepractice service delivery model for the high school students the SLP would gain time for intervention that was previously spent traveling between schools and preparing for services. In addition, the SLP may find that she can utilize the school day more efficiently by transitioning between telepractice and traditional therapy sessions to take advantage of differences in the elementary and high school daily schedules.

A needs assessment is best conducted in collaboration with key district employees, which may include the information technology coordinator or technician, special education director, SLP, and/or classroom teachers. To begin the needs assessment process, answer these questions:

- Does your state licensure law allow for the provision of speech-language therapy services through telepractice?
  - What other agencies may be involved? (e.g., school Medicaid program)
  - Are you licensed in the state where the client/patient resides?

- Why are you considering a telepractice project?
  - Are there currently unmet needs that could be met with this project?
  - Are there new or additional services that could be provided with this project?
  - Have you considered other alternatives to meet these needs?
  - What do you hope to accomplish with this project?
- What telepractice service delivery model would best meet the identified needs?
  - Are you considering live, interactive videoconferencing, use of e-mail or instant messaging, telephone contact, completion of online activities that record student responses?
- Do you have a short-term (1 year) and a long-term (3 year) plan for the project?
  - What is a possible start date?
  - Do you want to pilot the project for 1 year, and then re-evaluate to determine continued involvement?
- Is the telepractice model sustainable?
  - What are possible threats or challenges to the project?

These five questions were used to guide the initial development of the KSU telepractice project. The state of Ohio permits the provision of speech and language services through telepractice. However, to ensure compliance with state regulations, the Ohio Board of Speech Language Pathology and Audiology was invited to participate in the early discussions of the project as there were no known instances of speech-language services delivered through live interactive videoconferencing in the state of Ohio prior to the KSU telepractice project.

The motivation for the KSU telepractice project was the shortage of SLPs in Ohio, in particular in the rural school districts, which historically had difficulty recruiting and retaining qualified SLPs. In the spring of 2007, an informational letter introducing the project was sent to over 600 public school superintendents while state SLPs were introduced to the program at the state speech-language-hearing association convention. To encourage participation, the

ODE agreed to cover the entire cost of the project during the first year. Despite these efforts, no school districts initially expressed interest in the project. Eventually, through repeated contacts, the Hardin County Educational Service Center and four rural school districts agreed to participate. The service center had previously experienced difficulty providing required speech-language pathology services to the districts and wanted to explore alternatives for future anticipated SLP shortages. After discussion and a review of caseloads with the SLPs who served these rural districts, it was decided that the project would be a trial of intervention using live, interactive videoconferencing. Participants would be students in first through fifth grade with a speech and/or language impairment or specific learning impairment with a co-occurring communication disorder that were currently receiving services. Caution due to the newness of the model, and concerns about the effectiveness of telepractice, led the team to decide that the children would receive speech-language therapy services by telepractice for only half of the school year. They received their services through a traditional service delivery model for the other half of the school year.

Live, interactive videoconferencing delivered using desktop computers and Web cameras was selected as the telepractice method because the project intended to provide the students with their weekly speech-language intervention services. The use of readily available equipment was used deliberately to encourage sustainability of the project after the initial pilot was completed. Initially, the project was funded for a 2-year period. The team anticipated but did not know if the telepractice project as designed would be a sustainable model. It was determined to collect data as well as complete satisfaction surveys following the first year of implementation to determine the effectiveness and sustainability of the project.

After determining the viability and initial scope and focus, the next step is to identify the specific components of the intended project. The School-Based Telepractice Needs Assessment (SBTNA) contained in Appendix A can be used to guide this developmental process. Each of the seven sections of the assessment contains guiding questions to facilitate the planning process among the telepractice project team members. During this initial stage challenges to implementation can be identified, and differences of opinion on implementation can be discussed and resolved.

The first section of the SBTNA considers the equipment and infrastructure needs for the project. Many options exist, from computer-based telepractice applications to dedicated videoconferencing equipment and specially equipped videoconferencing rooms. Chapter 3 contains helpful guidelines for making the best technology choice.

The KSU telepractice project utilizes desktop computers with 22-inch monitors, add-on Web cameras and a Web-based videoconferencing application. In addition, a scanner, fax machine, copier, and telephone are available at each site. Unexpectedly, room selection played an important role in the KSU telepractice project. At the university where the speech-language therapy services originated, it was found that light from office windows interfered significantly with the clarity of the picture that was being projected to the students. Interior office space with no windows provided a much better video result. Also, a neutral, nondistracting background for the SLP has been very helpful in maintaining the students' focus on the computer and therapy activities. At the school site, participants encountered difficulties with sound reverberation and echo due to the cinder block construction of the school buildings. In some rooms it was necessary to install fabric covered partitions to reduce reverberation.

The videoconferencing originated from the university and was completed through Kent State University's Optical Connection-3 to the Ohio Academic Resources Network (OARnet). The OARnet is an integrated technology infrastructure that provides support and services to all academic institutions in Ohio. Student privacy was maintained through 128-bit AES Internet signal encryption that meets Federal Information Processing Standards (FIPS) and is HIPAA (Health Information Portability and Accountability Act of 1996) compliant (Grogan-Johnson, Alvares, Rowan, & Creaghead, 2010). At the school site, peak bandwidth usage became an issue during teacher planning times. During those periods, many individuals were logging onto Internet-based radio, and as a result the audio and video signal for the telepractice sessions was impacted. Restricting access to online radio during telepractice service delivery hours eliminated this interference. Because many equipment and software choices exist, it is helpful for the telepractice team to research different options and complete trials when possible to address the individual and unique needs and preferences of the individuals involved in the project.

The second category of the SBTNA involves the selection and training of the SLP and paraprofessional. Chapter 3 contains helpful information related to the skills needed by telepractioners. Also, continuing education courses are available from ASHA and the American Telemedicine Association (ATA), which provide training in the delivery of speech-language therapy services through telepractice. When the KSU telepractice project began, the SLPs learned how to provide telepractice services by reviewing the then available ASHA documents including: *Speech-Language Pathologists Providing Clinical Services Via Telepractice: Position Statement (ASHA 2005b), Speech-Language Pathologists Providing Clinical Services Via Telepractice: Technical Report (ASHA 2005c),* and *Knowledge and Skills Needed by Speech Language Pathologists Providing Clinical Services Via Telepractice (ASHA 2005a).* At that time the SLPs were not aware of any training programs in the provision of telepractice speech-language intervention and learned how to provide the services through trial and error. During the first 2 years of the program the SLPs documented what they were learning and developed a training guide that is now utilized with new SLPs joining the program and also with graduate students who complete a clinical training experience with the project. Since then, ASHA and the American Telemedicine Association (ATA) have developed training programs that are readily available.

The KSU project found that selection and training of the paraprofessional is critical to the success of a telepractice project. During the 5 years that the KSU project has been in existence, participants have had the opportunity to work with exceptional paraprofessionals that contributed significantly to the success of the project as well as paraprofessionals that actively worked to sabotage the project.

The KSU project asks the school district to interview and hire the telepractice paraprofessional. A job description was created by adapting the school district's classroom paraprofessional job description to include the specific duties of the telepractice position, such as assisting with scheduling student therapy times, copying and sending required paperwork, downloading homework for students, and ensuring the technology is functioning during telepractice sessions. The KSU project suggests to the district that the paraprofessionals who are most successful in the position possess the qualities of organization, punctuality, attention to detail, willingness to accept direction, a friendly outgoing personality, adequate reading, writing, and speaking skills, and willingness to learn the technology for the project. Traits to avoid include fear of technology, lack of flexibility, inability to problem solve, and individuals who are easily frustrated.

Training for the paraprofessional is jointly conducted by the school district and the KSU telepractice project. The district reviews information related to rules and regulations of the school district, student confidentiality, and specific job expectations (e.g., starting and ending times, absence reporting). A member of the KSU telepractice project travels to the district to provide hands-on training in the use of the equipment and a review of the project and its focus. The paraprofessionals in the KSU telepractice project do not function as speech-language assistants. They do not provide intervention services, provide feedback regarding student responses, or carry out therapy activities. The duties of the paraprofessional may vary based on the nature of the telepractice project and state regulations regarding the use of speech-language assistants. The roles of both the SLP and the paraprofessional will be refined as the intervention program (the next category in the SBTNA) is developed.

Chapter 2 contains a review of available research suggesting that telepractice has been successfully implemented with children in grades preschool through high school with a variety of communication impairments. Although clinical experience suggests that a wide variety of students are capable of successfully participating in a telepractice service delivery model, there are some situations where use of telepractice is not indicated. It is likely that there are some children who cannot participate in telepractice service delivery (e.g., those unable to attend to or see the monitor, or unable to sit or stand for an intervention session). In the past 5 years, the KSU project has provided services to approximately 300 different students with a variety of communication impairments ranging from preschool through high school. Services have also been provided to students with cognitive impairment, hearing impairment, autism, emotional/behavioral disorder, and specific learning disabilities. To date, one student was removed from the project as the clinicians could not provide adequate services through telepractice. This student had a cognitive and communicative impairment and was transitioning to the use of an augmentative alternative communication device. The clinicians were not able to easily access the device to program it or effectively work with the student and the paraprofessional to use the device in functional communication activities. In addition, four parents requested that their students be removed from telepractice and returned to a traditional service delivery model, and two middle school students refused to attend therapy services.

It is not yet known whether or not this service delivery model is equivalent to traditional service delivery models. Initial pilot data suggests that school-age children make similar amounts of progress in telepractice as compared to traditional service delivery models (Grogan-Johnson et al., 2010; Grogan-Johnson et al., 2011), but further study is needed. As a starting point, it may be helpful to identify minimum selection criteria for potential participants in the project.

Therapy material and activity selection for the telepractice sessions is an important consideration and is affected by the technology and software selected for use. The KSU telepractice project determined from the outset that materials utilized in the therapy session would consist primarily of on-line interactive web sites and/or the use of an interactive white board. It was determined that use of such materials would be more motivating to students and would provide greater access to materials that would relate to the classroom curriculum. For example, if the fifth grade class is studying endangered animals of the rain forest, a student with a language learning impairment may view a short video clip or read a portion of a student online newspaper about this topic during a therapy session. The SLP will then mentor the student through the process of recalling the main elements from the story by filling in a graphic organizer on the white board, and then writing or telling a summary of the information. Finally, the student could select a picture of an endangered animal and write or tell a descriptive novel or cause and effect expository paragraph. The final product could then be saved as a document and emailed to the student or to the paraprofessional to print and send with the student. Some videoconferencing software or equipment does not have the capability to share data as described previously. Instead, the SLP may utilize a document camera to show objects or pages of a book to a student, or hold pictures or cards up to the web camera for the student to see. Alternatively, the SLP and the student can each have a physical copy of a game, book, or activity and utilize the materials during the session much as they would in a traditional side-by-side session. It is important to consider that as videoconferencing technology improves and telepractice service delivery becomes more commonplace, additional options may become available for the SLP telepractioners in the future.

Integration and collaboration of the telepractice project into the school program is critical to the effectiveness and sustainability of any school-based telepractice project. Using the guiding questions in the SBTNA, a telepractice team can carefully craft and implement a plan for integrating the telepractice project. Consider providing a letter of introduction and an invitation to visit the project and watch a demonstration. Then provide separate informational sessions/demonstrations to the faculty, parents, and students. These orientation sessions can be conducted in person or through videoconferencing. During the first year of the KSU telepractice project, the telepractice SLP traveled to the four rural school districts to meet the district SLPs, faculty, administrators, students, and parents. The telepractice SLP explained the project, provided contact information, and attempted to engender enthusiasm for the project.

The importance of these informational sessions and demonstrations cannot be overestimated. The KSU project personnel discovered that parents, and in particular faculty members, often have misconceptions about the delivery of telepractice services. If not identified and corrected, these misconceptions may be communicated to students, parents, and other faculty members. The information sessions can disseminate general information about the project and answer particular questions, which is helpful in reducing the spread of misinformation.

Category five of the SBTNA asks the telepractice team to consider how it will measure the satisfaction of students, parents, and faculty as well as determine the success of the students and establish plans for continuous improvement. Evaluating your telepractice project through satisfaction surveys and data review can be instrumental in improving the service delivery model. Satisfaction surveys tailored to the specific telepractice project can be created for students, parents, and faculty. A sample student survey utilized by the KSU telepractice project is contained in Figure 5–1. It is helpful to determine how performance will be measured prior to initiating the project. Results of the satisfaction surveys from the KSU telepractice project as well as plans for continuous improvement are reviewed in the "How do I know it is working?" section later in the chapter.

In the funding/reimbursement/cost of service delivery category of the SBTNA, the telepractice team considers the cost of the project as well as the potential for reimbursement for the services. Chapter 8 contains detailed information regarding the cost-benefit of providing telepractice services as compared with traditional service delivery. During the first 2 years of the KSU telepractice project, the ODE provided funding for the project, which resulted in no direct cost to the school districts for the speech-language therapy telepractice project. Beginning in the third year of the project, the school districts began to share the cost of the project, and beginning in the fifth year, ODE funding was no longer available. To date, the school districts involved in the project are contracting directly with the university for the telepractice speech-language therapy services. In addition, the school districts are requesting reimbursement from the Ohio Schools Medicaid Program for students who qualify. Medicaid reimbursement for speech-language therapy services provided by telepractice in Ohio schools became available in 2011 after state senators from the counties where speech-language telepractice services are delivered, along with the school district superintendents, successfully lobbied the Ohio Department of Jobs and Family Services to make this a reimbursable service.

Student Satisfaction Survey

Speech Language Therapy Telepractice Project
Student Satisfaction Survey

Date: ____________ Site Location: ____________________

I am _______ years old. I am a ______ Boy ______ Girl

Survey completed with assistance from: ______________________________

	Yes www.emofaces.com	I don't know or I am not sure	No
I like coming here.			
I like having speech therapy with (insert SLP's name) on the computer.			
Speech therapy helps me learn to talk better.			
I would like to do speech therapy using the computer again next year.			
I could see and hear (insert SLP's name) during my therapy sessions.			
What did you like best about having speech therapy using the computer?			
What do you wish we could change about having speech therapy using the computer?			
Other Comments:			

Instructions: Place a copy of the evaluation form in front of the student. The evaluator should have a second copy of the evaluation form to record student responses. Read the following directions:
"We want to know how you liked the speech therapy program on the computer. I will ask you to answer some questions. First, please tell me how old you are."

"Now, I am going to ask you some more questions. After I ask you the question please answer by saying 'yes, I don't know, or no'." (Simultaneously point to the pictures representing the answers on the student copy of the evaluation form)

After completing the yes/no questions ask the student the remaining questions on the form and write their responses.

Source: Grogan-Johnson, S. (2012). *Providing school-based speech-language therapy by telepractice: A brief tutorial.* Copyright 2012 Rockville, MD: American Speech-Language-Hearing Association. Reprinted with permission.

Figure 5–1.

The final category of the SBTNA relates to the safeguards that are in place for the provision of speech-language therapy services delivered by telepractice. Because telepractice is a service delivery model, it must comply with the rules and regulations for maintaining student security and privacy under the Individuals with Disabilities Education Act (IDEA), HIPAA, and The American Recovery and Reinvestment Act of 2009, which included revisions to HIPAA regarding the privacy and security issues associated with electronic transmission of health information under the Health Information Technology for Economic and Clinical Health Act (HITECH Act) (Lazzarotti, 2009). Undoubtedly, the students' school district has policies and procedures in place to ensure student security and privacy that the SLP and the telepractice paraprofessional must follow. Additional potential threats to student privacy occur when services are provided by telepractice (Cohn & Watzlaf, 2011; Watzlaf, Fahima, Moeini, & Firouzan, 2010; Watzlaf et al., 2011; Watzlaf, Rhia, & Ondich, 2012). To minimize these risks, a beginning telepractice team is urged to complete a checklist for privacy and security information such as the one developed by Watzlaf et al. (2010). Maintaining these boundaries will be an ongoing and challenging responsibility for the telepractice team.

Completing the needs assessment process may give rise to the notion that a school-based telepractice project cannot or should not be implemented until all possible factors have been identified and accounted for. Although it is important to adequately prepare, no amount of planning will account for all difficulties or possible factors that will arise in implementing a telepractice project. The KSU project found it important to determine a start date and make every effort to initiate the project on that date, understanding that adjustments and project corrections will need to be made. In the next section, implementing the actual project is considered.

How Do I Implement the Telepractice Project?

The first step in implementation is to use the completed SBTNA to generate a prioritized task list and assign responsibilities to team members. While accomplishing the task list, provide regular progress reports to the district. Another important task to accomplish early in the implementation phase is to conduct a trial telepractice session. The trial helps to identify malfunctions in technology, assess the video and audio quality of the transmission, and identify any unexpected glitches.

The first needs assessment process was completed by the KSU telepractice project in May 2007, and an estimated start date was set for August at the beginning of the 2007–2008 school year. During the next 3 months, the needs assessment task list was completed (e.g., videoconferencing software and applications were tested, equipment was selected, purchased and installed, an SLP was hired, and trials with the telepractice equipment were conducted). Early telepractice trials identified firewalls that needed to be reconfigured in order to permit the videoconferencing sessions to occur. Troubleshooting also took place to improve the acoustic qualities in one of the four classrooms at the school sites and to establish better lighting at the university telepractice office. During trials with data sharing, it was discovered that not all desired Internet activities were able to be shared and, at a particular time each afternoon, we experienced diminished audio and video quality at one of the school districts. Many of the technology issues were resolved in anticipation of an August start date. However, delays in obtaining parent permission forms and hiring support personnel in the districts pushed the start date back to October 2007.

In addition to actually implementing a telepractice project, a second goal of the project was to investigate the effectiveness of telepractice services delivered to school-age children. A study was devised to measure the progress of children who received services in telepractice as compared to children who received services in a traditional service delivery model. Thirty-four students with speech sound disorders and/or language impairments participated in the study. They were divided into two groups with the first group of 17 children receiving intervention services by telepractice for 4 months followed by traditional intervention for 4 months. The second group of students received conventional intervention services for 4 months followed by telepractice intervention for 4 months. Outcome measures included student progress in accomplishing IEP goals and objectives during each treatment period, and results on standardized test scores. Results as measured by student progress reports indicated that the children made similar amounts of progress regardless of the intervention method. Also, there was no significant difference in test scores for either group before or after intervention in either service delivery model. Although standardized test results cannot be utilized as a measure of progress, the similarity in test scores pre- and postintervention suggests that the children performed similarly in both service delivery models (Grogan-Johnson et al., 2010).

How Do I Know It Is Working?

Measuring student progress is one critical component of determining the effectiveness of a telepractice service delivery model. As with traditional service delivery, it is essential for the SLP to regularly assess a student's performance in intervention and determine if adequate progress is being accomplished. It is also important to complete the self-assessment and satisfaction surveys identified in the SBTNA. After reviewing the survey and self-evaluation results, create a prioritized list of revisions and make any needed changes to the program.

At the completion of the first year of the KSU telepractice project, the students, parents, faculty, SLPs, telepractice support personnel, and building principals were surveyed (Grogan-Johnson et al., 2010). Results from 29 of 38 students and 22 of 33 parents surveyed revealed that 93% of students liked receiving speech and language intervention by telepractice and 82% of parents rated their satisfaction with the telepractice delivery model as "above average" or "very good" on a six-point rating scale ranging from "do not know" to "very good." In addition, 95% of parents believed that the telepractice services provided "above average" or "very good" results in improving their student's communication functioning based on the same rating scale.

Faculty survey results (15 of 27 possible surveys) revealed that the teachers reported they did not know their satisfaction level with the delivery model and did not understand the program or the students' progress in intervention. One exception was that teachers rated the students' attitude toward telepractice as "very good," which was consistent with the student satisfaction survey results. Three of four district-placed SLPs and all four telepractice support personnel reported "above average" or "very good" satisfaction with the program. Two building principals did not know their level of satisfaction and two were satisfied with the program. One principal in particular was dissatisfied with the program, citing faculty comments indicating that limited amounts of intervention were provided. However, upon reviewing attendance data from the telepractice SLP and support personnel, it was found that the telepractice students received the amount of treatment required by their Individualized Education Programs (IEPs) and were able to provide this data to the principal.

In addition to the student progress measures and satisfaction surveys, attendance data was also kept. There were 704 possible intervention sessions during the project period. Of the total possible sessions, 148 sessions were missed (21%). The types of cancellations were similar to those reported in traditional service delivery models such as student absence, inclement weather, assemblies, and special classroom projects. During the project period only seven sessions (.01%) were canceled due to technology issues (e.g., Internet access unavailable), all of which occurred at the school sites.

Based on the satisfaction survey results, the areas for improvement included increasing awareness and understanding of the project among faculty and school administrators, and increasing collaboration and integration into the curriculum. To improve these areas, several revisions to the telepractice project were instituted. First, a faculty presentation that included an actual demonstration of the telepractice equipment for use during the faculty orientation meetings at the start of the school year was developed. In addition, a weekly checklist to provide teachers and parents with a summary of each student's intervention session was implemented. The team reserved a half-hour faculty consultation time slot in the weekly telepractice schedule and increased the frequency of e-mail and phone contact with faculty members while documenting the number of contacts and faculty responses. Finally, the team implemented a monthly newsletter to provide information about telepractice and communication disorders, and to provide general speech sound and language stimulation activities for parents and students to enjoy at home.

How Do I Sustain the Project?

Many factors will impact the continuation of a telepractice project. Commitment to the process of continuous improvement can increase the opportunity for the project to continue. The KSU telepractice project has completed 5 years of telepractice service delivery and four cycles of evaluation and revision of the program. One of the most important factors related to sustainability relates to faculty and related district personnel acceptance, or "buy in." The project has worked with seven different school districts over this 5-year period and in each instance faculty acceptance has been a gradual process. Even with live demonstrations and in-service training prior to the initiation of the project, faculty surveys at the end of the first year of telepractice reflect limited knowledge and awareness of the program and student progress. Beginning in the second year and continuing in subsequent years, faculty surveys reflect increased awareness, acceptance, and recognition of student progress in the program.

We have not achieved faculty acceptance in all of the school districts we have worked with. One notable exception was a district where the team chose to discontinue the project after 1 year. During the initial planning stages and throughout implementation, the team faced varying levels of opposition and unwillingness to collaborate from several faculty members and IT staff. Although the majority of students in the telepractice project met or exceeded their IEP goals, collaboration with faculty was minimal, it was difficult to troubleshoot technology-related issues, and participants were not able to establish even a basic level of integration with the building staff.

Another factor that relates to the sustainability of the project is the ability to integrate the telepractice speech-language services into the general education curriculum, resulting in student gains in grade level indicators and benchmarks. This is a challenge faced by SLPs who provide traditional intervention services as well. By design, telepractice service delivery is often conducted by pulling the students out of the classroom for services. Also, because the telepractice SLP may not be physically present in the school district it can be challenging to determine current curriculum objectives and/or themes utilized in the classroom. Communication with faculty must occur through email and phone calls, rather than in-person conversations, and it has been found that faculty are not always responsive when using these communication methods. The KSU project is currently working to identify effective solutions to this challenge. The team is piloting the provision of telepractice speech-language therapy services in the classroom. Also, the recent adoption of the common core content standards by many states should provide ready access to accepted grade level indicators and benchmarks, which should facilitate this integration (Blosser et al., 2012).

Summary

This chapter described a five-step process for successfully implementing a school-based telepractice project. Focus questions, including, "How do I get started?" "How do I develop the telepractice program?" "How do I implement the program?" "How do I know it is working?" and "How do I sustain the program?" were utilized to introduce each step. A useful needs assessment tool, the SBTNA, was provided to help with defining scope and sequence in developing the telepractice project, and examples and practical illustrations from the clinical experience of the KSU telepractice project illustrated key points.

References

American Speech-Language-Hearing Association. (2005a). *Knowledge and skills needed by speech-language pathologists providing clinical services via telepractice* [Knowledge and skills]. Retrieved from http://www.asha.org/policy.

American Speech-Language-Hearing Association. (2005b). *Speech-language pathologists providing clinical services via telepractice: Position statement* [Position statement]. Retrieved from http://www.asha.org/policy.

American Speech-Language-Hearing Association. (2005c). *Speech-language pathologists providing clinical services via telepractice: Technical report* [Technical report]. Retrieved from http://www.asha.org/policy.

Blosser, J., Roth, F. P., Paul, D. R., Ehren, B. J., Nelson, N. W., & Sturm, J. M. (2012, August 28). *Integrating the core. ASHA Leader*.

Boswell, S. (2007, March 6). Ohio grant addresses personnel shortage: Innovative strategies meet short-and long-term goals. *ASHA Leader*, *2*(3)1, 14–15.

Cohn, E., & Watzlaf, V. (2011). Privacy and Internet-based telepractice. *Perspectives on Telepractice, 1*, 26–37. doi:10.1044/tele1.1.26

Grogan-Johnson, S. (2012). Providing school-based speech-language therapy services by telepractice: A brief tutorial. *Perspectives on Telepractice*, *2*, 42–48. doi:10.1044/tele2.1.42

Grogan-Johnson, S., Alvares, R., Rowan, L., & Creaghead, N. (2010). A pilot study comparing the effectiveness of speech language therapy provided by telemedicine with conventional on-site therapy. *Journal of Telemedicine and Telecare, 16*(3), 134–139.

Grogan-Johnson, S., Gabel, R., Taylor, J., Rowan, L., & Alvares, R. (2011). A pilot exploration of speech sound disorder intervention delivered by telehealth to school-age children. *International Journal of Telerehabilitation, 3*(1), 31–41.

Health Insurance Portability and Accountability Act of 1996, Public Law 104-191, 104th Congress. (1996). Retrieved July 20, 2011, from Centers for Medicare and Medicaid Services, HIPAA General Information, http://www.cms.gov/HIPAAGenInfo/

Individuals with Disabilities Education Act. (2004). Section 800 [c]8. Retrieved July 8, 2009, from http:// idea.ed.gov

Lazzarotti, J. (2009). *HIPAA enforcement regulations updated for penalty increases and enhancements under the HITECH Act.* Retrieved September 29, 2012, from http://www.workplaceprivacyreport.com/2009/11/articles/hipaa-1/hipaa-enforcement-regulations-updated-for-penalty-increases-and-enhancements-under-the-hitech-act/

Watzlaf, V., Fahima, R., Moeini, S., & Firouzan, P. (2010). VoIP for telerehabilitation: A risk analysis for privacy, security, and HIPPA compliance. *International Journal of Telerehabilitation, 2*(2), 3–14. doi:10.5195/IJT. 2010. 6056

Watzlaf, V., Fahima, R., Moeini, S., Matusow, L., & Firouzan, P. (2011). VoIP for telerehabilitation: A risk analysis for privacy, security, and

HIPPA compliance–Part II. *International Journal of Telerehabilitation*, *3*(1), 3–10. doi:10.5195/IJT. 2011. 6070

Watzlaf, V., Rhia, R., & Ondich, B. (2012). VoIP for telerehabilitation: A pilot usability study for HIPPA compliance. *International Journal of Telerehabilitation*, *4*(1), 25–32. doi: 10. 5195/IJT 2012. 6069

6

Telerehabilitation: Adult Speech and Swallowing Disorders

Farzan Irani and Rodney Gabel

Overview of Benefits and Limitations of Telerehabilitation

Telerehabilitation (used synonymous with telepractice and telehealth in this chapter) is defined by the American Speech-Language and Hearing Association (ASHA, 2005a) as, "the application of telecommunications technology to deliver professional services at a distance by linking clinician to client, or clinician to clinician for assessment, intervention, and/or consultation" and is deemed an appropriate model of service delivery for speech-language pathologists (SLP). The primary goal of using telerehabilitation is to overcome barriers related to access of services.

ASHA (2005b) lists a number of benefits and limitations to the use of telerehabilitation as a means of service delivery for SLPs. Some of the commonly recognized benefits of telerehabilitation include:

a. Improved and increased access to services previously not available due to physical distance or lack of specialized clinicians in the area;

b. Reduced travel to receive services can decrease fatigue and thereby increase a client's desire to seek services and derive benefits from services that would otherwise be unavailable;
c. Ease of scheduling and less disruption to the clients' work schedules or those of working family members;
d. Time is not lost by long travel to health care facilities;
e. Opportunity to receive services in the client's natural environment, thereby making a treatment more functional by including family/caregivers and the client's real-life situations.

As with all methods of service delivery, there are certain limitations. This also holds true for telerehabilitation. In the case of telerehabilitation, a primary limitation is the inability of the clinician to have direct physical contact with the client to provide cues, reinforcement, tactile stimulation and manipulation, and to assess strength and tone (ASHA, 2005b). It is also difficult to make changes to the environment during telerehabilitation interventions and make/maintain direct eye contact with the client (ASHA, 2005b). Finally, telerehabilitation can limit the ability to engage in real-world transfer activities. This is particularly important when providing services to an adult with a speech or swallowing disorder.

Role of Telerehabilitation in Adult Speech and Swallowing Disorders

In recent years, especially since ASHA's endorsement of the use of telerehabilitation as a means to providing SLP services (ASHA, 2005a) there has been an increase in the use of telerehabilitation. Over the years with refinement of technology and increased access to technology it can only be expected to grow and improve. To help with efforts to establish efficacy for services offered via telerehabilitation, ASHA recently established the Special Interest Group 18: *Telepractice*. The goal of SIG 18 is to provide education, leadership, and advocacy for issues in telepractice, telespeech, and teleaudiology (ASHA, 2012). Thus, it is evident that with improvements in technology, and increased accessibility, one will notice tremendous growth in the application of telerehabilitation for all SLP services. The method of service delivery though will vary based on client needs, which take precedence within the model of evidence-based practice (EBP; ASHA, 2004). Any practitioner considering the use of telerehabilitation must first and foremost adhere to the principles of EBP, which includes consideration for: (a) research evidence, (b) client preferences, and (c) clinical expertise. The remainder of this chapter focuses on the application of telerehabilitation for adults with speech and swallowing disorders with a focus on fluency disorders. The chapter is structured to account for available research evidence, considerations for client preferences, and clinical expertise in service delivery. The chapter ends with a detailed case study of the application of telerehabilitation for stuttering therapy.

Preliminary Considerations for Telerehabilitation for Adult Speech and Swallowing Disorders

In the case of adult speech and swallowing disorders, telerehabilitation has been utilized as a means of service delivery for clients with neurogenic communication disorders, fluency disorders, voice disorders, and dysphagia. The role and extent of application of telerehabilitation will vary from one individual client to the next, with no cookie cutter approach. Mashima and Doran (2008) provide an excellent review of candidacy of clients and the application of telerehabilitation. They list 12 criteria a SLP must consider when determining the client's candidacy:

1. The client's ability to sit in front of a computer and attend to the clinician;
2. The ability to see and understand material presented on a computer;
3. The ability to understand and follow direction to operate the equipment/computer;
4. The ability to minimize extraneous movements when sitting in front of the camera, thereby reducing any compromise to image resolution;
5. Manual dexterity required in operating a keyboard;

6. Hearing acuity;
7. Cognitive ability;
8. Speech intelligibility;
9. Overall comfort level with the use of technology;
10. Client or family/caregivers' willingness to participate;
11. Cultural/linguistic considerations for some clients including the availability of an interpreter if needed; and
12. Access to and availability of technical resources if needed.

In addition to the 12 criteria listed previously, an SLP must also take into consideration individual client preferences, the purpose of the telerehabilitation session, and be aware of any technological challenges that might present themselves during the session. It is ultimately up to the practitioner to determine the client's eligibility for telerehabilitation services and the best application of telerehabilitation for each client. Furthermore, the SLP also needs to consider confidentiality and privacy as outlined by the Health Insurance Portability and Accountability Act (HIPAA) and the Health Information Technology for Economic and Clinical Health (HITECH) Act (ASHA, 2010; Cason & Brannon, 2011; Cohn & Watzlaf, 2011; Denton, 2003; Logan & Noles, 2008; Watzlaf, Moeini, Matusow, & Firouzan, 2011). Any SLP offering services via telerehabilitation needs to consider online security of each session in addition to the security and privacy of all electronic documentation and health records for individual clients. Although describing and discussing specific risk analysis is not within the scope of this chapter, these topics are covered in greater detail in Chapter 9 of this textbook.

Models for Telerehabilitation Application

With the rapid advancement and increased accessibility to technology that facilitates telerehabilitation, we now have multiple options for service delivery. First, it is important to differentiate synchronous from asynchronous service delivery (ASHA, 2005c). Synchronous service delivery can be likened to a replacement for face-to-face assessment/treatment where the clinician and client meet in real time. Asynchronous service delivery, also called store and forward, on the other hand does not involve real-time communication between clinician and client. Asynchronous service delivery is more beneficial to obtaining client records, assessment data, and for consultations. Data from an asynchronous transmission can be gathered by another profession or the client/caregiver themselves.

In many situations, SLPs using telerehabilitation would benefit from the use of both synchronous and asynchronous service delivery. Often, synchronous services are used to obtain objective and perceptual assessment data and conduct live therapy whereas asynchronous models are used to obtain client/caregiver completed assessment information such as standardized scales, audio/video clips of clients in their natural environment, and any self-reported data.

Finally, when considering either synchronous or asynchronous service delivery, the SLP needs to evaluate the security of all information transmitted in keeping with HIPAA and HITECH Act. This includes the selection of appropriate technology to facilitate synchronous communication or securely transfer data for asynchronous communication. A review of the literature on the use of telerehabilitation (used synonymously with telehealth and telerehabilitation) indicates that various devices and platforms have been used successfully for synchronous communication with acceptable to good treatment outcomes.

Setting Up a Telerehabilitation Program

Synchronous telerehabilitation can be achieved by the use of various modalities including the telephone, dedicated videoconferencing devices such as those provided by Polycom Inc. (http://www.polycom.com), and the use of Web conferencing software such as Skype (http://www.skype.com), Oovoo (http://www.oovoo.com), Cisco Webex (http://www.webex.com), Adobe Connect Pro (http://www.adobe.com/products/adobeconnect.html), and so forth. Each platform has certain benefits and limitations that must be determined prior to offering services.

For example, the use of a telephone is the most simple and accessible means of providing services; however, it is not feasible when a clear video transmission is required for effective therapy. Thus, although its ease of use and access make it a convenient method of providing services, it is not the best choice for sessions where a clear audio-visual signal is required. In many cases, a telephone cannot function as a stand-alone replacement for face-to-face services. In some instances when a program manual with audio-visual stimuli can be supplied asynchronously to clients, the telephone can be used for synchronous service delivery (e.g., Carey et al., 2010; O'Brian, Packman, & Onslow, 2008).

Dedicated devices such as Polycom provide a good quality audio and video signal and meet security standards to maintain client confidentiality in keeping with HIPAA and the HITECH Act. However, to use a dedicated device such as this all users need to purchase the hardware and software to facilitate. Thus, such dedicated devices are used primarily to facilitate consultations with experts, or require clients to travel to a facility that has the hardware and software required to facilitate services.

More recently, Voice Over Internet Protocol (VoIP) web conferencing software such as Skype and ooVoo have become freely available and provide a good quality audio-visual signal. In order to access services via these software programs, a computer with a web camera and a DSL Internet connection is required. In addition, users need to download the software to their personal computer and create a user account. However, many VoIP services are not clear with their privacy policy and could be at risk of violating HIPAA confidentiality requirements (Cohn & Watzlaf, 2011).

In addition to the free VoIP services, software such as Adobe Connect Pro and Cisco Webex provide the ability to transmit audio-visual signals in addition to the ability to record sessions and share documents on either users' computer with a paid subscription. These software programs are cross-platform and only the service provider (SLP) is required to purchase a subscription to invite participants/clients to their secure "room" to attend a therapy session. However, these software programs require a high-speed Internet connection, and one can often notice significant delays in the transmission of audio-visual signals.

Application and Evidence for the Use of Telerehabilitation

As discussed in detail in Chapter 8 of this book, numerous pilot studies evaluating the effectiveness of telerehabilitation to evaluate and treat various adult speech and swallowing disorders have yielded promising outcomes. This section focuses on a few select studies reporting methods and outcomes for the use of telerehabilitation for adult speech and swallowing disorders.

Hill et al. (2006) completed a comparative study to evaluate the assessment of motor speech disorders using a telerehabilitation system versus a face-to-face evaluation conducted by an on-site SLP. Overall they found the use of the telerehabilitation system to yield positive outcomes with most measurements of severity to fall within clinically acceptable criteria. However, a few subtests on the Frenchay Dysarthria Assessment protocol did not match with face-to-face evaluations. This could be attributed to multiple factors including the severity of the motor speech disorder as well as technical issues such as the placement of the camera capturing the movements.

In a similar study, Palsbo (2007) explored the equivalence of functional communication assessment of poststroke patients using the Boston Diagnostic Aphasia Examination (BDAE) via videoconferencing and face-to-face assessment. The study was a randomized, double-crossover agreement study where pairs of SLPs independently gave each client a face-to-face assessment. Thus two SLPs completed a face-to-face assessment, and two other SLPs completed the assessment online from a remote site. The results indicated high agreement on results between the SLPs conducting a face-to-face assessment in comparison to the SLPs conducting the assessment via videoconferencing. The study found good agreement (95%) with regard to directing patients to all tasks irrespective of service delivery (videoconferencing versus face-to-face). The discrepancy in scoring might be a result of a methodological weakness because the SLPs were not randomized between remote and face-to-face assessment.

Cherney, Kaye, and Hitch (2011) present a novel method of combining both synchronous and asynchronous telerehabilitation for the treatment of aphasia. They used a custom developed program, web-Oral Reading for Language in Aphasia (web-ORLA™), for asynchronous telerehabilitation combined with constant monitoring of patient performance by an SLP at a distant geographic location. The web-ORLA™ included a virtual therapist who provided models and feedback similar to a real SLP. At the same time, all sessions were monitored either synchronously or asynchronously by an SLP at a distant site. The SLP made adjustments to the program and provided feedback as needed based on the patient's performance. In general they found the telerehabilitation program to be advantageous and effective in their initial pilot report. However, they also highlight disadvantages related to technology. It was time-consuming to develop and deliver the program, troubleshoot technological issues, the cost of the equipment, and cost of the therapist time (Cherney et al., 2011). Furthermore, technical difficulties related to data transfer could potentially increase therapist time to a degree that it could diminish the advantages of telerehabilitation. However, one must note that with improvement in technology, especially related to data transmission and videoconferencing, these difficulties can be expected to reduce over time, making telerehabilitation a more viable and beneficial option for many clients. Cherney and van Vuuren (2012) further expand on future directions with the use of virtual therapists such as the web-ORLA™ to work across a broad range of devices and access modalities and encourage peer-to-peer support to build a community.

Theodoros and Ramig (2011) explored the telerehabilitation delivery of the Lee Silverman Voice Treatment (LSVT® Loud) to clients with Parkinson's disease (PD). They provided a review of a program that was delivered synchronously via videoconferencing with the capacity to transmit and display written stimuli, measure sound pressure level, frequency, and duration of the voice in real time, and the ability to record and play back the client's speech online. In addition to the synchronous delivery, Halpern and colleagues (2005; cited in Theodoros & Ramig, 2011) have also developed an asynchronous program to deliver LSVT® Loud for clients to practice independently that can be used in conjunction with face-to-face treatment. Overall, the synchronous and asynchronous delivery of the LSVT® Loud was found to be effective, help reduce caregiver burden, and result in high patient satisfaction. However, like all other programs adapting to this new technology and service delivery method, Theodoros and Ramig also list numerous challenges to the delivery of this program that include patient selection, audio delays, video quality, and the treatment environment.

Telerehabilitation and Stuttering Therapy

With regard to the treatment of stuttering, telerehabilitation has been used to either (a) deliver therapy entirely; or (b) provide follow-up services after completion of an intensive stuttering therapy program. Studies such as the initial research exploring the telehealth adaptation of the Camperdown Program for the treatment of chronic stuttering in adolescents and adults (Carey et al., 2010; O'Brian et al., 2008) utilized the telephone as a means to conduct therapy in real time. Although this method lacked the ability to see the client directly throughout the therapy process, both a phase I trial and a randomized controlled trial indicated that this method of conducting therapy over the telephone was an evidence-based alternative to face-to-face therapy for clients who are unable to attend therapy. Carey et al. (2012) similarly extended the telehealth delivery of the Camperdown Program with the use of a Webcam to facilitate face-to-face interaction. In their Phase I trial, Carey et al. reported the Webcam delivery of the Camperdown Program to be efficient and efficacious, recommending a phase II trial of this delivery model.

Similar to the Camperdown Program, the Institute for Stuttering Treatment and Research (ISTAR) has also utilized videoconferencing to provide telerehabilitation services to clients who lived in remote areas and did not have access to services (Haynes & Langevin, 2010; Kully, 2000). In the case of ISTAR, telehealth delivery was often used to provide follow-up services to clients who had attended an intensive workshop at one of their centers. The ISTAR also employed the use of asynchronous services to send and receive test protocols to gather attitude inventories (Haynes & Langevin, 2010). Similarly, Dahm (2010) describes the application of telehealth to provide stuttering therapy online to a wide range of participants from a dispersed geographic area.

Case Study in Fluency Disorders

The use of telerehabilitation in the treatment of fluency disorders is particularly advantageous because of the lack of specialized centers for treating stuttering (Gabel et al., 2010; Mashima & Doran, 2008) and the need for long-term maintenance after discontinuation of the intensive therapy (Gabel et al., 2010; Gabel & Irani, 2012; Irani & Gabel, 2011; Irani, Gabel, Daniels, & Hughes, 2012).

A model of treatment commonly applied in the case of stuttering therapy for adolescents and adults is an intensive clinic. Intensive clinics traditionally offer approximately 75–80 hours of direct therapy over a span of approximately 3 weeks (Andrews, Guitar, & Howie, 1980; Gabel et al., 2010; Irani et al., 2012; St. Louis & Westbrook, 1987). However, research indicates that although intensive programs are effective in inducing rapid changes for most clients, these changes are often not maintained without regular follow-up therapy to help with the generalization, transfer, and maintenance of changes made during the intensive program (Andrews et al., 1980; Irani et al., 2012; St. Louis & Westbrook, 1987). The intensive programs offered throughout the United States are primarily residential programs and attract clients from far and wide. Often, clients attending such programs are not within driving distance from the clinic where intensive therapy was received, further, they do not have appropriate services available within close proximity to their residence (Gabel et al., 2010). Thus, it is of importance to seek innovative means to provide clients attending the intensive programs with follow-up therapy to help with maintenance of gains made during the intensive clinic (Irani et al., 2012).

A telerehabilitation model seems to be one avenue for doing this follow-up therapy. Thus, the authors initially started offering follow-up services to select participants attending Bowling Green State University's (BGSU) Intensive Stuttering Clinic for Adolescents and Adults (ISCAA) on a trial basis in 2008. Since the initial pilot offering, the intensive therapy+telerehabilitation follow-up model is now offered at the University of Toledo's (UT) ISCAA and at Texas State University's (TXSTATE) Comprehensive Stuttering Therapy Program (CSTP). Both programs, the ISCAA and the CSTP, are 10-day intensive programs that offer 60 hours of direct therapy.

This includes 20 hours of group therapy and 40 hours of individual therapy. In addition to the intensive program, clients are encouraged to continue receiving follow-up therapy via telerehabilitation on an "as-needed" basis immediately following the completion of the intensive program. The goal of the telerehabilitation follow-up provided is to help with transfer, generalization, and maintenance of skills learned during the intensive program. The ultimate goal for all clients attending the program is to help them become their own clinicians and effectively manage their stuttering. Previous research by the authors (Gabel et al., 2010; Irani & Gabel, 2011; Irani et al., 2012) indicated a need for structured regular follow-up. Due to the nature of the intensive program, telerehabilitation was the only option available for many of the clients.

Case Study of the Intensive+Telerehabilitation Model

We now present a single-subject case study of a 20-year-old male who was involved with the initial pilot testing of the telerehabilitation follow-up therapy. This particular case has been selected for discussion in this chapter to provide the readers with a deeper understanding of the process, initial limitations, and troubleshooting procedures to help make the service delivery model successful for their clients. For the purpose of this chapter, the client is called "Joe."

Description of Participant

At the time of the pilot study, Joe was a 20-year-old adult male who stuttered. At the time of completing the program, Joe was an undergraduate student. He reported that he had stuttered since childhood and had tried various types of therapies including intensive programs in the past. He mentioned that while most therapy programs he attended were effective for a short duration, he experienced relapse soon after being discharged from therapy. Joe had also previously attended the ISCAA at BGSU in 2005 and 2006. He observed that therapy was effective for a short duration after completing the intensive clinic, but his stuttering would worsen over time and he felt the need to "re-take" the program the following year. This is a theme not uncommon with stuttering therapy experiences (Gabel et al., 2010; Irani et al., 2012; St. Louis & Westbrook, 1987). At the time of the initial diagnostic, before beginning the intensive clinic, the participant displayed severe stuttering as measured by the Stuttering Severity Instrument, Third Edition (Riley, 1994; SSI: 3 score = 36). Stuttering severity was also measured based on frequency in percentage of syllables stuttered (%SS) in four speaking situations: monologue, conversation, reading, and phone calls. In addition to stuttering severity, the Locus of Control of Behavior Scale (LCB; Craig, Franklin, & Andrews, 1984), the Modified Erickson Scale of Communication Attitudes (S-24; Andrews & Cutler, 1974), and the Overall Assessment of the Speakers Experience of Stuttering (OASES; Yaruss & Quesal, 2006, 2008) were also administered to evaluate the effect of stuttering on Joe's communication attitudes and Quality of Life (QOL). Because Joe had initially attended the ISCAA in 2006, the draft version of the OASES (Yaruss & Quesal, 2006) was administered to allow for comparative data analysis. All scores indicated that stuttering had a profound impact of Joe's communication attitudes and QOL (LCB = 30; S-24 = 20; OASES Total Impact Score/Rating = 63.7/Moderate-to-severe). All measures of stuttering severity and the impact of stuttering on Joe's life were measured at regular intervals throughout the therapy program and formed the primary outcome measures to inform treatment effectiveness for Joe.

Candidacy for Telerehabilitation

Joe's candidacy for telerehabilitation was based on multiple factors. Joe was selected as a candidate for the telerehabilitation pilot, and as a suitable case description for this chapter because of his willingness to participate in the pilot project, determined by the informed consent. Also, Joe expressed an eagerness to volunteer as a participant and demonstrated the technical knowledge to facilitate the telerehabilitation sessions with relative ease. Based on his current living conditions in a university dormitory, Joe also had access to high-speed Internet to facilitate telerehabilitation. In the past, Joe had expressed the need for continued follow-up therapy after completion of the ISCAA, which made him a prime candidate for an initial pilot of the program. Joe also volunteered to complete a couple "mock" telerehabilitation sessions to identify any technical glitches and learn how to independently troubleshoot while still at the residential program. Third, Joe's past experiences with therapy and relapse following therapy indicated that he would benefit from a regular follow-up program aimed at maintenance of skills learned during the ISCAA. Thus, based on the factors described previously, Joe was deemed a suitable candidate for the initial pilot testing of the telerehabilitation follow-up program to the ISCAA.

Selecting a Telerehabilitation Platform/Program

At the time of this pilot study, Skype was selected as a tool to conduct preliminary testing and pilot of this program. Skype was selected because of its ease of use and ability to stream audio and video. However, since the initial pilot, the ISCAA has employed the use of more secure platforms such as CISCO's Webex, Adobe Connect Pro, and SCOPIA. The decision to discontinue the use of Skype was made in keeping with privacy/confidentiality standards in conducting telerehabilitation as per HIPAA and HITECH guidelines. Each program does come with its benefits and limitations and it is up to individual service providers to determine the best product for their specific needs.

Additional benefits the authors have noted regarding the use of paid platforms such as Adobe Connect Pro, CISCO Webex, and SCOPIA (http://www.radvision.com/Products/Video-Conference-Systems/Desktop-Video-Communications/SCOPIA-Desktop-Video-Conferencing/default.htm) are the ability to record live sessions for later analysis, ability to share documents and screens in real time, and better interactive tools such as the whiteboard that allows all users to share text/drawing. In the authors' experience, these programs have been found effective for conducting group therapy sessions as and when needed. An extension to this feature could include the involvement of family members/caregivers during the telerehabilitation sessions even if they are not physically present at the same site as the client and/or clinician.

Preliminary Testing and Troubleshooting

As mentioned previously, Joe volunteered to assist with preliminary testing and troubleshooting for the telerehabilitation program while completing the ISCAA residential program. During the preliminary testing and troubleshooting sessions, Joe was provided with a tutorial for effective use of the telerehabilitation software. Following the initial tutorial, two brief sessions were conducted using the telerehabilitation software. During this initial testing phase Joe and his clinician were seated in separate rooms within the University's Speech-Language and Hearing Clinic's premises. This allowed the clinician and Joe to maintain physical contact if required to troubleshoot any technological glitches that may arise. The one "glitch" that seemed to be a recurrent problem was the overall quality of the audio/video signal and a time delay. The clinicians decided to keep their phones available to help with improving the audio signal if required. They also used the initial testing sessions to acclimate themselves to the delay in the signal. The clinicians found it very important and helpful to acclimate to the signal delay that was initially very disruptive to the therapy process. It should be noted that most telerehabilitation programs do suffer from a minor delay and it is important for clinicians and clients to be aware of these delays. A good option to deal with this technological glitch is the use of an agreed upon rule where each individual (clinician or client) inserts a 5-second pause before responding. Another very common issue with the conduct of telerehabilitation is feedback noise. It is very important that all individuals participating in the telerehabilitation program use headphones and a microphone to avoid any feedback noise, which can be very disruptive to the smooth flow of a therapy/assessment session. At the bare minimum, the use of headphones will reduce chances of feedback.

Description of the Program

The ISCAA has been described previously (Gabel et al., 2010; Gabel & Irani, 2012) and has been found to have positive outcomes including a reduction in stuttering severity and self-reported positive changes in participants' attitudes, feelings, and beliefs about stuttering. Participants also reported an increased sense of control of their stuttering as a result of therapy.

For this pilot, the program combined the on-site intensive therapy with nonintensive follow-up sessions via telerehabilitation. The intensive therapy portion was conducted by a graduate student SLP supervised by a licensed SLP under the mentorship of a Board Recognized Fluency Specialist (BRSFD). A clinical fellow under the mentorship of the same BRSFD conducted the follow-up sessions.

The intensive portion of the program lasted 3 weeks for a total of 75 hours of direct contact time with the client. Several areas were addressed during this intensive portion: (1) educating the client about stuttering including identifying stuttering behaviors, (2) acceptance of stuttering focusing on attitude change (cognitive restructuring), (3) modifying stuttering, and (4) increasing fluency.

The telerehabilitation program lasted a total of 12 months and focused on maintenance of gains made during the intensive clinic. This service allowed the client to attend therapy in the privacy of his home using his personal computer. Approaches used during the follow-up portion remained the same as those used for the intensive portion. In essence, the intensive program was recycled based on client needs over a 1-year period. The structure of the follow-up sessions was as follows: (1) two therapy sessions a week for 1 hour each during the initial 6 months and; (2) one therapy session a week for 1 hour for the next 6 months. This was done in order to provide additional support to the client and help transition from the residential program to a regular follow-up program during the first 6 months. Therapy was reduced during the last 6 months to help limit the client's dependence on the therapist and assist the client in his journey toward becoming his own clinician.

Program Outcomes

Program outcomes were meticulously measured at regular intervals. The ISCAA utilizes an eclectic approach to stuttering therapy and addresses stuttering severity in addition to the affective and cognitive aspects of stuttering (Bennett, 2006). Thus, program outcomes were measured using a variety of instruments described earlier, including the SSI-3, S-24, LCB (Figure 6-1), OASES (Figure 6-2

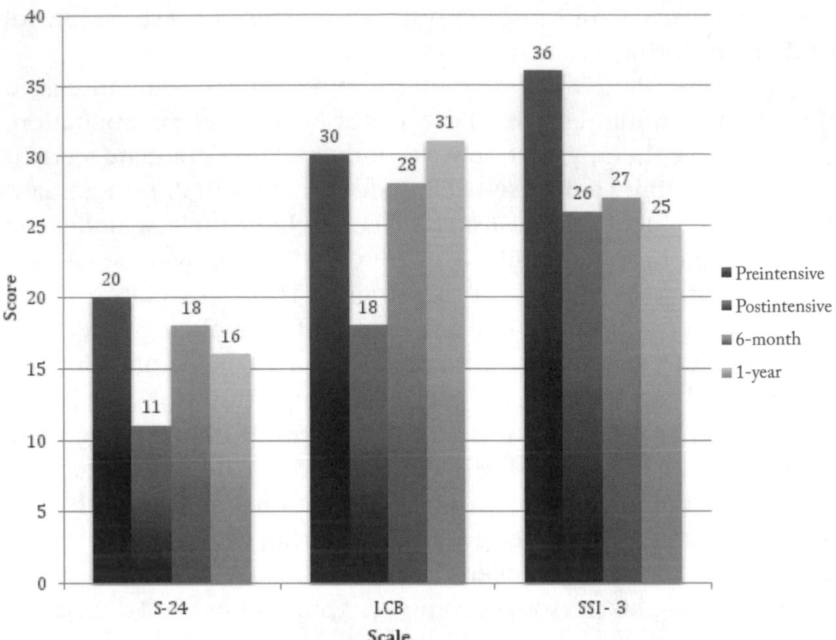

Figure 6–1. Joe's scores related to stuttering severity measured by the SSI-3 and communication attitudes measures by the LCB and S-24.

and Table 6–1) and %SS in a variety of speaking situations (Figure 6–3). All outcomes measures were administered before the start of the intensive program (Pre-Intensive), at the conclusion of the intensive program (Post-Intensive), 6 months after the telerehabilitation program (6 month), and at the end of the telerehabilitation program (1 year).

Overall, the results of the telerehabilitation follow-up program indicated Joe maintained all positive changes made during the intensive portion of the ISCAA. As seen in Figure 6–1, Joe demonstrated a decrease in outcome measures related to stuttering severity (decreased severity) 6 months after initiation of follow-up therapy. Outcome measures for the LCB scale indicated that Joe was not able to maintain the changes over the period of follow-up therapy.

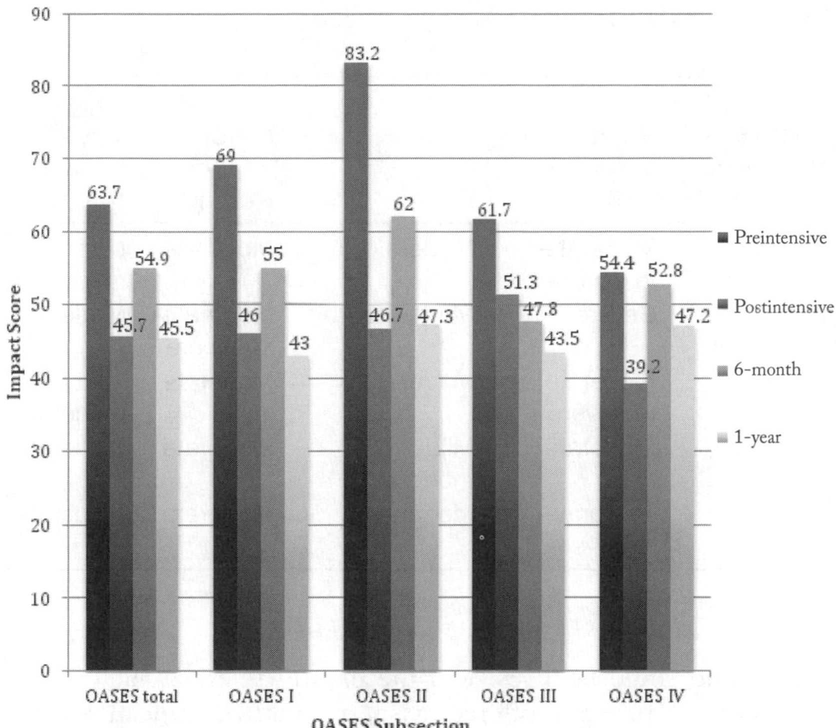

Figure 6–2. Joe's scores reported on the OASES.

Outcome measures related to attitudes toward communication, as measured by the S-24, however, indicated that Joe reported an increase in scores 6 months following initiation of follow-up therapy, followed by a gradual decrease in those measures at the conclusion of therapy. As seen in Figure 6–2, a similar trend was noticed on the OASES. Joe reported a positive impact at the end of the intensive clinic as measured by the impact scores on the OASES. At 6 months of the telerehabilitation program Joe reported a negative impact of stuttering on his life, as measured by increased impact scores on all sections of the OASES. However, at the conclusion of the telerehabilitation program, Joe reported an overall positive outcome with impact scores and ratings similar to those reported at the end of the intensive clinic. Results for the LCB and S-24 follow an interesting

Table 6–1. OASES Impact Ratings for Joe

OASES Subsection	Preintensive Impact Rating	Postintensive Impact Rating	6-month Impact Rating	1-year Impact Rating
I	Moderate-to-severe	Moderate	Moderate	Mild-to-moderate
II	Severe	Moderate	Moderate-to-severe	Moderate
III	Moderate-to-severe	Moderate	Moderate	Mild-to-moderate
IV	Moderate	Mild-to-moderate	Moderate	Moderate
Total	Moderate-to-severe	Moderate	Moderate	Moderate

pattern and could be a result of the nature (telerehabilitation) of the follow-up program offered. Also, it could be indicative of issues the client was experiencing as a part of transferring therapy skills into his life. Results on the OASES could indicate an increased awareness of the impact stuttering has on the participant's life, especially after returning to his "natural environment" after completion of the intensive program; however, this assumption was not corroborated by any report from the participant. Overall, this pattern could indicate that either intensive therapy is a more effective means to working on the attitudinal component of therapy and/or physical proximity and the ability to complete a variety of "real life" activities during therapy plays a positive role in maintenance of attitudinal changes. It should be noted that all follow-up therapy was via videoconferencing and there were no opportunities to complete extra clinical activities related to desensitization during the follow-up phase. One could assume that the changes reflected on the LCB, S-24, and OASES scales were facilitated by the completion of desensitization activities conducted during the ISCAA residential

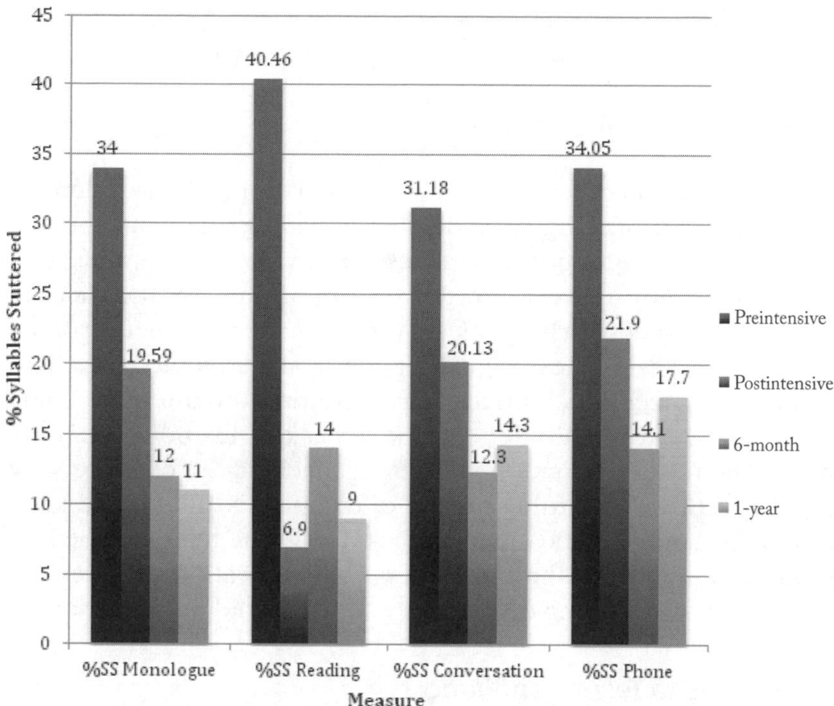

Figure 6–3. Joe's stuttering frequency measured in percent syllables stuttered (%SS).

component. It was not possible to complete similar activities during follow-up thereby causing a negative shift in attitudes but not severity of stuttering. Clinical evidence does not corroborate this assumption and will need to be investigated further in a separate study before any causal relationships can be established.

All measures related to stuttering severity and attitudes toward communication (except the LCB) were found to be lower at the conclusion of follow-up therapy when compared to scores reported before the start of therapy, indicating that the participant appeared to make clinically significant gains during the course of therapy and maintained these gains afterward. It is important, however, to obtain follow-up measures 6 months, 1 year, and 2 years posttherapy to assess the long-term effectiveness of this model.

Benefits to Telerehabilitation

Based on the outcomes presented for Joe, it appears that telerehabilitation is a promising approach for providing follow-up therapy to clients who might not have access to services in their area. This model of therapy delivery afforded the opportunity for the client to remain in contact with his clinician for a year after completion of the intensive program. These regular online sessions allowed the client to practice speech techniques learned during the intensive clinic and apply them to daily life situations back in his home environment. The telerehabilitation sessions also helped the client receive regular feedback regarding his use of techniques and helped keep him "accountable." The clinicians also found the telerehabilitation model an effective method to address communication attitudes and the impact of stuttering on everyday activities and participation.

Limitations to Telerehabilitation

In addition to the numerous benefits to using telerehabilitation as a means for providing follow-up therapy, it is also important to discuss the limitations associated with this model of service delivery.

The first and most pressing limitation is that of technological glitches. The clinicians found that sessions often needed to be canceled and/or conducted via telephone because of poor Internet connection and difficulty connecting to the service. Often service would be interrupted during an important discussion thereby reducing the overall effectiveness of therapy. It is important to discuss this limitation with the client, and recommend the client invest in a high-speed Internet connection.

A second limitation worth noting is the lack of physical proximity to the client. It was often difficult to demonstrate different techniques and provide the client with timely audio/visual cues when practicing techniques. Furthermore, this also limits the ability for the clinician to model certain behaviors and effectively conduct desensitization activities. Desensitization activities often require the clinician to accompany the client and model stuttering behaviors, including disclosure, in a public setting.

A third limitation was the physical restriction. Because both clinician and client need to be sitting in front of their respective computers for the duration of the telerehabilitation session, it was not possible for the clinician to monitor the client's use of techniques for transfer and generalization purposes to new settings. The clinician would assign transfer activities to the client and then discuss the same without the ability to observe the client in real time. With the recent advances in technology, however, it will soon be possible to overcome this particular limitation.

Conclusions and Future Directions

Overall, based on initial research reports on the use of telerehabilitation services, both synchronous and asynchronous, it appears that this is a model found to be effective for clients with various communication disorders. As discussed earlier in this chapter and elsewhere in the book, telerehabilitation is an effective and efficacious means of providing therapy. Nonetheless, similar to all other models, telerehabilitation has certain limitations that need to be addressed in future research and clinical work. Some of the most common limitations to providing assessment and therapy via telerehabilitation are associated with the use and current state of technology. Of course, telerehabilitation is not an option when the therapy protocol requires direct physical contact with a client, except in cases where consultation with an expert is required.

Based on the authors' experiences with using telerehabilitation as a means to provide follow-up services after an intensive stuttering therapy program, despite its numerous benefits, limitations with respect to technological glitches continue to persist and will need to be overcome in the future to make this a more effective and viable model for service delivery.

Certain technological glitches, as discussed in earlier sections, can be ameliorated by advance preparation on the part of the SLP. It is important for practitioners to familiarize themselves with the technology and potential technological glitches prior to offering services via telerehabilitation. This would include a thorough pilot of the selected platform with a list of potential breakdowns and a comprehensive troubleshooting guide that can be shared with clients. A second procedure is to complete a thorough consultation with potential clients to determine their eligibility for service via telerehabilitation. This would include addressing factors concerned with the individual client such as their ability to access a computer, cognitive ability, motor abilities, attention span, the home environment, availability of a caregiver when needed, and proficiency with technology. Furthermore, a practitioner must also determine whether a broadband Internet connection is available to the participant to facilitate the transmission of audio-visual data. It is the duty of the practitioner to assess each individual client's ability to benefit from telerehabilitation based on these personal factors (discussed earlier in this chapter; Mashima & Doran, 2008) as well as the availability of the hardware, software (when required), and appropriate Internet connection speed. Lastly, the authors also recommend that practitioners provide their clients with a comprehensive list of instructions and troubleshooting information before accessing the services. In many instances, videoconferencing services experience a slight delay in the transmission of audio-visual signals; the practitioner must also account for that delay and develop appropriate cues to help reduce interference during the session. This can include testing different scenarios with a colleague and providing clients with a list of "do's" and "do not's" prior to starting the session. In their own practice, the authors have found the use of such troubleshooting procedures to be very helpful in ameliorating a majority of technical glitches. The authors also provide clients with basic training for the use of the videoconferencing program when possible.

In the case of stuttering, as discussed in the case study, the authors have found it difficult to replicate all therapy procedures, especially those related to transfer and generalization using a telerehabilitation model. During the initial pilot studies, providing clients with regular homework assignments related to desensitization activities, for example, raising your hand and asking a question in class on three occasions this week, or asking a stranger for directions four times this week, addressed this limitation. In practice, it has been observed that clients often do not complete such homework activities and would benefit from the presence of a clinician when completing these activities. More recently with the advancements in mobile technology, VoIP programs such as Skype, ooVoo, Cisco Webex, and Adobe Connect Pro (to name a few) have developed mobile applications that support videoconferencing on smartphones and tablets running either Google's Android or Apple's iOS. This has opened up new possibilities within the realm of telerehabilitation. Furthermore, the availability of free wireless Internet at numerous public locations (at least in the United States) has also opened up avenues not available before. The authors are currently piloting the use of such devices to conduct therapy sessions with clients at different public locations to simulate transfer activities generally carried out during a face-to-face session. Although the clinician is not physically present with the client, it does help ensure that therapy is conducted in a variety of different locations there facilitating the transfer and generalization process.

Currently, the ISCAA provides all clients with a manual that describes various aspects of therapy, cues for specific procedures, and worksheets to facilitate transfer and generalization activities. With the availability of electronic books (e-books), authors can now incorporate audio and visual materials within a book/manual that can be accessed from several tablet devices and smartphones. Thus, in the future, the goal would be to convert the ISCAA manual to an e-book that includes audiovisual cues to guide clients through the program. This combined with the synchronous delivery of services via videoconferencing to a client's smartphone or tablet can help convert the ISCAA to an online program in the future.

As is evident from the current discussion and review of literature, the use of telerehabilitation is a viable model for the delivery of SLP services. At this time, advances in technology have made it possible to provide such services to a larger population effectively. However, the same technology continues to also be the greatest limitation to offering telerehabilitation services. Fortunately, with the rapid advancement in technology, and increased accessibility to such technology, the future possibility of telerehabilitation will expand manifold. One can expect to see a rise in the use as well as the efficacy of telerehabilitation services for adolescents and adults with speech and swallowing disorders in the future.

References

American Speech-Language-Hearing Association. (2004). *Evidence-based practice in communication disorders: An introduction* [Technical report]. Retrieved from http://www.asha.org/policy.

American Speech-Language-Hearing Association. (2005a). *Speech-language pathologists providing clinical services via telepractice: Position statement* [Position statement]. Retrieved from http://www.asha.org/policy.

American Speech-Language-Hearing Association. (2005b). *Speech-language pathologists providing clinical services via telepractice: Technical report* [Technical report]. Retrieved from http://www.asha.org/policy.

American Speech-Language-Hearing Association. (2005c). *Knowledge and skills needed by speech-language pathologists providing clinical services via telepractice* [Knowledge and skills]. Retrieved from http://www.asha.org/policy.

American-Speech-Language-Hearing Association. (2010). *Professional issues in telepractice for speech-language pathologists* [Professional issues statement]. Retrieved from http://www.asha.org/policy.

American Speech-Language-Hearing Association. (2012, September 21). *About special interest group 18, telepractice*. Retrieved from http://www.asha.org/SIG/18/About-SIG-18/

Andrews, G., & Cutler, J. (1974). Stuttering therapy: The relation between changes in symptom level and attitudes. *Journal of Speech and Hearing Disorders, 39,* 312–319.

Andrews, G., Guitar, B., & Howie, P. M. (1980). Meta-analysis of the effects of stuttering treatment. *Journal of Speech and Hearing Disorders, 45*(3), 287–307.

Bennett, E. (2006). *Working with people who stutter: A lifespan approach*. Upper Saddle River, NJ: Pearson Education, Inc.

Carey, B., O'Brian, S., Onslow, M., Block, S., Jones, M., & Packman, A. (2010). Randomized controlled non-inferiority trial of a telehealth treatment for chronic stuttering: The Camperdown Program. *International Journal of Language and Communication Disorders, 45*(1), 108–120. doi: 10.3109/13682820902763944

Carey, B., O'Brian, S., Onslow, M., Packman, A., Menzies, R., Nippold, M., et al. (2012). Webcam delivery of the Camperdown Program for adolescents who stutter: A phase I trial. *Language, Speech, and Hearing Services in Schools, 43*(3), 370–380. doi: 10.1044/0161-1461(2011/11-0010)

Cason, J., & Brannon, J. A. (2011). Telehealth regulatory and legal considerations: Frequently asked questions. *International Journal of Telerehabilitation, 3*(2), 15.

Cherney, L. R., Kaye, R. C., & Hitch, R. S. (2011). The best of both worlds: Combining synchronous and asynchronous telepractice in the treatment of aphasia. *Perspectives on Neurophysiology and Neurogenic Speech and Language Disorders, 21*(3), 83–90.

Cherney, L., & van Vuuren, S. (2012). Telerehabilitation, virtual therapists, and acquired neurologic speech and language disorders. *Seminars in Speech and Language, 33*(3), 243–257.

Cohn, E. R., & Watzlaf, V. J. M. (2011). Privacy and internet-based telepractice. *Perspectives on Telepractice, 1*(1), 26–37.

Craig, A., Franklin, J., & Andrews, G. (1984). A scale to measure locus of control of behaviour. *British Journal of Medical Psychology*, 57, 173–180.

Dahm, B. (2010, October). In Judith Kuster (Chair). *Stuttering therapy online*. Paper presented at the International Stuttering Awareness Day Conference.

Denton, D. R. (2003). Ethical and legal issues related to telepractice. *Seminars in Speech and Language, 24*(4), 313.

Gabel, R., Irani, F., Palasik, S., Swartz, E., & Hughes, C. (2010). Treatment outcomes of the intensive stuttering therapy for adolescents and adults. In A. E. Harris (Ed.), *Speech disorders: Causes, treatment and social effects* (pp. 139–159). New York, NY: Nova Science Publishers, Inc.

Halpern, A., Matos, C., Ramig, L., Petska, J., & Spielman, J. (2005, March). *LSVTC-A PDA supported speech treatment for Parkinson's disease.* Paper presented at 9th International Congress of Parkinson's Disease and Movement Disorders, New Orleans, LA.

Haynes, E., & Langevin, M. (2010, October). In Judith Kuster (Chair). *Telepractice at the institute for stuttering treatment and research (ISTAR)*. Paper presented at the International Stuttering Awareness Day Conference.

Hill, A. J., Theodoros, D. G., Russell, T. G., Cahill, L. M., Ward, E. C., & Clark, K. M. (2006). An Internet-based telerehabilitation system for the assessment of motor speech disorders: A pilot study. *American Journal of Speech-Language Pathology, 15*(1), 45–56.

Irani, F., & Gabel, R. (2011). Intensive stuttering therapy with telepractice follow-up: A case study. *Perspectives on Fluency and Fluency Disorders, 21*(1), 11–21. doi: 10.1044/ffd21.1.11

Irani, F., Gabel, R., Daniels, D., & Hughes, S. (2012). The long term effectiveness of intensive stuttering therapy: A mixed methods study. *Journal of Fluency Disorders, 37*, 164–178. doi: 10.1016/j.jfludis.2012.04.002

Kully, D. (2000). Telehealth in speech pathology: Applications to the treatment of stuttering. *Journal of Telemedicine and Telecare, 6*(2), 39–41.

Logan, P., & Noles, D. (2008). Protecting patient information in outsourced telehealth services: Bolting on security when it cannot be baked in. *International Journal of Information Security and Privacy, 2*(3), 55–70.

Mashima, P. A., & Doran, C. R. (2008). Overview of telehealth activities in speech-language pathology. *Telemedicine Journal and E-Health: The Official Journal of the American Telemedicine Association, 14*(10), 1101–1117.

O'Brian, S., Packman, A., & Onslow, M. (2008). Telehealth delivery of the camperdown program for adults who stutter: A phase I trial. *Journal of Speech, Language and Hearing Research, 51*(1), 184–195.

Palsbo, S. E. (2007). Equivalence of functional communication assessment in speech pathology using videoconferencing. *Journal of Telemedicine and Telecare, 13*(1), 40–43.

St. Louis, K. O., & Westbrook, J. B. (1987). The effectiveness of treatment for stuttering. In L. Rustin, H. Purser, & D. Rowley (Eds.), *Progress in the treatment of fluency disorders* (pp. 235–257). London, UK: Whurr.

Theodoros, D., & Ramig, L. (2011). Telepractice supported delivery of LSVT®LOUD. *Perspectives on Neurophysiology and Neurogenic Speech and Language Disorders, 21*(3), 107–119.

Watzlaf, V. J. M., Moeini, S., Matusow, L., & Firouzan, P. (2011). VOIP for telerehabilitation: A risk analysis for privacy, security and HIPAA compliance: Part II. *International Journal of Telerehabilitation, 3*(1), 3–10.

Yaruss, J. S., & Quesal, R. W. (2006). Overall assessment of the speaker's experience of stuttering: Documenting multiple treatment outcomes. *Journal of Fluency Disorders, 31*(2), 90–115.

Yaruss, J. S., & Quesal, R. W. (2008). *Overall assessment of the speakers' experience of stuttering.* Minneapolis, MN: Pearson.

7

Initiating and Sustaining a Telepractice Program for Individuals with Aphasia

Lyn R. Tindall

Introduction

Medical, technological, and rehabilitation advances have improved the quality of health care at a time when the prevalence of chronic diseases has increased due to the aging of the population. Chronic disabling conditions significantly limit an individual's activities of daily living and quality of life (Kobb, Hoffman, Lodge, & Kline, 2003). Although multiple effective treatments are available to reduce the effects of chronic diseases, many individuals experience barriers in accessing these treatments.

Traditional systems of health care delivery, including speech-language pathology services, may be difficult to access, yielding results that are inadequate or compromised for many individuals with aphasia. For example, those who reside in remote settings with limited health care options either travel great distances to medical facilities or do not receive care (Lacy, Paulman, Reuter, & Lovejoy, 2004). Travel to medical facilities is not only inconvenient but also generates expenses and creates caregiver burden and client dependency. Even individuals with aphasia who live close to medical facilities may experience travel difficulties that limit their ability to access care. As a result, clients who are not transported for evaluations or treatment are in essence denied access to speech-language pathology services or receive partial and incomplete treatment (Perlman & Witthawaskul, 2002).

To achieve the objective of delivering health services that meet the needs of individuals with aphasia, it is incumbent on speech-language pathologists to seek alternative ways to provide effective, less expensive care (Wilson, Onslow, & Lincoln, 2004). This care must include consideration of environmental characteristics that increase/decrease disability such as setting or treatment delivery method.

Recovery of function after brain damage may be more possible than previously realized (Bayles & Tomoeda, 2010). Neuroplasticity is the ability of the brain to reorganize, lay down new pathways, and rearrange existing ones (Kolb & Gibb, 2008). Principles of neuroplasticity include many factors (Kleim, 2006). Repetition, intensity, and duration are three factors that can be enhanced through telepractice. Repetition and intense stimulation are crucial for triggering neuroplasticity processes and recovery of brain function (Bayles & Tomoeda, 2010). Aphasia assessment and treatment can be provided through telepractice with more intensity than in-person treatment due to travel constraints and time associated with speech-language pathology sessions. In turn, telepractice can provide treatment to those who otherwise may forgo initiating treatment or cannot complete an intense aphasia program. Reducing or eliminating the burden of travel may increase the number of treatment sessions for those needing more intense treatment. Additionally, telepractice provides a way to deliver speech and language services to individuals in their natural environment, and in many cases with family members present. Evidence supports the notion that interventions are more effective when delivered to individuals in their own environment (McCue, Fairman, & Pramuka, 2010).

However, use of telecommunication technology should not be recommended solely on convenience and cost savings. The notion that delivery of speech-language pathology services via telecommunication technology is "better than nothing" must be avoided (Tindall & Huebner, 2009). A successful telepractice program includes thorough and careful planning as well as continued management to provide the best care for clients. Such a program should include the following strategies for success: *Planning and Start Up, Choice of Technology, Continued Management,* and *Special Consideration for the Client Encounter.*

Planning and Start Up

Initial stages of program planning provide opportunities to identify and analyze client care issues and develop realistic goals. To accomplish this, the selection of a team of individuals to guide the process is important to the development of a successful telepractice program. Suggestions for members of this team include:

- A clinical lead
- A support person from executive leadership
- A representative from Information Technology (IT)
- Others may be added depending on the setting.

If these individuals are not available, as in a small private practice, collaboration may be necessary to assist in the initial planning stages.

A needs assessment should be the first step in developing a telepractice program. This could include collection of data on underserved clients, costs of providing care (including costs of implementing the telepractice program), missed opportunities, no-show rates, and so forth. This step will provide a clear understanding of the how the program will be expected to meet the needs of clients and the organization, and these data will be a guide for developing quality improvement measures. The development team should then identify resources and barriers relevant to the program within the organization. Barriers to be considered include monetary barriers such as third-party reimbursement issues, licensure, credentialing and privileging barriers, training of clinicians, scheduling difficulties, and technology problems. Identification of barriers and resources at the initial phase of implementation will eliminate or minimize problems that may arise during implementation of a telepractice program. Return on investment analysis will provide information about cost effectiveness of the investment. Finally, continuous quality improvement methods to evaluate the program will help sustain and improve the quality of services.

Technology

The dilemma in choosing a technological system is that technology is ever-changing. With the goal of sustainability in mind, technology must be flexible beyond the initial funding stage. Therefore, in choosing a system, decisions must be made about specific equipment, identification of types of services, and client needs before deciding on technology options (Bashshur & Shannon, 2009). Decisions must also be made concerning peripheral accessories. The entire system may be purchased from a single vendor or separately if it results in a better quality system. The first consideration in choosing technology is to determine the telepractice modality. This decision will depend on the options of live interaction (real-time) with a client or review of clinical data (store-and-forward).

Telepractice Modalities

1. Real-Time (Synchronous): This encounter is similar to an in-person clinic visit. Use of this modality will require scheduling for all parties involved and allocation of space and time for both the client location and the clinician site.
2. Store-and-Forward (Asynchronous): Data are recorded then sent to a supporting site for review. These data may be recorded images (e.g., a modified barium swallow or videostroboscopy) or client files.

After choosing the modality of an encounter, the place of service delivery must be determined. Clients can receive services in their homes, within a clinic, or at distant sites, such as other clinics, hospitals, or offices. Room videoconferencing and/or desktop conferencing systems are available for these applications. These decisions will guide the choice of equipment needed and help in setting up the environment. The quality of service of a network is significant. Interrupted video or audio signals are not acceptable in clinical videoconferencing; therefore input from IT personnel will assist in making informed decisions about technology for each application.

Concern for security and privacy is a high priority when choosing telecommunication equipment. Manufacturers should be able to discuss available security features to protect client's privacy and comply with regulations. Bandwidth refers to the data rate supported by a network connection or interface. It represents the capacity of the connection. The greater the capacity, the more information it can carry. A low-bandwidth connection, such as a dial-up modem, may be best used for store-and-forward applications. High-bandwidth connections are preferred for real-time videoconferencing and are associated with better quality of video and smoothness of motion.

There are several telecommunication networks available. They include the following:

- POTS—"Plain Old Telephone Service" is synonymous with basic telephone service over the public telephone network. These connections are low bandwidth and are available through dial-up modems.
- ISDN—"Integrated Services Digital Network" are group systems in large-scale settings, such as conference rooms and classrooms, that use videoconferencing over integrated services digital network (ISDN), which is an all-digital replacement for plain old telephone service (POTS).
- IP—"Internet Protocol." Each device on an Internet or intranet has an IP address that enables systems to communicate with each other.

All of these systems have limitations. The best strategy is to make certain a knowledgeable network engineer is consulted during the planning stages of development to determine which telecommunication equipment will best meet the needs identified. Each setting is different, each caseload is unique; therefore, practitioners should avoid the notion of "one size fits all" when it comes to choosing a telecommunication system for telepractice.

Environment

Careful consideration must be given to the environment of both the client's and clinician's space to be used in a telepractice application. The environment should be set up to maximize client comfort and ease of accessing services, and be private and secure. Ease of access to a quiet room convenient to clients with aphasia, who may also have movement disabilities, provides the best setting. This includes doorways that are wide enough for wheelchairs and rooms that are large enough to accommodate telecommunication equipment and additional staff if needed. Keep in mind the type of clients served when choosing furniture. Tables and chairs should be at comfortable levels for children and adults.

In addition to telecommunication equipment required for transmission of the speech-language therapy application, other equipment should minimally include a telephone and fax machine. A computer may also be necessary to use during a speech therapy session. A telephone is essential if problems arise during the therapy session. A fax machine can be used to transmit therapy materials, letters, and so forth. A light or sign placed outside the treatment room will indicate that the room is in use and will protect the privacy of clients.

Lighting and décor are important factors to consider when planning a room designed for telepractice. Lighting on the face of clients and clinicians should be adjustable to minimize shadows on their faces. If the room has exterior windows, they should be covered with room darkening blinds or draperies. Objects such as mirrors, artwork, plants, fans, and wallpaper with patterns should be eliminated as they may cause reduced video quality of the signal. The best wall color is a neutral nonwhite color such as light gray, blue, or beige.

Audio quality is another important factor to consider. If possible, room reverberation and echo should be eliminated. An IT or audio-visual (AV) person can provide advice on optimal placement of microphones to achieve the best audio quality and eliminate feedback. Camera placement is crucial for the best video image of the client and clinician. The camera image ought to display the head and shoulders of a client and clinician, but also include the capability to zoom in and out so that others in the room can be identified or to zoom in on therapy materials.

Business Plan

Development of an appropriate business infrastructure will enhance technical and clinical aspects of telepractice. Evaluation of progress and outcomes are critical components of a successful program. Establishment of measureable goals and timelines will allow tracking of accomplishments and identification of obstacles to success. Communication concerning performance to leadership, providers, and clients will encourage their support and participation.

An effective business plan should include:

- Policies, procedures, and standards of practice (SOP)
- A memorandum of understanding (MOU) with sister facilities
- Financial goals to maximize resources
- Quality indicators
- A marketing plan
- A backup plan for technical difficulties.

Staff Preparation

Competent staff is essential and may present a challenge to the development and maintenance of a program. Clinicians must obtain education and training on all aspects of a telepractice endeavor. They must also complete credentialing and privileging when required. Licensure in the state where a client is located is required and supported by the American Speech-Language Hearing

Association guidelines (ASHA, 2005). According to the ASHA position statement, "The use of telepractice does not remove any existing responsibilities in delivering services, including adherence to the Code of Ethics, Scope of Practice, state and federal laws (e.g., licensure, HIPAA, etc.)," and ASHA policy documents on professional practices. Therefore, the quality of services delivered via telepractice must be consistent with the quality of services delivered in person.

Organizations such as ASHA and the American Telemedicine Association (ATA) provide workshops and short courses during their annual conferences. Additionally, the ASHA Special Interest Group (SIG) 18 offers opportunities to obtain continuing education units (CEU). Local and statewide professional organizations may also offer training programs in telepractice.

Staff preparation may also include rehabilitation technicians, such as speech-language pathology aids (SLP-A) or family members to assist in the presentation of stimulus items or pictures. Staffing issues must be paired with the abilities of clients in order to assure a successful encounter. Thus, careful assessment must be made of a client and identification and training of support staff is needed.

Marketing

Marketing is the activity, set of institutions, and processes for creating, communicating, delivering, and exchanging offerings that have value for customers, clients, partners, and society at large (American Marketing Association, 2007). Marketing strategies are used to convince a clientele to use services or products. To do this, the first step is to identify a particular client base, then direct marketing strategies toward them.

A telepractice marketing plan should include the following:

- Description of telepractice services
- Identification of clients, physicians, and rehabilitation personnel that might be interested in telepractice services

- Promotion and dissemination of information about the program
- Evaluation of marketing performance.

The Patient Encounter

As in all other aspects of telepractice, planning and preparation of the client encounter are critical for the success of a telepractice therapy session. Client-centered care must be the goal with results comparable to a traditional in-person visit. Awareness of all facets that will affect the outcome of a session ought to be considered prior to the encounter, during the telepractice session, and follow-up after the session has ended with preparation for the next encounter. Follow-up should include feedback from clients and family members about their experience using telecommunication technology to receive speech pathology services.

Planning

Planning and preparation include selection of an appropriate candidate for this type of service delivery system. Client selection should include:

- Evaluation of sensory deficits of a client such as vision and hearing and if the telecommunication equipment can accommodate these deficits
- Client's cognitive ability to attend and focus on a therapy task
- Client's capability to detect stimulus items presented by clinician
- Client's ability to manipulate objects during a session if appropriate.

Deficits in any of these areas may necessitate recruitment of an aid or family member to assist in presentation of stimulus items, encouragement of the client to stay on task, or providing information to the distant clinician about the appropriateness of a response. If there is uncertainty about whether a client would be able to summon help in an emergency, then another person should always be present in the therapy room with him or her, with a way provided to summon help. Staff roles and responsibilities should be defined and accepted by all persons involved in a telepractice session.

Prior to a telepractice session, a process should be in place to educate and orient a client about the session, technology, and what to expect, and the client should be allowed to consent or decline. Therapy materials may be mailed ahead of time or faxed just before a session begins. When a client arrives, a staff person should be charged with the responsibility of greeting, checking in the client, and escorting him or her to the therapy room.

During the therapy session, a light or "do not disturb" sign outside of the treatment room door will alert others that speech therapy is in session and protect the privacy of clients. Clients should receive the same level of privacy as if they were present in the telepractice therapy room. A split-screen view that includes the client and clinician will allow a clinician to see what the client sees. This enables a clinician to determine if a stimulus item is in focus and within camera range for the most effective presentation. Everyone in the room at the time of the treatment session must be identified, and the client informed when someone leaves or enters the room. Clinicians should look into the camera and try to reduce extraneous movement during a session to avoid pixilation of the image. Slow deliberate movements work best when switching from one stimulus item to another. For safety reasons, at the conclusion of therapy, wait until the client has left the treatment room and is in the company of others before disconnecting equipment.

After the therapy session is completed, a mechanism for assessing satisfaction of both the clinician and client should be used. Outcome measures taken during therapy will be beneficial in determining progress, comparing to traditional in-person outcomes, and assessing quality improvement. Information gathered using these methods will help plan the next telepractice session. If technical problems arise during the treatment session, troubleshooting may be necessary by technical support personnel.

The Evidence

Studies have investigated comparisons of telepractice assessments and treatment of aphasia outcomes to traditional in-person outcomes. Results indicated that telepractice is an effective method of delivery of speech services. In addition to traditional treatment outcomes, studies of effectiveness have also considered other client, caregiver, provider, and health care facility issues. For example, loss of quality of life of clients with aphasia generally includes loss of perceived control and struggles with coping (Keers et al., 2005). The introduction of telepractice technologies has the potential to facilitate the restoration of empowerment and self-determination among clients and care providers (Levy, Bradley, Morison, Swanston, & Harvey, 2002). Evaluation of outcomes of treatment traditionally includes client satisfaction with therapy techniques and delivery of services. Satisfaction with telepractice reflects individuals' values and expectations regarding delivery of services in this manner (Yip, Chang, Chan, & Mackenzie, 2003). Much of the telepractice satisfaction literature reports on studies with a small sample size or descriptive feasibility studies (Guillen et al., 2002; Gustke, Balch, West, & Rogers, 2000; Hilty, Marks, Urness, Yellowlees, & Nesbitt, 2004; Huston & Smith, 1996; Taylor, 2005; Whitten & Love, 2005). As telepractice technology becomes a more widely accepted health care delivery system, the perspective of user satisfaction and clarification of their experiences will be increasingly important in the evaluation process. Evaluating the costs and benefits of telepractice should include the perspectives of providers, clients, payers, and society. Service providers are affected by missed appointments and truncated treatment, and facilities may fail to achieve maximum client and financial outcomes related to poor attendance and follow through. Costs of care are important to providers of health services and include such cost-benefit analysis as the cost of missed appointments. Recent studies address the economic impact of telepractice and demonstrate that missed appointments result in loss of clinician time and translate into lost revenue for the facility (Dansky, Palmer, Shea, & Bowles, 2001; Deyo & Inui, 1980; Magnusson & Hanson, 2005; Noel, Vogel, Erdos, Cornwall, & Levin, 2004; Stensland, Speedie, Ideker, House, & Thompson,

1999). Speech-language pathologists are interested in the use of telepractice methods for service delivery; however, they share the same concerns identified by other medical professionals: reimbursement, licensure, and patient confidentiality issues (Denton, 2003). Efficacy studies will help meet the challenge of identifying the aspects of telepractice that are best suited to the delivery of speech and language services. Studies are emerging with promising results for these types of service delivery systems.

Telepractice technology options include the capability of delivering service to clients in their homes or to a telehealth clinic located close to their home. There are benefits and challenges of delivering speech pathology assessments and interventions to each of these locations. Home telepractice provides services to clients in their natural environment and includes caregivers and significant others in treatment sessions. Assessments are more difficult in this setting due to lack of testing materials available in a patient's home. Providing services to a client in a telehealth clinic may ensure that testing materials are available and a trained technician can assist in the administration of aphasia tests. Interventions delivered to clients at both sites are well suited to telepractice technology.

Telepractice Assessment of Aphasia

Studies of the use of telepractice technology to deliver speech and language services to clients with aphasia historically focused on assessment (Georgeadis, Brennan, Barker, & Baron, 2004; Lemaire, Boudrias, & Greene, 2001; Nakamura, Takano, & Akao, 1999; Wertz et al., 1987; Wertz et al., 1992). Online assessment of adult neurogenic communication disorders demonstrated good strength of agreement when compared to in-person assessments. These researchers found that telepractice-delivered assessments were comparable to in-person evaluations. Provision of speech pathology services appears to be well suited for telepractice technology as clients can see and hear a clinician give instructions and then responses can be judged through visualization and auditory output provided by this technology.

For many clients, it may be beneficial to conduct speech and language assessments in a traditional in-person manner especially if the patient will receive services in his or her home. The availability of testing materials and objects, and someone to present stimulus items, may make it impossible to assess clients in their homes. For clients receiving assessments in a telehealth clinic, aphasia tests and a trained technician to present items should be available for this purpose.

In order to provide assessments to a telehealth clinic, aphasia tests and objects should be purchased for that purpose. Training should be provided to speech-language pathology aids (SLP-A) or technicians (usually a licensed practical nurse) to present stimulus items used in testing. The remote clinician administering the test can record responses. Written responses by the patient can be faxed to the clinician for scoring or a document camera can be used to transmit the responses. As previously described, careful attention should be given to lighting, acoustics, and camera placement for both the patient and remote clinician.

Telepractice Aphasia Treatment

Research that compares outcomes of telepractice to in-person therapy in the treatment of communication disorders is promising (Hauber & Jones, 2002; Nakamura et al., 1999; Scheideman-Miller et al., 2002). A review of these studies revealed improvement in functional outcomes and/or satisfaction measures for the treatment of communication disorders via telepractice technology. Using telepractice technology, researchers investigated the assessment and treatment of adults with communication disorders using pre- and posttests, comparisons to in-person service delivery, and satisfaction surveys, and many included clinician satisfaction measures. The study of telepractice outcomes is in the early descriptive stage. To advance the science, studies on various populations of individuals with communication disorders need to be carefully designed and implemented. The presumed convenience and cost savings to persons with diagnoses of stroke, traumatic brain injury, progressive neurological diseases, or congenital speech disorders need to be further investigated.

Case Presentations

Anomia refers to difficulties retrieving words and is a common symptom of aphasia. Cueing is an established method of treating naming disorders. The cueing strategy used in the following case studies is based on two principles. First, as detailed by Geshwind (1967), Luria (1966), and Benson (1979), five varieties of anomia are associated with aphasia and five are nonaphasic in nature. Therefore, this cueing strategy includes motor, paraphasia, semantic, and category-specific cues. Secondly, according to Marshall (1976), delay, semantic association, phonetic association, and description were followed by their intended targets. Sentence completion is almost always easier when providing the correct response. The cueing hierarchy was designed to progress from hardest to easiest in eliciting the correct picture name.

Telepractice sessions were the same for the following three case presentations. After a video connection was established, a split screen was used in order to see both client and stimulus picture. A split screen will enable you to determine if the stimulus is in focus or has enough light for the client to be able to see it. After a picture was presented, clients were given 6 seconds to respond. Marshall (1976) reported that delay was most frequently followed by successful production of the target. Subsequent cues from the cueing hierarchy in Figure 7–1 were presented until the correct target was produced.

Client A

Client A was a 57-year-old college-educated retired mining engineer. He was 1 year post-onset of a left cerebrovascular accident (CVA). His diagnosis was Broca's aphasia and his aphasia quotient (AQ) on the Western Aphasia Battery (Kertez, 1979) was 40.06. After an initial assessment, the Televyou TV 500SP® from Wind

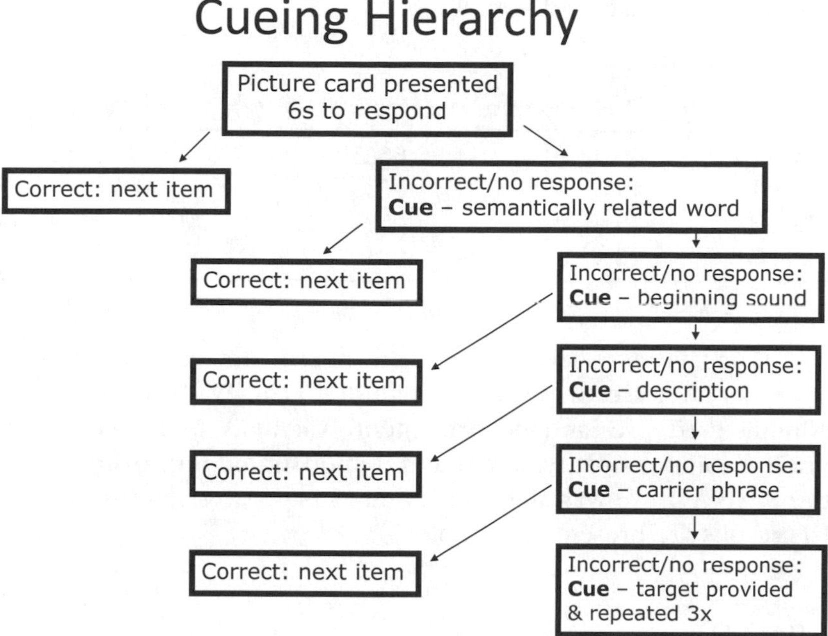

Figure 7–1. A diagram representing the cueing hierarchy used for case presentations.

Currents Technology was installed in his home to receive therapy. The TV 500SP® is a stand-alone plug-and-use videophone with duplex speakerphones that use plain old telephone service (POTS) lines. It has a 5-inch active matrix display with adjustable color and brightness and transmits and receives voice and simultaneous video. Clients were able to independently answer the videophone and a connection was made between the client and clinician.

Speech therapy was provided three times weekly for 4 weeks. Three lists of ten items each were targeted for intervention. Randomly selected Snodgrass pictures (Snodgrass & Vanderwart, 1980) were used in treatment. This is a standardized set of 260 pictures that provide consistency of pictorial representations. Each picture was presented to the client using the cueing hierarchy previously described.

Table 7–1. Results for Client A

	Pretreatment	Posttreatment	Maintenance
WABAQ	40.6	86.2	
List A	10%	100%	90%
List B	10%	100%	100%
List C	20%	90%	90%

Data were collected pre- and posttreatment and then at 4 weeks after treatment was concluded. The WAB AQ was also administered pre- and posttreatment. Client A increased word-finding abilities posttreatment and demonstrated improvement on the WAB AQ. He was able to maintain his progress after 4 weeks. His results are presented in Table 7–1.

Client B

Client B was a 63-year-old farmer with a high school education. He was evaluated at 3 months post-onset of a left CVA. His score on the WAB AQ was 83.5. He also used the Televyou TV 500SP® for therapy three times a week for 4 weeks. The Snodgrass word list and cueing hierarchy previously described were used as stimulus items during treatment. Improvement in naming was observed after treatment and maintained at 4 weeks. See Table 7–2 for results.

Table 7–2. Results for Client B

	Pretreatment	Posttreatment	Maintenance
WABAQ	83.5	85	
List A	50%	90%	80%
List B	70%	90%	90%
List C	40%	80%	80%

Table 7–3. Results for Client C

	Pretreatment	Posttreatment	Maintenance
WABAQ	6.9	6.9	
List A	0%	30%	
List B	0%		
List C	0%		

Client C

Client C was an 80-year-old farmer with a high school education. He was 3.5 years post-onset of a left CVA. His diagnosis was Broca's aphasia. Although his WAB AQ score was 6.9, it was felt that he might benefit from therapy. He completed only four sessions using equipment and cueing hierarchy previously described. Word list A was the only list treated. Even with so few treatments, Client C was able to improve naming on that list from 0% to 30%, demonstrating that even individuals with severe aphasia are able to use telepractice equipment and achieve gains in therapy. His results are presented in Table 7–3.

Conclusions

All the clients responded well to therapy delivered via videophones. They could participate independently at home. No assistance was needed for these clients to ambulate to the room where the videophone was located and operate the equipment. Feedback from clients and spouses indicated that they liked not having to drive to the clinic for speech therapy sessions and speech therapy sessions motivated clients to get out of bed and get dressed for each treatment session. Telepractice reduces or eliminates travel costs for clients and clinicians, increases compliance with scheduled therapy sessions, and provides for more frequent therapy sessions.

Lessons Learned

The following items are "pearls of wisdom" gleaned from many years of delivering speech-language pathology services to clients with aphasia. Telepractice can be a rewarding experience by enabling many individuals to have access to speech pathology services who would otherwise not be able to benefit from speech intervention.

- Planning ahead and anticipation of all possible scenarios cannot be emphasized enough.
- Telepractice should never be undertaken alone. Experts in the field of telecommunication technology and delivery of telerehabilitation services are a valuable asset.
- Cultivate a good relationship with your technical support. Success or failure may hinge on that person.
- Know what your equipment is capable of doing and be an expert on how to use it.
- Have a thorough understanding of your client's abilities and level of acceptance in using telepractice to receive services.
- Accept that there will always be individuals for whom telepractice is not well-suited.
- Always have a backup plan for when things don't go according to plan.

Summary

Research supports the effectiveness of telepractice for assessing and treating aphasia. Though investigations of treatment are emerging with promising results, further investigations are needed to confirm the efficacy of this therapy delivery approach. Carefully planned and delivered interventions enhance patient outcomes and optimal recovery. Based on evidence from treatment studies, there is a need for enhanced treatment intensity in chronic aphasia (Meinzer, Rodriguez, & Gonzalez, 2012). Telepractice can address the need for massed practice and relevant treatment settings, especially in areas with limited health care resources and therapists.

If clients are denied services, opportunities for enhancing quality of life for these individuals with aphasia are lost. Telepractice technology may bridge the gap in the delivery of health care by enabling some clients who would otherwise not receive services to participate in treatment. This technology may be beneficial to clients and their families by empowering older chronically ill individuals to participate in their own care.

Disclaimer: These contents do not represent the views of the Department of Veterans Affairs or the United States government.

References

American Marketing Association. (2007). *Definition of marketing*. Retrieved December 30, 2010, from http://www.marketingpower.com/AboutAMA/Pages/ DefinitionofMarketing.aspx

American Speech-Language-Hearing Association (2005). *Speech-language pathologists providing clinical services via telepractice: Position statement.* Retrieved December 30, 2010, from http://www.asha.org/practice/telepractice/

Bashshur, R., & Shannon, G. (2009). *History of telemedicine.* New Rochelle, NY: Mary Ann Liebert.

Bayles, K., & Tomoeda, C. (2010, November). *Neuroplasticity: Implications for treating cognitive-communication disorders.* Paper presented at the American Speech-Language-Hearing Association Convention, Philadelphia, PA.

Benson, D. (1979). Neurological correlates of anomia. In H. Whitaker & H. A. Whitaker (Eds.), *Studies in neurolinguistics, 4*, 293–328. New York, NY: Academic Press.

Dansky, K., Palmer, L., Shea, D., & Bowles, K. (2001). Cost analysis of telehomecare. *Telemedicine Journal and e-Health,* 7(3), 225–232.

Deyo, R., & Inui, T. (1980). Dropouts and broken appointments: A literature review and agenda for future research. *Medical Care, 18*(11), 1146–1157.

Georgeadis, A., Brennan, D., Barker, L., & Baron, C. (2004). Telerehabilitation and its effect on story retelling by adults with neurogenic communication disorders. *Aphasiology, 18*(5/6/7), 639–652.

Geshwind, N. (1967). The varieties of naming errors. *Cortex, 3,* 97–112.

Guillén, S., Arredondo, M., Traver, V., Valero, M., Martin, S., Tragantis, A.,

Robinson, S. (2002). User satisfaction with home telecare based on broadband communication. *Journal of Telemedicine and Telecare, 8,* 81-90.

Gustke, S., Balch, D., West, V., & Rogers, L. (2000). Patient satisfaction with telemedicine. *Telemedicine Journal, 6*(1), 5-13.

Hauber, R., & Jones, M. (2002). Telerehabilitation support for families at home caring for individuals in prolonged states of reduced conciousness. *Journal of Head Trauma Rehabilitation, 6,* 535-546.

Hilty, D., Marks, S., Urness, D., Yellowlees, P., & Nesbitt, T. (2004). Clinical and educational telepsychiatry applications: A review. *Canadian Journal of Psychiatry, 49*(1), 12-23.

Huston, J., & Smith, T. (1996). Evaluating a telemedicine delivery system. *Topics in Health Information Management, 16*(3), 65-71.

Keers, J., Links, T., Bouma, J., Scholten-Jaegers, S., Gans, R., & Sanderman, R. (2005). Diabetes rehabilitation: Effects of a multidisciplinary intensive education programme for diabetic patients with prolonged self-management difficulties. *Journal of Clinical Psychology in Medical Settings, 12*(2), 117-126.

Kertez, A. (1979). *Aphasia and related disorders.* New York, NY: Grune and Stratton.

Kleim, J. (2006, November). Can understanding the basic principles of neural plasticity improve Rehabilitation? *Academy of Neurologic Communications Sciences and Disorders.* ANCDS Annual Meeting, Miami, FL.

Kobb, R., Hoffman, N., Lodge, R., & Kline, S. (2003). Enhancing elder chronic care through technology and care coordination: Report from a pilot. *Telemedicine Journal and e-Health, 9*(2), 189-195.

Kolb, B., & Gibb, R. (2008). Principles of neuroplasticity and behavior. In: Stuss, Winocur, & Robertson (Eds.), *Cognitive neurorehabilitation.* Cambridge, UK: Cambridge University Press.

Lacy, N., Paulman, A., Reuter, M., & Lovejoy, B.. (2004). Why we don't come: Patient perception of no shows. *Annals of Family Medicine, 2*(6), 541-545.

Lemaire, E., Boudrias, Y., & Greene, G. (2001). Low-bandwidth, Internet-based videoconferencing for physical rehabilitation consultations. *Journal of Telemedicine and Telecare, 7,* 82-89.

Levy, S., Bradley, D., Morison, M., Swanston, M., & Harvey, S. (2002). Future patient care: Tele-empowerment. *Journal of Telemedicine and Telecare, 8*(2), 52-54.

Luria, A. (1966). *Higher cortical functions in man.* New York, NY: Basic Books.

Magnusson, L., & Hanson, E. (2005). Supporting frail older people and their family careers at home using information and communication technology: Cost analysis. *Journal of Advanced Nursing, 51*(6), 654–657.

Marshall, R. (1976). Word retrieval behavior of aphasic adults. *Journal of Speech and Hearing Disorders, 41,* 444–451.

McCue, M., Fairman, A., & Pramuka, M. (2010). Enhancing quality of life through telerehabilitation. *Physical Medicine and Rehabilitation Clinics of North America, 21*(1), 195–205.

Nakamura, K., Takano, T., & Akao, C. (1999). The effectiveness of videophones in home healthcare for the elderly. *Medical Care, 37*(2), 117–125.

Noel, H., Vogel, D., Erdos, J., Cornwall, D., & Levin, F. (2004). Home telehealth reduces healthcare costs. *Telemedicine Journal and e-Health, 10*(2), 170–183.

Perlman, A., & Witthawaskul, W. (2002). Real-time remote telefluoroscopic assessment of patients with dysphagia. *Dysphagia, 17*(2), 162–167.

Scheideman-Miller, C., Clark, P., Smeltzer, S., Cloud, A., Carpenter, J., Hodge, B., & Prouty, D. (2002). Two-year results of a pilot study delivering speech therapy to students in a rural Oklahoma school via telemedicine. *Proceedings of the 35th Hawaii International Conference on System Sciences.*

Snodgrass, J., & Vanderwart, M. (1980). A standardized set of 260 pictures: Norms for name agreement, image agreement, familiarity, and visual complexity. *Journal of Experimental Psychology, 6*(2), 174–215.

Stensland, J., Speedie, S., Ideker, M., House, J., & Thompson, T. (1999). The relative cost of outpatient telemedicine services. *Telemedicine Journal, 5*(3), 245–256.

Taylor, P. (2005). Evaluating telemedicine systems and services. *Journal of Telemedicine and Telecare, 11*, 167–177.

Tindall, L., & Huebner, R. (2009). The impact of an application telerehabilitation technology on caregiver burden. *International Journal of Telerehabilitation, 1*(1), 3–8.

Wertz, R., Dronkers, N., Bernstein-Ellis, E., Shubitowski, Y., Elman, R., Shenaut, G., ... Deal, J. L. (1987). Appraisal and diagnosis of neurogenic communication disorders in remote settings. In R. H. Brookshire (Ed.), *Clinical aphasiology, 17,* 117–132. Minneapolis, MN: BRK Publishers.

Wertz, R., Dronkers, N., Bernstein-Ellis, E., Sterling, L., Shubitowski, Y., Elman, R., ... Deal, J. L. (1992). Potential of telephonic and television technology for appraising and diagnosing neurogenic communication disorders in remote settings. *Aphasiology, 6* (2), 195–202.

Whitten, P., & Love, B. (2005). Patient and provider satisfaction with the use of telemedicine: Overview and rationale for cautious enthusiasm. *Journal of Postgraduate Medicine, 51*(4), 294-300.

Wilson, L., Onslow, M., & Lincoln, M. (2004). Telehealth adaptation of the Lidcombe program of early stuttering intervention: Five case studies. *American Journal of Speech-Language Pathology, 13,* 81-93.

Yip, M., Chang, A., Chan, J., & Mackenzie, A. (2003). Development of the telemedicine satisfaction questionnaire to evaluate patient satisfaction with telemedicine: A preliminary study. *Journal of Telemedicine and Telecare, 9,* 46-50.

8

Evaluating Telepractice: Measuring Success, Cost-Benefit, and Outcomes

Scott T. Palasik and Farzan Irani

Introduction

With the rapid advancement in technology over the past few years, telepractice has now become a feasible and popular option of service delivery for speech-language pathologists (SLP). This significant increase of interest in telepractice has been supported by the American Speech-Language-Hearing Association (ASHA) as noted by the ASHA position statement and technical report on telepractice (ASHA, 2005a; ASHA, 2005b). In addition, ASHA has established a Special Interest Group (SIG) with a focus in telepractice (http://www.asha.org/SIG/18/). As a result, it is evident that a large number of SLPs are now adopting telepractice as a model of service delivery. Keeping the rapid growth of telepractice within the field of audiology and speech-language pathology in mind, it is important for practitioners to develop a system to effectively measure communication outcomes of patients being served as well as the cost-benefit of telepractice models used in comparison to traditional face-to-face service delivery.

The objective of this chapter is to provide the reader with an overview of current research and trends in the measurement of communication outcomes of patients served via telepractice. Furthermore, this chapter also provides practitioners with helpful tips to determine the cost-benefit of a telepractice service delivery in comparison to traditional service delivery for their own individual practice.

Preliminary Considerations

When developing a telehealth program, the practitioner must, first and foremost, determine the needs and benefits of telepractice to the population served. Due consideration must be given to the materials used in live treatment sessions and whether they translate to the online medium. Furthermore, investigating whether there are any such tools already available (or adapted) for telepractice is a vital step when setting up a program dealing with any clientele. Often, a practitioner might need to be creative and develop new materials or adapt readily available materials to assess treatment outcomes and provide the best quality care to their patients.

After determining the need and feasibility of offering telepractice services, the practitioner must consider the overall cost of setting up and offering services via telepractice. In making this determination, the practitioner needs to consider the initial upfront investment as well as recurring costs. The initial upfront investment includes equipment required to conduct telepractice successfully. This includes (and is not limited to) a computer with a high-quality web camera, headset with microphone, external storage devices, suitable furniture, and reconfiguration of the room if required. Included in this initial investment, the practitioner must also incorporate a contingency budget to pay for replacing malfunctioning equipment, as well as to upgrade equipment as needed.

In addition to the initial investment and contingency, the practitioner must also factor in recurring expenses including a stable high-speed wired (Ethernet) Internet connection, telepractice software that meets privacy and security standards, antivirus software subscriptions, and encryption software for all computers and external storage devices used for telepractice delivery.

Based on the clientele served, needs might vary. It is strongly recommended that the practitioner first create an inventory of all hardware and software required to effectively conduct telepractice to help determine the total cost of offering this service prior to purchasing equipment and offering the service. Based on the patient's needs, some practitioners may need more equipment (e.g., encrypted storage drives) whereas others might require more investment in software to facilitate training or data collection. It is important to note that telepractice is a business, so as a practitioner's business grows using this delivery model, further cost-benefit analysis might be suggested to expand and improve treatment.

Measuring Outcomes

In the new world of telepractice, the primary objective guiding any skilled speech-language pathologist is the gathering of outcome data to assess patients' progress in order to tailor and deliver effective and efficient treatment. The adaption of materials typically used during traditional face-to-face treatment to the telepractice environment may not be as difficult as one may initially perceive.

First, it is important to talk about the research examining the use of formal and informal assessment tools used with telepractice technology. At this time, there are limited studies investigating the use of standardized and nonstandardized assessment tools with telepractice in communication sciences and disorders. One study outside of the field of speech-language pathology looked at the accuracy of using standardized assessment tools during telemedicine delivery with older adults with dementia, depression, and delirium (Loh et al., 2004). All adult clients were serviced through face-to-face and videoconferencing telemedicine delivery. Loh et al. (2004) examined the use of the Mini Mental State Exam (MMSE) and the Geriatric Depression Scale (GDS). The importance of this study was that the researchers compared face-to-face administration of these two assessment tools with the videoconference delivery. They found there did not appear to be a systematic bias between delivery methods, and telepractice delivery of the two measures could be effective when diagnosing dementia and depression. This is encouraging information when certified speech-language pathologists may desire to use similar evaluation questionnaires with adult clients via a telepractice delivery model.

Another study looking at assessment procedures with telepractice was Waite, Cahill, Theodoros, Busuttin, and Russell (2006). This study examined six children between 4 and 7 years old diagnosed with speech disorders. The purpose of the study was to gather pilot data on how efficacious videoconferencing telepractice is when using the following speech measures: single word articulation test (SWAT), intelligibility rated on connected speech samples, and an oromotor assessment of function and structure. The results indicate adequate agreement between face-to-face and telepractice SWAT assessment. However, agreement on the perceptions of fricatives and the rates for the oromotor examination were low between the two service delivery models. Waite et al. (2006) reported that these lower agreement ratings could be due to technical and methodological challenges. The importance of this study was that it showed that outcome measures based on audio and visual perceptions can be influenced by the quality of Internet connection and hardware (cameras) and the effectiveness of the delivery of directions to clients.

In a follow-up project, Waite, Theodoros, Russell, and Cahill (2010) investigated the use of the CELF-4 standardized language assessment tool. They compared conventional face-to-face delivery and videoconferencing telepractice with 5- to 9-year-old children previously diagnosed with language impairments. No significant differences were found between the results gathered from the telepractice delivery of the CELF-4 and the conventional face-to-face delivery model. This study once more demonstrated that standardized assessment tools can be adapted to telepractice programs with little adjustment of the stimuli being delivered.

Further support for the delivery of assessment materials through videoconferencing has also been seen in the area of motor speech disorders. Hill et al. (2006) examined 19 adult dysarthric clients using the perceptual assessments battery. The battery consisted of the following measures: speech samples from conversational speech and reading, a 9-item version of the Intelligibility of Dysarthric Speech (Yorkston & Beukelman, 1981) and the Frenchay Dysarthria Assessment (Enderby, 1983). Hill et al. (2006) found administration of the perceptual assessment battery via telepractice to be an effective means for assessing motor speech disorders. They also noted that some of the subtests of the Frenchay Dysarthria Assessment could not be administered due to logistical challenges of the clinician being unable to see internal oral structures for accurate assessment. This brings in an important point for telepractice assessment and treatment, *not all assessment tools can be effectively administered.* This relatively obvious point is useful when clinicians may be picking and choosing which evaluation tools are appropriate for conventional face-to-face assessment versus videoconferencing. A nice rule of thumb to ensure diversity in tools and accuracy of outcomes is to try and perform a mixture of telepractice and face-to-face interactions when assessing any disorder. Additionally, some state licensure laws require that the assessment be conducted face-to-face. Practitioners must always be knowledgeable about their individual state requirements and have their clients' best interests at heart.

The use of remote computer technology has been reported to be an effective telepractice delivery model in the field of audiology as well. Krumm (2007) clearly explained the procedure of performing pure tone and speech audiometry via remote access to computerized equipment. This study indicates that with the proper equipment, clients can effectively participate in basic assessment tools for the diagnosis of hearing disorders. The notion of using remote computing for audiology assessment was confirmed when Krumm, Huffman, Dick, and Klich (2008) performed distortion product otoacoustic emissions (DPOAE) and automated auditory brainstem response (AABR) screening on 20 infants less than 45 days old. Test results for both the DPOAE and the AABR screenings were not significantly different when face-to-face or telepractice delivery models were used. This study further demonstrates that telepractice can be an effective and reliable tool for performing assessments, even with infants during hearing evaluations. The importance of this research is the use of videoconferencing with application sharing software that can control a remote computer, presenting another option for clinicians. This setup also provides more control to the skilled practitioner when delivering computerized evaluation tools and visual imagery that require a high level of audio and/or visual accuracy and clarity during presentations. This is especially beneficial in sparsely populated or underserved locations where a trained expert might not be accessible on site.

When talking about treatment outcome measures in speech-language pathology, it might be helpful for practitioners to start with some of the basic outcome data used in live face-to-face treatment settings that can be easily adapted to telepractice delivery. Collecting speech samples from patients with speech and language and audiological concerns is a relatively simple task and is not that much different during telepractice delivery as compared to the traditional service delivery model. Some telepractice programs, like the Lidcombe Program of Early Stuttering, have utilized the fundamental treatment component of collecting speech samples as their primary outcome measure to compare short-term and long-term outcomes (Lewis, Packman, Onslow, Simpson, & Jones, 2008). This program asks parents to collect three speech samples for each assessment period; one sample at home, one away from the home environment with child's awareness, and one at home without the child's knowledge. The Lidcombe Program has demonstrated that during telepractice services, gathering speech samples as the primary assessment procedure to gauge client progress can be an effective treatment delivery system for children who stutter and their families when the traditional face-to-face treatment model is not available.

The retrieval of speech samples as outcome measures via telephone telepractice conversations was further supported by the Phase 1 research performed with adults who stutter involved in the Australian-based Camperdown Program (O'Brian, Packman, & Onslow, 2008). Unplanned telephone calls were made by clinicians to clients before and after treatment. During these telepractice phone calls, three 10-minute recordings were performed consisting of a conversation between the client and clinician and two conversations between the client and strangers. From these speech samples percentage of syllables stuttered and syllables per minute (SPM) were measured. The study suggested that telepractice services via telephone conversations for adults who stutter have the potential to be an efficacious treatment. This program provides further support for gathering speech samples during telepractice telephone calls as a vital form of outcome measures that can be manipulated in the same way as conventional face-to-face recordings of speech samples. With advances in technology, many traditional telepractice software options such as Adobe Connect Pro are available as a free application for mobile platforms such as iOS and Android. When a client has the required device and has provided consent, clinicians can monitor the client's performance via videoconferencing as well, thus adding to the quality and efficacy of the data gathered. This provides another option to clinicians, in addition to videoconferencing telemedicine treatment, while still having the ability to gather appropriate samples with conversational speech in novel situations such as communicating with strangers.

One of the assets of telepractice delivered through video technology, as compared to telepractice via the telephone, is that videoconferencing provides both video and audio components. With the use of video and audio, skilled practitioners in speech-language pathology can assess vocal performance and any visual elements related to communication disorders. Mashima et al. (2003) randomly assigned voice-disordered patients to be treated in either a traditional face-to-face individual therapy program or in a remote videoconferencing telepractice treatment program. Patients received the same treatment in both groups. Vocal samples were collected by skilled speech-language pathologists for pre- and posttreatment outcome measures. Acoustic measures of the patients' voice quality were then conducted with speech samples. These samples were recorded from live samples prior to telepractice treatment, and then used for acoustic analysis. Even though the speech samples from this study were not taken online, this study is important because it opens up the discussion about gathering vocal samples from patients with voice disorders. With the free acoustic analysis software, Praat (Boersma & Weenink, 2013), patients could be educated through telepractice about how to record speech samples and then send sound files to certified practitioners (i.e., a store and forward model of sharing data). Clinicians could then use the same acoustic software to perform spectral analysis as outcome measures related to vocal changes. This is a low-cost way to perform outcome measures for voice patients using telepractice and does not require patients to drive to a physical location for vocal sample performances.

Again, the use of speech samples and vocal samples is a foundational component of outcome measures to track treatment progress with many communication disorders. These can be fairly easily recorded using digital technology within videoconferencing software programs such as ones developed by companies including Adobe, Cisco, Logitech, and Microsoft. With the expanding technology encapsulated in cell phones, patients and families could record themselves during day-to-day conversations using both audio and video recordings. These recordings of speech samples could then be sent to their practitioner. Along the same lines, patients and families can use cell phone live Webcam video technology including, but not limited to, Adobe Connect Pro or Cisco Webex to stream live conversational speech samples to skilled treatment providers to assess speech and language samples in real time. If they do not have access to cell phone technology such as those discussed previously, clients can purchase a basic digital hand recorder to capture speech samples, download those samples onto a computer, and send those sound files to their skilled treatment providers for analysis of speech, language, and vocal skills. Alternatively, certain web conferencing programs also allow participants to record audio/video both online as well as offline that can be stored to a server. If a practitioner subscribes to such a program, clients could also complete audio/video recordings through the telepractice program and submit them to the clinician either synchronously or asynchronously.

Another common outcome measure typically used in the field of speech-language pathology is self-reporting perceptional measures. These self-report measures gather vital data about personal attitudes regarding specific disorders collected from patients, families, teachers, and skilled practitioners. Some of the previously mentioned research that used speech samples for outcome measures also utilized perceptual ratings as another form of data collected during telepractice. O'Brian et al. (2008) used self-report measures of stuttering severity from adult patients along with a self-reported 9-point Speech Naturalness Scale. Lewis et al. (2008) collected questionnaires from parents of children who stutter to evaluate their satisfaction and acceptability of the telepractice treatment. In addition to vocal samples, Mashima et al. (2003) used perceptional judgments of vocal quality and collected patient satisfaction about their vocal improvement. Collecting self-report measures can be as easy as sending patients an email with an attached (with prior consent from the patients) document including Likert questions, open-ended questions, and different perceptional questions to be answered and returned to the skilled practitioner via email. As well, there are perceptional measures like the Overall Assessment of Speaker's Experience of Stuttering (OASES) (Yaruss & Quesal, 2008) that can be mailed to the client with a postage-paid return envelope. This provides the skilled therapist more options and ease of delivery in telepractice to a variety of clients.

Thus, to summarize and review some salient points with regard to measuring treatment outcomes using the telepractice service delivery model, it is most important for the clinician to be creative and resourceful. First, treatment outcomes can be measured either synchronously or asynchronously. In the case of synchronous administration of outcome measures, it is important for the practitioner to ensure a good quality audio and video connection with the patients. It is also helpful for the practitioner to complete an audio and video recording of the live session for later review to determine reliability and validity. Asynchronous outcome measure assessments can involve the administration of a patient-completed questionnaire (e.g., the OASES), which, depending on copyright, might need to be mailed to the client or can be administered as an online form using software such as Adobe Acrobat Pro or Survey Monkey (http://www.surveymonkey.com). Additionally, clients can also share audio and/or video samples of their speech and language with the clinician asynchronously. This can be done if the patient (or caregiver) completes a recording of the speech/language sample and then shares the sample with the practitioner either via email or by uploading the sample to a secure server accessed by the clinician.

Determining Cost-Benefit

The cost to benefit ratio of telepractice is a defining component when assessing the success of this service delivery model. Medical settings, universities, school districts, and private clinics need to be conscious of the expenses they may incur delivering therapy in both the traditional face-to-face or through telepractice service delivery models. Information regarding cost can be a determining factor for facilities and clients with respect to the overall efficiency of treatment. For the individual practitioner, it is important to complete a thorough cost-benefit analysis by considering both the initial investment (and contingency funds) and the recurring expenses of telepractice.

Facility and Family Costs of Telepractice

There is limited research in the field of speech-language pathology with respect to evaluating costs related to providing telepractice services. Yet, with the increased use of telepractice in public schools across the country, some of these facilities have produced research about the cost benefits of telepractice delivery. One study by Doolittle, Williams, and Cook (2003) aimed to estimate how much it would cost for telemedicine clinical consulting at school clinics for the pediatric population as compared to ambulatory medical settings over the span of one school year. They determined expenses to each of the 10 telepractice sites using standard cost-accounting measures. The salary and benefits of the staff doing the consulting and the length of the time of each consult determined the direct labor cost. Furthermore, all costs related to equipment and supplemental tools were factored in to the expenses per site with 6% depreciation over 3 years. The physical space utilized by all sights was considered by multiplying the square footage of the office by the going rent rate. The cost to medical settings was determined by how long telepractice consultants would have occupied space at a hospital facility. Expenses were then analyzed with a regression curve to chart the changing longitudinal cost to the facility over the year. The results revealed that prior to 165 consults, the cost of telemedicine was greater than the projected cost of conventional face-to-face medical consultations. However, following this number of consults, telemedicine consults became more cost effective. At 200 consults, the telemedicine consults were predicted to be nearly

10% cheaper than conventional face-to-face consults conducted in a medical setting. This study suggests that facilities looking to offer telepractice delivery should look at several expenses in order to judge short- and long-term cost-effectiveness of using telepractice, especially the overall volume of usage of the model.

Young and Ireson (2003) further corroborate the benefit of telemedicine in school-based settings by investigating the cost-benefit of this model for parents receiving consultations from skilled medical personnel provided by two elementary schools. The cost to the schools was calculated by factoring the expense of the equipment, training, the service delivery personnel's salary, and time of each consult with parents. Cost to the patient was calculated by factoring the parents' self-reported cost of traveling to a hospital, potential physician costs, and loss of work time for traditional consultations. Young and Ireson suggested that telemedicine could save parents a potential of \$101.00 to \$224.00 per visit per child in addition to significant time missed at work. It is important to note that the medical practitioners providing the telemedicine services in this study were hesitant at first about the use of telepractice delivery for reasons of sacrificing the physical presence of the client for digital video contact. However, these same medical personnel later reported satisfaction with the telemedicine technology. This study offers support for the use of telepractice provided in school-based facilities. This can translate to speech-language pathology in that communication with parents can be performed effectively and at a low cost. In turn, more effective communication with parents can connect treatment needs with home follow-up, resulting in improved outcomes for the children served.

Follow-up outpatient treatment is a valuable part of treating individuals with a variety of health-related disorders. One study by Zissman, Lejbkowicz, and Miller (2004) compared medical costs of multiple sclerosis patients using telemedicine and conventional face-to-face treatment. They found the telemedicine group experienced lower deterioration of their disability and an improvement in six of ten multiple sclerosis symptoms, thus resulting in 67% of these participants saving 35% of medical costs. Patient costs are an important expense component skilled professionals need to consider when preparing to perform telepractice delivery. It is an indicator of greater treatment efficiency when a service provider can deliver equally effective treatment at a lower cost.

Fauchier et al. (2005) also examined how to cut patient costs for health services using remote technology to monitor the medical needs of patients. This study examined the use of home monitoring implantable cardioverter defibrillators (ICD). Fauchier et al. (2005) found patients saved almost $1,000 in follow-up visits because of the remote technology related to the operation of the ICD. This study supports findings from an earlier research project by Jerant, Azari, and Nesbitt (2001), which also found that congestive heart failure (CHF) readmission frequency and costs were significantly decreased with the use of videoconferencing and telephone telemedicine. In the medical world, a major expense of clients is readmission for the same disease or disorder. The use of telemedicine delivery may reduce readmissions, which can save clients and hospitals money.

Another study concerned with cutting treatment costs to the patient was Ahmed et al. (2008). This research examined the cost of follow-up care for adult epileptic clients using telemedicine videoconferencing for 8 months from January to August. Forty-one patients were split between receiving conventional face-to-face follow-up treatment and telemedicine treatment. Each patient was seen one to two times a month. Expenses incurred by the client were recorded. These costs included travel expenses calculated as cost per kilometer traveled along with lost working hours, the use of a hotel if required, an escort to accompany them to visits if required, and whether the escort lost time working (similar to the parents taking off time from work to bring their pediatric children to a consultation visit in the Young and Ireson study shown previously). The cost analysis conducted by Ahmed et al. (2008) indicated that epileptic patients performing conventional face-to-face services paid an average of $466.00 for their treatment regimen as compared to the average out-of-pocket cost of $36.00 paid by patients receiving telemedicine services. The savings of more than $400 for patients receiving telemedicine services is appealing to say the least. Self-report surveys from patients indicated that almost all were satisfied with the services provided, and almost 76% of the traditional face-to-face delivery participants were willing to try telemedicine follow-up treatment. This study shows that the desire by patients to seek alternative means of health care is a real and valid perception. Keeping this in mind, speech-language pathologists looking to venture into telepractice can feel encouraged by the growing interest of individuals willing to seek treatment through this service delivery model. It is suggested that skilled practitioners judge interest of clients before undertaking the step of purchasing telepractice equipment. This first step of judging interest could save practitioners time and unwanted expenses.

The previously mentioned studies are foundational research demonstrating that educational and medical facilities can benefit financially from the use of telepractice service delivery models. Not only can a school save critical funds with increased use of telepractice, but this mode of consulting with parents also can be time-effective. Telemedicine technology can also be cost-effective for patients served in medical settings by reducing readmissions. These are important factors for medically based speech-language pathologists to evaluate when considering the provision of telepractice services. However, it is important to remember the limitations of telepractice and closely monitor individual clients to ensure every client receives the best possible therapy. Sometimes telepractice is not the best delivery method for treating specific patients. Speech-language pathologists treat individuals, and one form of treatment or service delivery does not always suit an entire population.

The Use of Telehealth for Home-Health Practitioners

The field of speech-language pathology, like many health care service disciplines, has a large number of providers who perform home health services. This type of treatment has different costs including travel expenses for therapists and a loss of time servicing patients due to traveling. Telepractice might help businesses save money in the long term by providing clients with videoconferencing treatment. Komet (2001) was one of the first to study the home-based telepractice delivery. With the growing number of individuals requiring home-based health services, Komet (2001) suggested that "by extending the reach of care providers, telehealth can enable home health care agencies to increase the number of patients they care for while maintaining or lowering costs" (p. 184). Komet further says that by providing telepractice home care, practitioners can conceivably reach three times as many people in need. Telepractice can also assist the process of monitoring patients to become more efficient and manageable while reducing costs related to traveling to home health clients. Furthermore, the use of telepractice can open up an endless supply of skilled medical personnel to be in contact with patients, with the use of remote technology monitoring vital signs from a distance.

As discussed previously, the use of remote technology is another way to decrease client need for constant personal contact with health care professionals. A study by Dinesen et al. (2012) examined the effectiveness of a home monitoring system for patients with chronic obstructive pulmonary disease (COPD). The study found hospital readmissions were lower and hospitalization costs were significantly reduced for clients who had the home monitoring system as compared to the control group that did not. The importance of this study for the speech-language pathologist is that by developing strategies that empower patients to monitor their own progress, less time may be needed for one-on-one therapy. In turn, patients can reduce expenses by not having to rely on a practitioner for all of their treatment success.

Cherney and van Vuuren (2012) suggested "Telerehab programs that allow participants to receive treatment sessions without the presence of an SLP at every session would increase cost effectiveness" from the provider's point of view (p. 247). By increasing self-reliance with encouraging independent use of treatment tools and techniques, practitioners are cutting costs related to seeing the client. This saves the client money and saves businesses the expense of personnel focused on one client. This allows for a business to see more clients, thus expanding its clinical practice.

Integrating technology into telepractice along with some creative thinking are vital components to a successful, cost-effective telepractice facility. The development of new software that patients can use at home to practice techniques has found booming success with computers, tablets, and smartphone applications (apps). The sheer volume of apps is beyond the scope of this chapter. However, if patients and skilled practitioners have access to technology supporting applications with smartphones and a variety of tablets (e.g., Apple iPad, Kindle Fire, Samsung Galaxy), performing simple searches through the many speech and language apps may yield wonderful telepractice treatment activities for clients to use independently. The use of smartphone and tablet apps also can decrease time skilled practitioners use to create therapy activities, thus potentially decreasing preparation time. Like anything new, time is needed to acquaint oneself with tablet technology and searching for applications. However, following the initial investment of time and money, preparation time per client may actually decline, thus opening up more opportunities for direct contact billing time to service more clients.

Although there is no research in the field of communication disorders to support this yet, Duesterhoeft (2012) suggests the field of telepractice can provide health games through the new world of tablets and smartphones, which can be monitored remotely by health care practitioners to assess patient progress. Again, there are many computer, tablet, and smartphone apps available for free to minimal costs, with more being developed every day. This may be an additional expense to practitioners and clients. However, with diligent research, therapists can surely develop a cost-effective program for clients by mixing various telepractice activities. Another way to encourage more client practice time, and thus less need for constant direct therapy with one client, is by integrating a system of reminders for clients to perform independent practice of treatment techniques. These type systems can be integrated with telepractice technology and keep clients accountable for their practice time. With patient consent, practitioners can ask patients to text them whenever they complete independent practice time. The skilled practitioner does not have to answer these texts, which is understood by both parties when this therapy practice is discussed. This simple form of telepractice contact via texting can also be another source of data practitioners can use to track patient performance without requiring face-to-face or even videoconferencing telepractice contact. If patients are not comfortable texting the practitioner, they can set up reminders in their phone to practice therapy techniques during the day. This again opens up more opportunities for practitioners to service more patients effectively.

The Cost of Telepractice

For any facility, whether it is a school, hospital, private clinic, or community center, it is important to perform a cost benefit analysis for both the financial benefits and perceived satisfaction from the clients and clinicians providing telepractice. Family and client satisfaction and their expenses are significant factors to consider when starting telepractice delivery. As indicated previously, some of the physical expenses incurred for telepractice appear to be similar to conventional face-to-face treatment. These similar costs include, but are not limited to, physical space required to deliver treatment, assessment, and therapy tools, and the salary of personnel providing services to clients and families. When doing a cost benefit analysis, it appears that these expenses are relatively consistent for both telepractice and face-to-face treatment.

Telepractice, while reducing general space requirements, does have additional equipment costs. This chapter will not detail exact costs of equipment, as that is a constantly changing and evolving component. Furthermore, health care practitioners need to perform thorough research with their needs associated with caseload size and personnel. That being said, for the small business speech-language pathologist, equipment costs can be as simple as getting a good desktop or laptop computer. Tablets can also be used for telepractice; however, for better streaming video and audio, clinicians may want to be hardwired (Ethernet) into a broadband Internet system. There is always a degradation of signal and Internet speed associated with the use of wireless Internet; hence, it is strongly recommended that practitioners utilize a wired connection (and also encourage their patients to do the same) in order to provide the highest quality services. Other costs to consider with videoconferencing telepractice are limited to Internet providers in some areas, detachable Web cameras for laptops without built-in cameras, software to deliver clear and effective therapy, recurring monthly costs for Internet and specialized software for conducting telepractice sessions, and a subscription to a professional software encryption service; patient data and any protected health records are to be stored electronically.

Again, each new telepractice business should evaluate the interest of telepractice services from patients, families, and the community before moving forward with purchasing the required equipment. This can be performed by simply asking current patients if they might be interested in piloting videoconferencing. Practitioners can also ask patients about their expenses to attend face-to-face treatment (travel cost, loss of time at work) along with what computer equipment they may have to perform effective telepractice treatment. It is also important to determine patient comfort (or familiarity) with the use of new technology. If patients and families show an interest, practitioners can move forward with researching equipment for their perceived needs and then perform a thorough cost-benefit analysis.

To summarize, conducting a cost-benefit analysis is important for any practitioner who plans to offer services via telepractice. The review of literature highlights that telepractice, when well planned, can be a very efficient service delivery model with significant cost savings for both the patient and the practitioner. However, it is important for the clinician and/or the facility to determine the cost-benefit of telepractice. After determining that there will be no degradation in the quality of services offered via telepractice, and all treatment outcomes can be measured effectively via this service delivery model, the practitioner must engage in a thorough cost-benefit analysis. Important factors to take into consideration when making this determination include: (a) the initial investment in both equipment and software/technology; and (b) recurring expenses that include Internet, software subscriptions to facilitate telepractice, data encryption services (including antivirus and antimalware), and mailing costs for sending and receiving patient-completed forms/questionnaires. Lastly, it is important for the practitioner to determine if the client has the necessary hardware, Internet connection, and skills to access services via telepractice.

Conclusion

This chapter provides an overview for determining communication outcomes for patients receiving therapy via telepractice as well as a cost-benefit analysis of this service delivery model. As discussed throughout this chapter, it is important for the practitioner to consider both of these factors when planning to offer services via telepractice.

First and foremost, practitioners must complete a survey of their clientele to ensure that the patients can easily access and will benefit from this service delivery model. If a majority of the patients (or their caregivers) do not have access to high-speed (wideband) Internet, a computer with a Web camera, and the technical knowledge to facilitate this model, these are strong contraindications.

Second, practitioners must survey the tools available to effectively evaluate communication outcomes for the majority of their clientele when offering services via telepractice. This can include tools that are already adapted for the telepractice service delivery model, or tools that can be easily adapted for use with telepractice. Adaptation of such outcome measures can be done either by administering the test/outcome measure synchronously online during a telepractice session or asynchronously via offline recordings of speech/language samples and/or mailing the form/questionnaire to the patient.

Third, the practitioner must engage in a thorough cost-benefit analysis for adopting this service delivery model. In order to do so, it is recommended the practitioner consider all costs involved in the initial setup as well as recurring costs to offer this service. Practitioners must assess their own individual needs (and needs of their clientele) to determine such costs. As noted in some research, telepractice becomes more cost-effective when a practitioner provides the service to a larger number of clients. For a patient, the benefit of telepractice is the savings in time required to travel to the practitioner, fuel costs, and the overall cost of therapy. Thus, for this model to be feasible, it must help reduce overall costs incurred by the patient as well as the practitioner, unless the purpose of telepractice is to provide services to a population in a geographically remote area who might not have access to specialized services.

Even though equipment costs for telepractice have dropped significantly over the years, doing a thorough cost-benefit analysis with a trained accountant would be advantageous to any business. With effective delivery of telehealth services, travel costs can be significantly reduced for patients, families of patients, and businesses that perform home-based health services. This cost alone may be a big selling point for some patients to participate in this form of treatment.

A final note for all practitioners to consider is that laws (both federal and state) governing the use of telepractice will continue to evolve. For instance, in January 2013, the Nebraska senate introduced a bill to provide telepractice services in public schools in order to save parents money and potential employment status when taking off time from work to see medical personnel. This is noted because it is important for practitioners to be conscious of the laws governing telepractice as they venture through the process of starting telepractice delivery. These types of laws encouraging telepractice delivery will and continue to be developed in order to service the greater good.

Acknowledgments

It is with great appreciation that we thank our wonderful graduate assistants Stephanie Davis, Kate Menzies, and Julianne Mier. We would also like the thank K. Todd Houston for inviting us to write this chapter. Additionally, we extend our appreciation to The University of Akron and Texas State University for their continued support. Finally, our appreciation goes out to the patients and families we have had the pleasure to service with telepractice and face-to-face delivery models. It is these individuals who continually inspire us to be better at the art of clinical practice.

References

Ahmed, S. N., Mann, C., Sinclair, D. B., Heino, A., Iskiw, B., Quigley, D., & Ohinmaa, A. (2008). Feasibility of epilepsy follow-up care through telemedicine: A pilot study on the patient's perspective. *Epilepsia, 49*(4), 573–585.

American Speech-Language-Hearing Association. (2005a). *Speech-language pathologists providing clinical services via telepractice: Position statement* [Position statement]. Retreived from http://www.asha.org/policy.

American Speech-Language-Hearing Association. (2005b). *Speech-language pathologists providing clinical services via telepractice: Technical report* [Technical report]. Retreived from http://www.asha.org/policy.

Boersma, P., & Weenink, D. (2013). *Praat: Doing phonetics by computer* [Computer program]. Version 5.3.40, Retrieved February 2, 2013, from http://www.praat.org/

Cherney, L. R., & van Vuuren, S. (2012). Telerehabilitation, virtual therapists, and acquired neurologic speech and language disorders. *Seminars in Speech and Language, 33*(3), 243–257. doi: 10.1055/s-0032-1320044

Dinesen, B., Haesum, L. K. E., Soerensen, N., Nielsen, C., Grann, O., Hejlesen, O., & Ehlers, L. (2012). Using preventive home monitoring to reduce hospital admission rates and reduce costs: A case study of telehealth among chronic obstructive pulmonary disease patients. *Journal of Telemedicine and Telecare, 18*(4), 221–225. doi: 10.1258/jtt.2012.110704

Doolittle, G. C., Williams, A. R., & Cook, D. J. (2003). An estimation of costs of a pediatric telemedicine practice in public schools. *Medical Care, 41*(1), 100–109.

Duesterhoeft, T. (2012). The road not traveled: The role of telehealth in the new era of mobile healthcare. *GAMES FOR HEALTH: Research, Development, and Clinical Applications, 1*(4), 254–256.

Enderby, P. (1983). *Frenchay dysarthria assessment*. San Diego, CA: College-Hill Press.

Fauchier, L., Sadoul, N., Kouakam, C., Briand, F., Chauvin, M., Babuty, D., & Clementy, J. (2005). Potential cost savings by telemedicine-assisted long-term care of implantable cardioverter defibrillator recipients. *Pacing and Clinical Electrophysiology: PACE, 28*(Suppl. 1), S255–S259.

Hill, A. J., Theodoros, D. G., Russell, T. G., Cahill, L. M., Ward, E. C., & Clark, K. M. (2006). An internet-based telerehabilitation system for the assessment of motor speech disorders: A pilot study. *American Journal of Speech-Language Pathology/American Speech-Language-Hearing Association, 15*(1), 45–56.

Jerant, A. F., Azari, R., & Nesbitt, T. S. (2001). Reducing the cost of frequent hospital admissions for congestive heart failure: A randomized trial of a home telecare intervention. *Medical Care, 39*(11), 1234–1245.

Komet, H. (2001). An analysis of the home health marketplace: How telehealth technology may assist home health agencies with changes in home care delivery under the prospective payment system. *Home Health Care Management and Practice, 13*(2), 142–148.

Krumm, M. (2007). Audiology telemedicine. *Journal of Telemedicine and Telecare, 13*(5), 224–229.

Krumm, M., Huffman, T., Dick, K., & Klich, R. (2008). Telemedicine for audiology screening of infants. *Journal of Telemedicine and Telecare, 14*(2), 102–104. doi: 10.1258/jtt.2007.070612

Lewis, C., Packman, A., Onslow, M., Simpson, J. M., & Jones, M. (2008). A phase II trial of telehealth delivery of the Lidcombe Program of early stuttering intervention. *American Journal of Speech-Language Pathology, 17*(2), 139.

Loh, P. K., Ramesh, P., Maher, S., Saligari, J., Flicker, L., & Goldswain, P. (2004). Can patients with dementia be assessed at a distance? The use of telehealth and standardised assessments. *Internal Medicine Journal, 34*(5), 239–242.

Mashima, P. A., Birkmire-Peters, D. P., Syms, M. J., Holtel, M. R., Burgess, L., & Peters, L. J. (2003). Telehealth: Voice therapy using telecommunications technology. *American Journal of Speech-Language Pathology, 12*(4), 432.

O'Brian, S., Packman, A., & Onslow, M. (2008). Telehealth delivery of the camperdown program for adults who stutter: A phase I trial. *Journal of Speech, Language and Hearing Research, 51*(1), 184.

Waite, M. C., Cahill, L. M., Theodoros, D. G., Busuttin, S., & Russell, T. G. (2006). A pilot study of online assessment of childhood speech disorders. *Journal of Telemedicine and Telecare, 12*(3), 92–94.

Waite, M. C., Theodoros, D. G., Russell, T. G., & Cahill, L. M. (2010). Internet-based telehealth assessment of language using the CELF-4. *Language, Speech, and Hearing Services in Schools, 41*(4), 445.

Yaruss, J. S., & Quesal, R. W. (2008). *Overall assessment of the speakers' experience of stuttering.* Minneapolis, MN: Pearson.

Yorkston, K. M., & Beukelman, D. R. (1981). *Assessment of intelligibility of dysarthric speech.* Austin, TX: Pro-Ed.

Young, T. L., & Ireson, C. (2003). Effectiveness of school-based telehealth care in urban and rural elementary schools. *Pediatrics, 112*(5), 1088–1094.

Zissman, K., Lejbkowicz, I., & Miller, A. (2012). Telemedicine for multiple sclerosis patients: Assessment using health value compass. *Multiple Sclerosis Journal, 18*(4), 472–480.

9

eSupervision and eMentoring: Professional Development for Current and Future Professionals

Charles H. Carlin, Emily L. Carlin, Jennifer L. Milam, and Tali R. Weinberg

Introduction

In a rural public school district in the Midwestern United States, a veteran speech-language pathologist (SLP) is about to retire. She is a long-time resident of the community and is dedicated to her students, families, and school district. In order to better ensure the school district has enough time to hire a suitable replacement, she submits her intent to retire paperwork to the human resources office months in advance. The school district immediately posts the vacancy announcement with the state department of education and calls area universities for job leads. Unfortunately, months go by and no qualified applicant calls the school district. To make matters worse, the school district cannot afford to pay well and is spread across a large geographical area. The new SLP needs to be assigned to one middle and two elementary schools, and it takes 30 minutes to drive between buildings. The caseload isn't high, but there are severely impaired students at each of the buildings, and there is no shortage of evaluations and meetings. Finally, in July and before the school year starts, a newly graduated SLP contacts the school district. She excitedly shares that she is getting married and moving back home near the school district. There is one hitch, the applicant is a new graduate, and she requires clinical fellowship (CF) supervision for her national certification with the American Speech-Language-Hearing Association (ASHA). The district cannot hire her; there is no SLP supervisor available who is appropriately credentialed and willing to travel to the school district for an entire academic year. Additionally, the union contract calls for new employees to be paired with district mentors from the same discipline. Because she will be the only SLP in the district, someone in the special education department will have to be assigned to her. This mentoring arrangement is far from ideal.

Impact of Supervisor and Mentor Shortages

This scenario is not unique to the public schools and CF supervision. The limited availability of SLP supervisors impacts recruitment of qualified applicants (Wright-Harp & Cole, 2008), access to desirable employment opportunities (Wood, Miller, & Hargrove, 2005), and retention of employees (Wright-Harp & Cole, 2008) across employment settings. Furthermore, supervisor shortages restrict the number of available off-campus clinical placements for graduate students (ASHA, 2008). When the number of clinical placements is restricted due to a lack of supervisors, graduate students and universities struggle to meet practicum requirements for graduation, state licensure, and national certification (ASHA, 2007; Dudding & Justice, 2004). When employers cannot recruit, hire, or retain qualified applicants due to supervisor shortages, the following have been observed:

- Speech-language vacancies remain unfilled.
- Underqualified or unqualified individuals fill speech-language vacancies.
- Novice SLPs receive inferior supervision and feel unproductive and ineffective.

- SLPs feel isolated.
- Quality professionals resign.
- Clients go without services or fail to make adequate progress.
- Employers contract with national companies or regional private practices to meet the needs for speech-language services.

During the 2006 Forum on Strategizing Solutions to Personnel Shortages in Speech-Language Pathology, a national group of stakeholders from higher education institutions, business and health care, school districts, state boards of education, governmental agencies, and recruitment firms convened. These stakeholders were asked to identify barriers to the recruitment and retention of SLPs and then brainstorm solutions to personnel shortages (McNeilly, 2006). Not only did they identify a shortage of supervisors as a contributing factor, but they also felt that the limited number of mentors served as a barrier to the recruitment and retention of SLPs across work settings. In order to address this lack of mentors, the stakeholders recommended the following:

1. Future SLPs should be mentored as early as possible (e.g., high school).
2. Mentoring should be regarded as a long-term collaboration that is supported by administrators.
3. Due to their busy schedules, mentors should receive release time to conduct mentoring activities.

Employers and graduate programs need to overcome barriers that are associated with access to supervisors and mentors in order to recruit the best graduate students and SLPs, retain them as long as necessary, and provide them with high-quality professional development and support. Access to high-quality speech-language supervisors and mentors is critically important to the professional development of pre- and in-service SLPs (ASHA, 2008), especially because learning does not and should not end upon receipt of the degree in speech-language pathology. Instead, SLPs are encouraged, and in some cases expected to engage in continuing education throughout their careers in order to acquire new work skills (e.g., third-party insurance billing requirements, compliance with special education law, universal precautions) and maintain and enhance clinical competencies (ASHA, 2010).

Access to Supervision and Mentoring Through Technology

In the not-so-distant past, SLPs hand wrote, photocopied, and mailed out treatment plans, progress reports, daily notes, and evaluations to supervisors and mentors for review and approval. Graduate students wrote term papers, research articles, and dissertations using typewriters or word processors. Therapy materials were largely created from scratch. Less experienced SLPs and graduate students primarily communicated with their supervisors and mentors through written or typed out notes, phone calls, or face-to-face interactions. Times have changed and technological advances now allow SLPs and graduate students the opportunity to engage in academic, work, and professional development activities in vastly different ways. SLPs complete paperwork and third-party billing on sophisticated computer programs. Clients receive individualized services and evaluations through the use of telepractice and interactive computer programs. High-tech augmentative and assistive communication devices are prevalent, smaller, and widely versatile. Applications (apps), tablets, and the Internet are easily infused into the therapeutic and diagnostic process in order to achieve goals and objectives, motivate students, elicit a multitude of responses, and generalize skills across communication partners and settings. Communication between professionals can occur instantly even at a distance. Technology is everywhere, and it continues to change how graduate students, SLPs, supervisors, and mentors operate.

As stated previously, technology helps professionals in our field become more efficient, effective, and connected during clinical placements and at work. Not only does technology connect friends and families across great distances, but it can also be integrated into supervisory and mentoring activities. E-supervision, which can also be called telesupervision or distance supervision, uses videoconferencing and other technologies to connect supervisors and supervisees so that high-quality responsive clinical supervision can occur. The e-supervisor, who is physically housed in a setting that is different from the supervisee, utilizes videoconferencing and other technologies to clinically supervise synchronously (i.e., directly in real time), asynchronously (i.e., indirectly at a different time), or through some hybrid combination of the two. E-supervisors are able to see, hear, and evaluate the supervisees' performance during the delivery of interventions, assessments, and other professional activities. Additionally, e-supervisors and supervisees meet virtually with the videoconferencing technology, talk by phone, instant message, text, share computer screens and documents, and email information in order to further develop clinical competencies. Technology greatly strengthens the supervisory relationship and allows clinical supervision to occur despite geographic and scheduling barriers.

E-mentoring, much like face-to-face mentoring, connects an expert SLP with a less experienced one (Anderson & Shannon, 1988), a faculty member with a student (Lechuga, 2011), and a more experienced student with a more novice student (Jackson & Woolsey, 2009). A feature that is unique to e-mentoring is the inclusion of technology as the vehicle to help educate, counsel, and direct a mentee (Apel, 2007). E-mentoring occurs synchronously, asynchronously, or through a hybrid combination and provides opportunities to increase a mentee's access to high-quality academic, professional, and personal support. The e-mentoring pairs collaborate virtually via online file sharing and cloud storage (e.g., GoogleDrive, Wikispaces), through video- or teleconferencing, and with texts, emails, and other store-and-forward technologies (e.g., Youtube video demonstrations).

Table 9–1 summarizes some of the various technologies and their applications that can be used during the processes of e-supervision and e-mentoring. The choice of technologies will depend on the goals of the project; amount of available funding; number of people involved; security needs; licensure, certification, employment, and third-party reimbursement regulations; and available resources (e.g., bandwidth, technology support) (Dudding & Carlin, 2012). The list of technologies is not exhaustive as it is expected to grow as new technologies are developed and incorporated into future supervision and mentoring projects.

Table 9–1. Technological Applications for E-Supervision and E-Mentoring

	Synchronous "Real-Time"	**Asynchronous "Store and Forward"**
Observation of direct client activities and professional interactions (e.g., meetings, consultations, grand rounds, presentations)	Mobile devices (e.g., smartphones, tablets), desktop (e.g., Elluminate, Gotomeeting, Skype) and midlevel videoconferencing technologies (e.g., Tandberg and Polycom systems)	Recordings stored on external devices (e.g., DVDs, flash drives, digital voice recorders), Internet-based sites (e.g., YouTube), and videoconferencing technologies.
Communication with e-supervisor or e-mentor	Teleconferencing, videoconferencing, and instant messaging (e.g., Skype).	Texting, emailing, voicemail, scanning, faxing, and social networking technology (e.g., Facebook, Twitter).
Sharing information (e.g., therapy materials, paperwork)	Desktop and midlevel videoconferencing technologies. Screen sharing (e.g., Skype, Adobe Connect).	Cloud storage services (e.g., Google Drive), e-mailing, faxing, scanning, online forums, blogs, screen shots (e.g., Microsoft Windows), and dedicated e-supervision or e-mentoring websites (e.g., Wikispaces) or platforms (e.g., Springboard, Blackboard).

The Process

E-Supervision

The process of clinical e-supervision borrows many elements from traditional face-to-face supervision. In keeping with Anderson's (1988) Continuum Model of Supervision, clinical e-supervision is a dynamic process that changes as the needs and skills of the supervisee change. The ultimate goal of clinical e-supervision is the achievement of complete supervisee independence from the e-supervisor. The supervisee moves along a continuum of supervisory support, and begins with the supervisee being completely reliant on the e-supervisor for direction and instruction. Over time, the e-supervisor provides less support as the supervisee develops clinical competencies, problem-solving skills, and self-evaluation. As the supervisee develops clinical competency, the amount of supervisory direction strategically decreases and the amount of supervisee participation and independence increases (McCrea & Brasseur, 2003).

The process of clinical e-supervision employs three stages of supervisory dependency: evaluation-feedback, transitional, and self-supervision (Anderson, 1988). In order to ensure the supervisee meets with success during the clinical e-supervision process, the supervisee is thoughtfully and systematically moved through the three stages. These stages are based on the supervisee's proficiency level within each course outcome, clinical competency, or work-related skill. During the evaluation-feedback stage, the e-supervisor is dominant and holds a direct and active style of supervision as the supervisee encounters many new types of disorders and clinical situations. As in any new situation, the supervisee is expected to be unfamiliar with expectations and standards of practice, and therefore needs a considerable amount of support and guidance (McCrea & Brasseur, 2003).

As the supervisee develops some level of proficiency and becomes better acquainted with the work setting, colleagues, caseload, and duties, clinical e-supervision progresses to the transitional stage. During this stage, the e-supervisor and supervisee participate in joint problem-solving and deliberation around a clinical problem, skill, or competency (Anderson, 1988). Although the supervisee is not working independently, some clinical independence begins to emerge. Midway through the transition stage, the supervisee self-evaluates clinical behaviors, plans certain future actions, and modifies some behaviors during ongoing interventions, diagnostics, meetings, and other professional endeavors. Toward the end of this stage, the supervisee and e-supervisor collaborate to develop lessons and solutions to clinical problems. In some instances, the e-supervisor starts functioning as a colleague and the supervisee acts as a self-supervisor.

The final stage of e-supervision is self-supervision. During this stage, the supervisee accurately analyzes clinical behaviors and outcomes and alters behaviors accordingly (McCrea & Brasseur, 2003). The supervisee no longer requires direct and active e-supervision, constant analysis, and feedback. The e-supervisor now functions as a mentor or colleague to the supervisee. It is important to note that movement through these stages is not a timed or rigidly arranged process; e-supervisors and supervisees move through the experience based on individual readiness and professional competencies being established.

E-Mentoring

Given that the field of speech-language pathology suffers from a dearth of e-mentoring literature, the process can be borrowed and adapted from traditional forms of mentorship. University programs, employers, for-hire private companies, colleagues, or professional associations can be enlisted to match mentees with appropriate and qualified e-mentors. E-mentors can elect to work 1:1 or with small groups of mentees. Once the match is made, Murray and Owen (1991) suggest that the e-mentor and mentee develop clearly defined professional, personal, and educational goals and ensure that these goals serve as the focus of the mentoring activities for the duration of the relationship. These goals should be tied to specific activities, be geared toward the attainment of skills or knowledge, and contain achievable time lines (Murray & Owen, 1991). The e-mentor and mentee should discuss how frequently they need to "meet" (McCrea & Brasseur, 2003) and agree upon the format of these meetings (e.g., Skype videoconference call, telephone call, instant messaging). The e-mentor and mentee should commit to the plan, almost as if it was a contract between them, and agree that someone could terminate the relationship without penalty or fault (Murray & Owen, 1991). In order to ensure a successful e-mentoring experience, ASHA (2005) recommends the following:

- Be clear about how often and how the mentoring pair will communicate and when follow-up can be expected. Even if the mentor cannot assist immediately, there must be acknowledgment that the mentor is working on it.
- Ensure confidentiality.
- Stay in frequent contact, especially during the first few weeks of the relationship.
- Establish a trusting relationship.
- Respect the views, experiences, and ideas of the other person.
- Honor commitments and take action.
- Be appreciative of the help that is offered or given. Provide a thank you note or sincere email; acknowledgment goes a long way.
- Make the relationship mutually beneficial. As the mentor comes across information or resources, it should be shared with the mentee.
- Demonstrate and allow flexibility.

It should be pointed out that ASHA's (2005) mentoring-mentee recommendations appear to have utility across most supervisory and mentoring experiences that occur at a distance through the use of technology. This is significant because while e-supervision and e-mentoring offer new possibilities, the core of the relationship and professional expectations must remain the same—built on trust and mutually defined goals and objectives.

E-Supervision and E-Mentoring Projects

When universities and employers first consider using technology to connect supervisors and mentors, many questions ensue. Which technologies should be used? How will the project be developed, implemented, and sustained. How can pitfalls be avoided and barriers removed? The success of the project depends on careful planning, thoughtful implementation, and supportive stakeholders and environments. Stakeholders, colleagues, or experts in the field can be brought together to brainstorm an effective plan that will support all phases of the project and generate strategies that can be put into place to avoid or alleviate potential roadblocks. Although e-supervision and e-mentoring are a relatively new concept in the field of speech-language pathology, much can be learned from past e-supervision and e-mentoring projects.

E-Supervision in Speech-Language Pathology

Several models of e-supervision exist in the field of speech-language pathology. These models use videoconferencing and other technologies to provide e-supervision to graduate SLP students who are enrolled in advanced clinical practica, school-based externships, or in school districts where they are acting as the sole provider services. Although no study has yet evaluated the use of e-supervision with ASHA-certified SLPs or CFs, important elements from the literature on graduate students can be applied to these in-service professionals. Readers are also encouraged to investigate a wide array of e-supervision models that were developed in the related fields of education, social work, counseling, psychology, and physical therapy. No matter the discipline, these examples can serve as models or starting points for future e-supervision projects.

OMNIE E-Supervision Project

Due to the persistent shortages of SLPs in Ohio school districts, superintendents lobbied for the licensing of speech-language pathology assistants (SLPA). In order to address the large volume of SLP vacancies across the state and avoid the use of SLPAs, the Ohio Department of Education established a funded collaboration with the Ohio Master's Network Initiatives in Education (OMNIE) and seven Ohio universities (Boswell, 2007). Through this collaboration, a specialized school-based graduate SLP internship was developed (i.e., the SLP Intern Model Graduate Program), which aimed to graduate enough SLP interns to fill the vacancies in speech-language positions. Graduate SLP students in the program completed an initial year of pediatric coursework and clinical practica and then were hired by school districts as their primary practicing professional (prior to graduation and certification). During the first year of employment, the graduate SLP students also completed their medical practica and online coursework focusing on adult patients, in the evenings, on the weekends, or during the summer. The graduate SLP students were allowed to have up to 50 children on their caseload and were required to be supervised by a district-provided SLP. This supervisor was required to observe the graduate SLP student at least 25% of the time during direct client interventions, assessments, and screenings.

Much as the school districts struggled to hire SLPs in the past, shortages of available supervisors now presented a new challenge to the school districts—who would supervise and support these graduate SLP students? In order to overcome the shortage in qualified SLP supervisors, the Ohio Department of Education intervened and provided funding for technology, e-supervisors, and research. Through the introduction of technology into the supervisory process, graduate SLP students were able to be placed in rural and hard-to-fill school districts while still being supported by high-quality SLPs. This innovative approach to supervision and staffing helped to meet the needs of many stakeholders and ensured high-quality professional standards of supervision were maintained.

Carlin, Milam, Carlin, and Owen (2012) investigated how weekly e-supervision supported the graduate SLP students. In this study, the Continuum Supervision Model (Anderson, 1988) was adapted for use with graduate SLP students during the yearlong public school-based internship. The model of clinical e-supervision that resulted incorporated desktop videoconferencing and other technologies into the supervision process. The e-supervisor and graduate SLP student met "virtually" to prepare lessons, discuss observations and paperwork, problem solve clinical situations, and review assessment and progress data. Through the use of the technology, observations occurred in real-time during individual, small-group and large-group therapy, assessments, screenings, and meetings.

Instead of physically demonstrating intervention and assessment techniques with the children on the caseload, the e-supervisor described what to do in detail, supplied example lesson plans, or provided premade video demonstrations. Information (e.g., assessment reports, test protocols, client progress, treatment plans) was shared through a dedicated website, e-mails, texts, screen sharing, and instant messages.

The study used data from surveys, supervision logs, and structured interviews from the 6 e-supervised and 46 face-to-face graduate SLP interns. Data were analyzed to determine the graduate SLP students' perceptions of e-supervision support and to compare these perceptions with past experiences with face-to-face supervision. The data showed e-supervision was positively regarded by the graduate SLP interns and they felt adequately supervised and supported. Carlin et al. (2012) found 83% of the graduate SLP students (n = 6) in the study agreed that e-supervision was a more convenient form of supervision when compared to face-to-face supervision. Of these graduate SLP students, 67% agreed e-supervision was less stressful because the supervisor was not physically in the room. All of the e-supervised graduate SLP students agreed e-supervision promoted their independence. These same students also showed some neutrality when they were asked to further compare face-to-face and e-supervision. Half of the e-supervised graduate students stated that e-supervision was more productive than direct supervision, whereas the other half remained neutral. Having experienced both forms of supervision, one student remarked that she has had good encounters with both e-supervision and direct supervision and does not prefer one method over the other (Carlin et al., 2012).

Although the e-supervised graduate SLP students were not widely observed during classroom-based lessons, they were observed across a wide array of other professional activities (e.g., pull-out interventions, assessments, screenings, parent meetings, consultations with teachers). The e-supervised graduate SLP students believed they were provided with more than an adequate amount of support and feedback from their e-supervisors, received timely feedback through the use of instant messaging and emails, and obtained access to helpful Internet-based resources related to intervention and assessment techniques. Finally, the study also found that the e-supervised students were supervised more frequently during assessments when compared to their face-to-face supervised peers.

Landro Play Analyzer

At the university level, clinical instructors supervise multiple graduate students at one time and therefore experience difficulty balancing the large volume of observations with other university duties (Tellis, Cimino, & Alberti, 2010). In order to maximize the clinical instructors' time, manage overlapping observations, and develop graduate students' clinical competencies, Tellis et al. designed a unique clinical observation laboratory. Through the use of the Landro Play Analyzer (LPA), clinical instructors were capable of remotely supervising multiple graduate students and recording these intervention and diagnostic sessions all at once.

Originally created to help football coaches collect statistics during a game, LPA Enterprise Edition Network System by IRIS Technologies was adapted for use by clinical instructors and graduate students in order to record and analyze client intervention and diagnostic sessions synchronously and asynchronously. The LPA not only allowed clinical instructors to observe multiple sessions in real time, but also permitted graduate students to store, view, pause, categorize, tag, and analyze prerecorded speech-language samples and critique their own performance. Bookmarked sections were quickly transferred to Microsoft Excel for analysis, saved the data on the central server or converted into MPEG movies, and then burned it on a CD or DVD. Sessions of past clients were further used to teach future graduate students how to collect case histories, baseline levels, and progress data. The LPA technology allowed the clinical instructors to view multiple clients and student clinicians, from various angles, in four treatment rooms. Supervisors had the option of viewing from the observation laboratory on a quad-screen computer monitor or from one of the four treatment rooms, with a tablet PC streaming the other three meetings in progress. During the sessions, clinical instructors tagged and catalogued specific segments for later review and discussion.

The use of LPA technologies provided numerous advantages for universities, clinical instructors, graduate students, clients, and caregivers/families. First, clinical instructors were able to observe multiple sessions simultaneously and at a distance as well as offer graduate students specific feedback on their performance. Second, the archived sessions allowed graduate students to evaluate their own performance after each session and over the span of a semester. Third, the recorded sessions provided speech-language clients with a unique opportunity to identify their own errors and increase their motivation during interventions. Fourth, the caregivers and family members were able to view the client's progress at home and observe potentially useful home carryover activities. Finally, recent advancements by IRIS Technologies (e.g., software enhancements) enabled any computer or laptop to become a Landro Workstation, which greatly reduced the cost, technological requirements, and training. Tellis et al.'s (2010) observation laboratory in combination with the LPA technology provided an excellent model of e-supervision for busy university SLP clinical instructors.

DLV-SLP

As mentioned earlier, e-supervision can be used to increase graduate students' access to highly qualified supervisors (Wood et al., 2005) and meet the needs of busy faculty members who are assigned to supervise graduate students across large geographical areas (Olson, Russell, & White, 2001). Another e-supervision model that was used to connect graduate students with a high-quality university supervisor was the Distance Learning in Virginia Educating Speech-Language Pathologists (DLV-SLP) program. DLV-SLP program contained an accelerated online graduate program and supervised clinical placements that aimed to increase the number of available master's level SLPs who could be hired to work in the Commonwealth of Virginia public school system (Dudding, 2004). A single university-based supervisor provided both e-supervision and face-to-face supervision to the graduate students' at their public school placements. E-supervision occurred from the e-supervisor's university office via the Polycom Viewstation SP and 512 models. Each graduate student received at least five sessions of face-to-face and five sessions of e-supervision, and each supervisory session lasted a minimum of 2 hours.

Dudding (2004) used survey research and interviews to compare the graduate students' perceptions of face-to-face and e-supervision. The results of the study showed that the graduate students viewed e-supervision as a successful method of supervision and felt that it met their needs as nontraditional graduate students. The e-supervision technology was easy to use, and the process of e-supervision was less stressful than face-to-face supervision in some instances. Despite the benefits, several weaknesses of e-supervision emerged. First, as was found in Carlin et al. (2012), e-supervision was primarily restricted to pullout interventions (one-on-one speech therapy outside of the classroom) despite being considered flexible enough to capture an entire classroom setting. Second, the graduate students felt that the technology reduced the e-supervisor ability to view intervention and diagnostic materials (e.g., books, test protocols/forms, worksheets). Last, issues with Internet connectivity and the lack of coordinated technology support were a source of frustration for the graduate students.

Despite the limitations that were identified by the graduate students, "the quality of the supervisory relationship [was] the key factor in the perception of the supervisory experience, regardless of the method" (Dudding, 2004, p. 75). If the graduate students and supervisor had a healthy working relationship, the students seemed able to look beyond any challenges associated with the specific form of supervision.

E-Supervision in Related Disciplines

E-supervision offers opportunities for increased engagement across several settings, in various disciplines, and in any number of configurations and combinations (i.e., teleconferencing, synchronous and asynchronous communication, and face-to-face and videoconferencing). However, in education, and specifically teacher education, the use of e-supervision to support clinical or "field-based" experiences for students is sparse and few instances of technology-engaged experiences—university-based, school-based, or clinical—have been documented; especially where field experiences are involved.

For nearly 75 years the typical student teaching experience (the primary and capstone field experience in teacher education) has relied on a triad approach (Alger & Kopcha, 2009), involving the student teacher, school-based mentor teacher, and university supervisor. "Supervisors and on-site cooperating teachers [are] assigned to observe and conference with the student teachers six times over the course of the semester. Feedback to the student teacher is both formative and summative" (Alger & Kopcha, 2009, p. 31). Each observation and conference is conducted face-to-face with the university supervisor visiting the school. Although this model presents some strengths, there are a significant number of challenges and, in turn, critiques of the practice. For instance, there is a lack of role-expectations among the university supervisor and school-based mentor teacher (Bullough & Draper, 2004) and poor communication between all three parties (Slick, 1998). Additionally, many education programs point out the issues of insufficient mentor training for classroom teachers (Rodgers & Keil, 2007) and lack of congruence between university teachings and expectations in the classroom (Walkington, 2005). Although the use of e-supervision has the potential to remediate many of these problems, as noted by Alger and Kopcha (2009), little is known about how to use technology to supervise and support student teachers.

Several studies explore the use of emerging technologies in teacher education including the delivery of professional development to practicing teachers through online learning communities and forums (e.g., Barnett, Harwood, Keating, & Saam, 2002) and using a variety of "teaching teleapprenticeships" (Levin & Waugh, 1998) throughout preservice education coursework. Computer-mediated communications (Simpson, 2006) are also becoming increasingly useful and feasible in learning environments. Technologies such as electronic discussion boards, Web-based forums, and asynchronous videos or lectures aim to extend learning, encourage community-building among participants, and enrich universities' abilities to reach student and practicing teachers, at a greater distance.

During a student teaching semester, Gruenhagen, McCracken, and Judy (1999) documented the use of real-time observations of a distance learning site via videoconferencing. Several benefits emerged, including university students being able to work in distant communities, rural schools receiving the benefit of having student teachers, and enhanced professional collaboration. However, student teachers cited missing the face-to-face interaction and difficulties with moving school children to a distance-technology capable site.

As previously noted, although the potential to engage technologies to support student teachers during their field experiences theoretically seems viable and beneficial, substantial documentation of real-time, video-based e-supervision in teacher education is scant. Teacher education remains poised to move forward with this technology and arguably would be well served to do so in an effort to meet the demands not only of its teacher candidates, but also of rural and traditionally difficult-to-staff schools. Perhaps, as Gruenhagen et al. (1999) noted, ". . . distance education is a presently used medium but will be an essential component of future communication technologies and educational endeavors" (p. 8).

E-Mentoring in Speech-Language Pathology and Related Fields

Mentoring Academic-Research Careers (MARC)

MARC, an online mentoring program for speech-language pathology and audiology PhD students, junior faculty, and postdoctoral scholars, was developed by ASHA as a part of the ASHA Focused Initiative on the PhD Shortage in Higher Education. Findings from surveys and focus groups in 2005 alerted ASHA of the lack of mentoring programs geared toward recruiting and retaining PhD students and junior faculty in the field.

Interested students are paired with audiology and speech-language pathology faculty who hold a PhD degree. The mentor assists the mentee with goals related to grant writing, the grant review process, job interviews, finishing a doctoral dissertation, and research. The pair establishes and maintains a relationship via email and phone for an average of 1 hour per week over an 8-month time period.

MARC offers mentees several advantages such as an online forum called MARC "Community," which enables collaboration between other mentees and faculty, valuable insight into the field beyond the mentee's current education and experience, inspiration, and networking opportunities. However, past participants of MARC noted several challenges including lack of follow-up on both ends due to busy schedules, trouble initiating a relationship due to poor introduction, little structure in terms of establishing goals and expectations, and lack of interest in the mentor's area of expertise.

Student to Empowered Professional (S.T.E.P.) Mentoring Program

This one-on-one online mentoring program was developed by ASHA to support mentoring relationships and the further recruitment of racial/ethnic minority students in audiology and speech-language pathology. Although preference is given to disadvantaged groups, S.T.E.P. is open to all undergraduate and graduate students enrolled in communication sciences and disorders programs. Matched with a mentor based upon similar professional interests, including clientele, work setting, and career goals, students receive advice from a professional audiologist or speech-language pathologist through e-mail, Skype, phone, text, or Facebook for a 3- or 6-month period.

S.T.E.P. offers students several advantages such as networking opportunities outside their home university, goal planning experience, access to the online S.T.E.P. Mentoring Community, which enables students and mentors to discuss specific issues, and resource sharing. However, S.T.E.P. presents several weaknesses including lack of overall structure, reliance upon the student to continue the relationship with further questions, and too little time to build rapport.

Connecting to Success

Compared to all groups of young adults, as a whole, youth with disabilities "have the highest unemployment rates, lowest participation in postsecondary training and education programs, and the highest likelihood of remaining dependent on public assistance programs following high school" (Connecting to Success, 2010). Connecting to Success was developed by the National Center on Secondary Education and Transition at the University of Minnesota (NCSET) to assist youth with disabilities through the transition into adult life. As an online mentoring program, Connecting to Success utilizes a combination of email and face-to-face meetings to link disabled and at-risk youth with mentors from schools, community organizations, and businesses for one school year. The program provides youth with the emotional and motivational support needed to remain in school and deter drug use, tools to overcome societal barriers, inspiration to follow dreams, access to needed resources, and information regarding critical interview and on-the-job skills. (http://ici.umn.edu/ementoring/)

MentorMatch

This online mentoring program connects blind and visually impaired persons with a similarly impaired mentor. Developed by the Canadian National Institute for the Blind (CNIB) and the American Foundation for the Blind (AFB), Mentormatch pairs individuals based upon the mentee's area of interest. The program is open to individuals of all ages and disciplines currently working or in search of employment in Canada or the United States. With a current database of over 1,000 mentors, MentorMatch provides individuals with the opportunity to speak to successful blind or visually impaired persons in the specific field of interest, prepare for upcoming job interviews, motivation, and practical skills.

E-mentoring programs provide a variety of benefits for graduate students and SLPs. These programs extend access to high-quality mentors and valuable resources and extend professional and emotional support to achieve goals. With the use of technology such as Skype and e-mail, traditional mentoring has evolved. Similar to e-supervision, e-mentoring enables people to connect with professionals in their fields of interest without having to deal with the factor of distance.

The Future of E-Supervision and E-Mentoring

Possibilities and Pitfalls of E-Supervision and E-Mentoring

"Unprecedented growth and technological advances associated with both the personal computer industry and the Internet"

(Panos, Panos, Cox, Roby, & Matheson, 2002) permit supervisors and mentors to observe and communicate with students in different locations. Therefore, it should come as no surprise that the use of technology is recommended as one means to overcome barriers associated with the shortages of and access to qualified SLP supervisors and mentors (Hallett, 2002; Robinson, Creaghead, Hooper, Watson, & McNeilly, 2007). A review of the literature provides guidance to individuals who are considering the use of technology during future supervision or mentorship projects.

Multiple forms of technology can be combined to support graduate SLP students and less experienced SLPs. In Carlin et al. (2012), e-supervisors used videoconferencing technology (i.e., Skype) to unobtrusively observe direct interventions and diagnostics at a distance. Next, the instant messaging feature on Skype was used during observations as a means to deliver synchronous supervisory feedback. Then, follow-up instant messages, texts, and e-mails were used to share the results of the observations, communicate recommendations for future client activities, and schedule future observations. Last, graduate SLP students were directed to access a dedicated e-supervision website that contained materials exchange database and summaries of evidence-based practices, resources on impairments of communication, examples of forms, information on assessments and screenings, and developmental milestones. The graduate SLP students positively regarded the combined use of technology because adjustments could be made while services occurred, an electronic paper trail of feedback was produced, communication was seamless, and the graduate SLP students were no longer limited to resources that were only available in their physical vicinity (Carlin et al., 2012). Wood, Miller, and Hargrove (2005) further discussed the combined benefit of using Internet-based resources, PowerPoint presentations, emails, and videoconferencing technologies for use when supervising clinical interns, trainees, and new psychologists in rural settings. It would seem future developers of e-supervision and e-mentoring projects would be wise to combine different forms of technology to provide comprehensive direct and indirect support.

Candidates for e-supervision and e-mentoring should be partially selected based on their comfort level with technology. It seems that the graduate students' and supervisors' amount of previous experience working with technology affects the quality of e-supervision. In a comparison of two groups of school counseling interns, one using only direct supervision and the other using a hybrid of face-to-face and e-supervision, it was noticed that "'high computer users'. . . have more positive attitudes toward technology than those not classified that way" (Conn, Roberts, & Powell, 2009, p. 303). Prior to beginning e-supervision, it might be necessary to offer supervisors and supervisees adequate training and time to familiarize themselves with the technology being used.

Finally, it has been acknowledged that a positive working relationship was necessary in order for the e-supervision (Conn et al., 2009) and e-mentoring projects to be successful. The development of a positive relationship may be slowed if there is a minimal amount of face-to-face contact during the project or there was a prior relationship before the distant project began. Psychiatry residents emphasized that e-supervision was an acceptable supplement to face-to-face meetings if the supervisor and supervisee "established a relationship and working alliance characterized by mutual respect and trust, before the project began (Gammon, Sorlie, Bergvik, & Hoifodt, 1998, p. 414). This sentiment was echoed by student teachers in rural Georgia who missed the personal contact they had with the university supervisors (Gruenhagen et al., 1999). Nonetheless, these student teachers felt that they were able to establish a connection with the e-supervisor because they previously took face-to-face classes with the supervisor and the pair had scheduled periodic on-site visits.

Despite the fact that studies have shown that multiple technologies can be used to professionally develop graduate students and SLPs, weaknesses need to be considered (Carlin et al., 2012; Dudding, 2004). This is especially true because technological limitations have the potential to negatively impact the e-supervisor-supervisee and e-mentor-mentee relationships (Dudding, 2004; Gammon et al., 1998). One such limitation relates to the integrity of the Internet connection and technology. In a study by Carlin et al. (2012), graduate SLP students and supervisors experienced dropped calls and frozen screens on Skype and were forced to make a new connection or refresh the screen. Once the Internet service was upgraded,

Ethernet cables were used (in lieu of wireless), and observations were scheduled outside of peak Internet usage times, the issues of dropped calls and frozen screens were greatly reduced. In a similar study of student teachers, Skype and iChat were used and problems with the public schools' firewalls, lack of Ethernet or wireless access, and low bandwidth created disturbances during e-supervision (Orr, 2010).

When videoconferencing technology was used to e-supervise psychiatry residents in Norway, the researcher found that reduced image quality impaired students' ability to read the e-supervisor's nonverbal cues (Gammon et al., 1998). Because they received a reduction in eye contact and other nonverbal cues from their e-supervisor, the psychology residents felt that the quality of communication was reduced and it was confusing to know when to start and finish talking. Due to the reduction in nonverbal feedback and communication, the psychiatry residents were forced to learn how to read other cues like changes in their supervisor's vocal intonation. Gammon et al.'s findings parallel the perceptions of graduate SLP students who were e-supervised in the public schools. In Dudding (2004), the graduate SLP students noted that there were differences in the communication processes that occurred during e-supervision when compared to face-to-face supervision. More specifically, graduate SLP students noted they received limited nonverbal feedback from the supervisor. Despite the fact that technological limitations impacted observations and communication between the e-supervisor and supervisee, when the pair were given an adequate amount of time to acclimate themselves to the technology and improvements were made, most graduate students responded positively to the technology (Carlin et al., 2012).

Security and confidentiality are often cited as concerns when e-supervision is used (Panos et al., 2002). Panos et al. recommended that safeguards be put into place to protect client information (e.g., use of initials or codes to describe clients during supervisory sessions) and that permissions should be obtained whenever recordings are made. Panos et al. further stressed the importance of selecting technologies that held the appropriate level of security to ensure the confidentiality and security of client information.

Making the Case for a Hybrid Approach to E-Supervision and E-Mentoring

Several disadvantages of e-supervision-only models have been noted in the research. Graduate SLP students noted it was difficult for e-supervisors to explain how to use specific therapy techniques over Skype (Carlin et al., 2012). Consequently, these graduate SLP students preferred to have the e-supervisor on site when a strategy or technique needed to be physically demonstrated. "The level of quality of e-supervision must be considered when comparing its equivalence and adequacy to face-to-face interactions" (Panos et al., 2002, p. 428). In the supervision of students, factors such as quality of equipment, the amount of contact between supervisee and supervisor, and the level of support provided by the supervisor, affect the efficacy of e-supervision. Panos et al. argued that due to the lack of quality control, e-supervision cannot be the sole method of supervision, but rather used to augment direct supervision.

Lending support to Panos et al. (2002), research found e-supervised graduate SLP students preferred that future projects incorporated a hybrid approach to supervision especially during the first month of the clinical experience (Carlin et al., 2012; Dudding, 2004). It appears that the graduate SLP students in both these studies believed they would benefit more and be supported most through a combination of face-to-face and e-supervision. "Technology-mediated relationships" can develop given adequate initial face-to-face time and, if needed, several meetings interspersed throughout the working relationship (Conn et al., 2009, p. 303). E-supervision and e-mentoring provide advantages that are not always available with traditional face-to-face only arrangements. These advantages appear to be compounded when face-to-face meetings and technology are combined to form a hybrid model of supervision and mentorship.

Conclusion

The growing use of e-supervision and e-mentoring in various education and health-related fields, to accommodate students and less experienced professionals, alleviate the burden of long distance travel and shortages of qualified supervisors and mentors. Although current research suggests e-supervision can be just as effective as face-to-face supervision given adequate technology and supportive supervisors (Carlin et al., 2012), more research is needed in order to determine the degree to which e-supervision and e-mentoring benefits all parties involved.

E-supervision and e-mentoring extend clinical and employment opportunities into remote, rural, and hard-to-fill locations where the support of an on-site experienced professional might not be available (Wood et al., 2005). They allow access to desirable clinical internships where supervision and mentorship are either limited or nonexistent (ASHA, 2008). E-supervision and e-mentoring enable higher education institutions and employers the opportunity to minimize travel time and reduce associated transportation costs (e.g., mileage reimbursement) while providing a valuable and necessary service to graduate students, less experienced professionals, and partnering stakeholders (i.e., OMNIE, the state SLP licensure board, the participating school districts, and universities) (Dudding & Justice, 2004).

For the busy supervisor and mentor, the use of technology allows graduate students or less experienced professionals to be supervised and mentored without sacrificing time for travel (Olson et al., 2001) and maximizing the focus on the individual's practice. The cost of the videoconferencing technology and equipment is often offset by the increase in productivity, expanded access to a broader spectrum of employment and externship sites, and reduction in travel time and associated costs (Dudding & Justice, 2004).

References

Alger, C., & Kopcha, T. J. (2009). eSupervision: A technology framework for the 21st century field experience in teacher education. *Issues in Teacher Education, 18*(2), 31–46.

American Speech-Language-Hearing Association (n.d.). *Mentoring academic-research careers (MARC)*. Retrieved from http://www.asha.org/students/gatheringplace/marc/.

American Speech-Language-Hearing Association (n.d.). *Student to em-*

powered professional (S.T.E.P.) mentoring program. Retrieved from http://www.asha.org/students/gatheringplace/step/.

American Speech-Language-Hearing Association. (2005). *The ASHA gathering place: Mentoring manual.* Retrieved from http://www.asha.org/students/gatheringplace/explore/.

American Speech-Language-Hearing Association. (February, 2007). *The subject is change: Creating a vision for the future education of speech-language pathologists.* Presentation made at the 2007 Speech-Language Pathology Education Summit, New Orleans, LA.

American Speech-Language-Hearing Association. (2008). *Clinical supervision in speech-language pathology* [Technical report]. Retrieved from http://www.asha.org/policy.

American Speech-Language-Hearing Association. (2010). *Code of ethics* [Ethics]. Retrieved from http://www.asha.org/policy.

Anderson, E. M., & Shannon, A. L. (1988). Towards a conceptualization of mentoring. *Journal of Teacher Education, 39*(1), 38–42.

Anderson, J. L. (1988). *The supervisory process in speech language pathology and audiology*. Austin, TX: Pro-Ed.

Apel, K. (2007). On mentoring. *Language, Speech, Hearing Services in Schools, 38*, 171.

Barnett, M., Harwood, W., Keating, T., & Saam, J. (2002). Using emerging technologies to bridge the gap between university theory and classroom practice: Challenges and successes. *School Science and Mathematics*, *102*(6), 1–15.

Boswell, S. (2007, March 06). Ohio grant addresses personnel shortage: Innovative strategies meet short- and long-term goals. *ASHA Leader, 12*(3), 1, 14–15.

Bullough, R. V., & Draper, R. J. (2004). Making sense of the failed triad. *Journal of Teacher Education, 55*(5), 407–420.

Carlin, C. H., Milam, J. L., Carlin, E. L., & Owen, A. (2012). Promising practices in e-supervision: Exploring graduate speech-language pathology interns' perceptions. *International Journal of Telerehabilitation*, *4*(2), 25–37.

Conn, S. R., Roberts, R. L., & Powell, B. M. (2009). Attitudes and satisfaction with a hybrid model of counseling supervision. *Educational Technology and Society, 12*(2), 298–306.

Connecting to Success. (2010). *Connecting to success.* Retrieved from: http://ici.umn.edu/ementoring/.

Dudding, C. C. (2004). *Perceptions of the use of videoconferencing for supervision: Differences among graduate clinicians*. Unpublished doctoral disscrtation, University of Virginia, Charlottesville.

Dudding, C. C., & Carlin, C. H. (November, 2012). *Telesupervision: Who's watching who?* Presentation made at the 2012 American Speech-Language-Hearing Association National Conference, Atlanta, GA.

Dudding, C. C., & Justice, L. M. (2004). An e-supervision model: Videoconferencing as a clinical training tool. *Communication Disorders Quarterly, 25*(3), 145–151.

Gammon, D., Sorlie, T., Bergvik, S., & Hoifodt, T. S. (1998). Psychotherapy supervision conducted via videoconferencing: A qualitative study of users' experiences. *Nordic Journal of Psychiatry, 52*, 411–421.

Gruenhagen, K., McCracken, T., & Judy, T. (1999). Using distance education technologies for the supervision of student teachers in remote rural schools. *Rural Special Education Quarterly, 18*(3/4), 1–10.

Hallett, T. L. (2002). The impact of technology on teaching, clinical practice, and research. *ASHA Leader, 7*(11), 4.

Jackson, C. A., & Woolsey, J. D. (2009). A different set of classrooms: Preparing a new generation of clinicians. *Forum on Public Policy Online, 1*, 1–10.

Lechuga, V. M. (2011). Faculty-graduate student mentoring relationships: Mentors' perceived roles and responsibilities. *Higher education: The International Journal of Higher Education and Educational Planning, 62*(6), 757–771.

Levin, J., & Waugh, M. (1998). Teaching teleapprenticeships: Electronic network-based educational frameworks for improving teacher education. *Interactive Learning Environments, 6*(1–2), 39–58.

McCrea, E. S., & Brasseur, J. A. (2003). *The supervisory process in speech-language pathology and audiology*. Boston, MA: Allyn & Bacon.

McNeilly, L. (2006). Stakeholders seek solutions to personnel shortages. *ASHA Leader, 11*(16), 12–30.

Murray, M., & Owen, M. (1991). *Beyond the myths and magic of mentoring*. San Francisco, CA: Jossey-Bass.

Olson, M. M., Russell, C. S., & White, M. B. (2001). Technological implications for clinical supervision and practice. *Clinical Supervisor, 20*(2), 201–215.

Orr, P. P. (2010). Distance supervision: Research, findings, and considerations for art therapy. *Arts in Psychotherapy, 37*, 106–111.

Panos, P. T., Panos, A., Cox, S. E., Roby, J. L., & Matheson, K. W. (2002). Ethical issues concerning the use of videoconferencing to supervise international social work field practicum students. *Journal of Social Work Education, 38*(3), 421–437.

Robinson, T., Creaghead, C., Hooper, C., Watson, J., & McNeilly, L. (2007). *Speech-language pathology education summit proceedings*. Rockville, MD: American Speech-Language-Hearing Association.

Rodgers, A., & Keil, V. L. (2007). Restructuring a traditional teacher education supervision model: Fostering enhanced professional development and mentoring within a professional development school context. *Teaching and Teacher Education*, *23*, 65-80.

Simpson, M. (2006). Field experience in distance delivered initial teacher education programmes. *Journal of Technology and Teacher Education, 14*(2), 241-254.

Slick, S. K. (1998). The university supervision: A disenfranchised outsider. *Teaching and Teacher Education, 14*(8), 821-834.

Tellis, G. M., Cimino, L., & Alberti, J. (2010). Current issues: Advanced digital technology for supervising graduate clinicians, *Perspectives on Administration and Supervision, 20*(1), 9-13.

The Canadian National Institute for the Blind & American Foundation for the Blind. (2004). *Mentor match.* Retrieved from: http://www.careerconnect.org/_cnib/home.asp.

Walkington, J. (2005). Becoming a teacher: Encouraging development of teacher identity through reflective practice. *Asia-Pacific Journal of Teacher Education*, *33*(1), 53-64.

Wood, J. A., Miller, T. W., & Hargrove, D. S. (2005). Clinical supervision in rural settings: A telehealth model. *Professional Psychology: Research and Practice, 36*(2), 173-179.

Wright-Harp, W., & Cole, P. A. (2008). A mentoring model for enhancing success in graduate education. *Contemporary Issues in Communication Sciences and Disorders, 35*, 4-16.

10

The Business of Telepractice

Marnee Brick

Introduction

Traditionally, speech-language pathologists have often sought new avenues of service delivery that improved outcomes for their patients. The American Speech-Language-Hearing Association (ASHA) has served as a leading resource for telepractice and an advocate for consistency of service delivery systems across the United States (Brown, 2011). Along with the development of preferred practices, the evolution of distance technology has provided speech-language pathologists (SLPs) with additional resources that provide new service delivery options (Theodoros, 2012). Research has supported the efficacy of services delivered through telepractice. A recent study indicated that students who received services through a telepractice platform demonstrated a greater mastering of their goals (Alvares et al., 2011). The field of speech-language pathology aligns itself well with telepractice and for that reason, many professionals in the field have chosen to embark on the journey of planning and developing their own private practices with a telepractice service delivery model. Quality performance indicators for a successful telepractice company include a sustainable business plan that encompasses professional practice standards. This chapter outlines the process by which SLPs can begin to plan and implement effective telepractice services.

Preparing to Start a Private Practice

Speech-language pathologists have the capacity to excel in private practice. The qualities that drive graduate students to achieve a master's degree define the characteristics that are necessary to establish a successful service-based business. Starting a private practice can be challenging; however, maintaining four key characteristics can drive successful outcomes: proactiveness, resourcefulness, resilience, and maintaining a "learner" perspective.

Proactiveness

Being proactive gives the statement, "I own this goal. I am the one who will make it happen. I will plan, prepare, and execute." Graduate students endure tremendous responsibilities under specific time boundaries. Taking ownership and following through with commitments are necessary for a successful outcome. When exploring private practice, the SLP has the responsibility to manage a multitude of factors related to professional, legal, financial, and service standards. A private practice is not sustainable without a consistent proactive approach.

Resourcefulness

Resourcefulness is the quality that states, "I am focused on solutions, and I will relentlessly seek strategies to improve the outcomes." Graduate students are immersed into an environment where the ability to be resourceful is a strong predictor of their success. Quality performance in clinical and academic scenarios, in addition to securing resources for maintaining a healthy lifestyle, requires students to work through new challenges and find unique solutions. Similarly, a successful private practice requires a leader who has the capacity to find solutions and maintain standards, while other challenges persist.

Resilience

Resilience is reflected by the statement, "I believe so strongly in my purpose that I will try longer, push harder, and reach further than anyone else would do in this scenario. I am the difference between success and failure." Students in graduate school understand what it means to feel discouraged and exhausted. To achieve their goal of earning a master's degree, students persist through challenges and recommit to their vision of becoming a speech-language pathologist. SLPs who start private practices may face barriers, disappointments, and setbacks. Resilience grows from recognizing opportunities in challenges and by gaining experience in overcoming obstacles.

A Learner

A learner asks, "What don't I know?" Before making a commitment to pursue the profession of speech-language pathology, students seek information, such as program requirements, qualifications, and perhaps opportunities that will exist upon graduation. Students make a conscious, informed decision to commit to the program. The same thoughtful diligence is necessary for studying the requirements, qualifications, challenges, and opportunities for private practice. Grodzi (2009) provides practitioners with an insightful self-assessment tool that articulates performance indicators for successful practice management. When starting a private practice, speech-language pathologists could benefit by incorporating the tool as a set of personal development goals to pursue.

Business Fundamentals

It is not typical for graduate programs in communication disorders to include courses on leadership and business management. Speech-language pathologists devote their careers to improving people's lives through service. Many speech-language pathologists feel disconnected from the business goals of a successful company, such as earning a profit (Grodzki, 2000). Professionals who are committed to establishing a successful practice need to seek resources for building a strong business foundation and reconcile that generating revenue is a solid strategy for continuing to serve people who need support (Grodzki, 2009).

The first step in exploring the business aspects of a private practice is to brainstorm a list of questions that fall under two categories: personal health and business health.

Personal Health

Personal health considers how starting a private practice will impact the SLP's wellness, priorities, and financial sustainability.

Personal Financial Considerations

What is my financial situation? How much income will allow me to stick with my private practice, rather than working elsewhere? How does this translate into billable hours? Am I willing to invest a tremendous amount of nonbillable hours? Do I have a transition plan where I can ease into private practice, yet not depend on the income right away? How much will I have to pay other people to assist me with my business? How much should I invest in tools and materials right away? How much risk am I willing to take with the unknown? What is my ultimate financial goal?

Personal Wellness Considerations

What are my priorities in life? Am I willing to adjust my priorities while I invest significant time and resources into starting my business? Can I still live in a value-based way or is this experience going to be toxic for me? If I can establish my practice, will it bring value to my life? What do I want from this? Will I be able to set my own timeline for making this happen? Do I have a support system so I can manage all of my responsibilities? Can I persist for 1,000 days before considering abandoning my vision? What is my ultimate purpose in doing this . . . why am I doing this? What will define success for me?

Business Health

Business health refers to the private practice being legally sound and sustained through quality systems and supports. Rather than feeling overwhelmed by the unknown, it is proactive to use uncertainty to generate useful questions. Examples of common start-up questions are below.

What type of business is best for me?

Sole ownership—The SLP is fully responsible for all debts, obligations, and profits related to the business. As a sole owner of the business, a creditor can make a claim against the SLP's personal or business assets to pay off any debt.

Partnership—Two or more SLPs combine financial resources and share profits based on the terms of an agreement.

Corporations—The SLP incorporates the business and is not personally liable for debts or obligations of the business.

Cooperatives—The business is owned by an association of members who have pooled their resources to create a service solution.

How do I legally set up a private practice in this community? Where do I name and register my business? Where do I obtain a business licence?

What do I need to know about taxes, payroll, billing, and expenses?

Are there financial supports for starting my private practice? How much income do I need to sustain my business?

How will I know if my services are needed? How will I find my clients? How will my clients find me? What services will bring the most value to the region? Who can I approach about referrals?

How much liability insurance do I need?

How do I grow my business? What is my plan?

The next step is to visit a community agency that specializes in small business development to consult with a business advisor. Through collaboration, the SLP will receive recommendations and be equipped to develop an action plan.

Common Action Plan Steps

Consult with a certified public accountant and a lawyer.

- Explore agencies that provide loans, investors, grants, tax credits, networking, and other financial supports for establishing a small business. When approaching potential lenders, SLPs should be prepared to explain how much money is required, how the funds will be used, and when the money will be repaid (Cope Grand & Stout, 2005).
- Study telepractice models, equipment, standards, expenses, and options for support such as having access to a technical advisor.
- Determine regulations for working with out-of-state clients or employees, which is a feasible option in a telepractice model.
- Learn about small business awards for new ventures. The application process often serves as a checklist for service excellence in business.

- Analyze the market and competitors to ascertain a clear target population that would find value in the services offered. Dunbar and McDonald (2004) shared three concepts for starting a market analysis: (a) Defining the market of interest, (b) Understanding what the customers in that market are seeking and what would bring them value, and (c) Identifying the differentiating components from the competitors that would draw customers toward the business.
- Explore tools and strategies that reach, inform, and invite potential clients from the target market.
- Work through the development of a business plan. The business plan facilitates a thorough exploration of the feasibility and sustainability of the business idea. It is often required to secure financial support and it serves as a helpful planning document (MacDonald, 2006). Using a business plan template (MacDonald, 2006, p. 50) guides the SLP in exploring and documenting key information about the company. Ultimately, the business plan should read as a story that provides clarity and elicits enthusiasm from the reader (Finch, 2010).

Company Framework

The company framework defines the culture, systems, and standards.

Culture

There are four initial steps to developing a cultural framework: a vision, mission, belief statement, and company values.

Vision

A vision answers the question, "What do I want to accomplish?" It describes what the triumph would be for the company or its cause.

An example of a vision is, "Our vision is to be the country's leading online speech therapy service provider."

Mission

A mission statement answers the question, "Why am I doing this?" It should resonate with potential clients and encourage solidarity for a common goal. An example of a mission statement for a company that focuses on children with cochlear implants might be, "Our mission is to help kids tell their own stories."

Although an early therapy goal may be for children to attach meaning to the sounds they hear, they are the path to becoming capable communicators who will confidently use their voice to tell their stories and impact their world. Families will celebrate this mission and become contributing partners to achieving the heart-warming and rewarding quest for their children.

As the company grows, additional staff members must learn the story behind the mission and commit to its achievement. Mission-driven services require that the actions of all team members contribute to the ultimate goal, which, in this example, is to help kids tell their own stories.

Belief

A belief statement drives team members toward achieving the mission and invites potential customers to say, "I believe that, too." The speech-language pathologists who serve children though TinyEYE's (the author's company) online platform, as seen in Figure 10–1, share the belief statement that reads, "We believe that all children should have equal access to quality therapy services, regardless of where they live."

Values

The company values define target behavior. Values contribute to making decisions and developing a brand, which will appeal to potential customers and ideal team members. The values should be evident in all employees and complete the sentences, "We are ___.

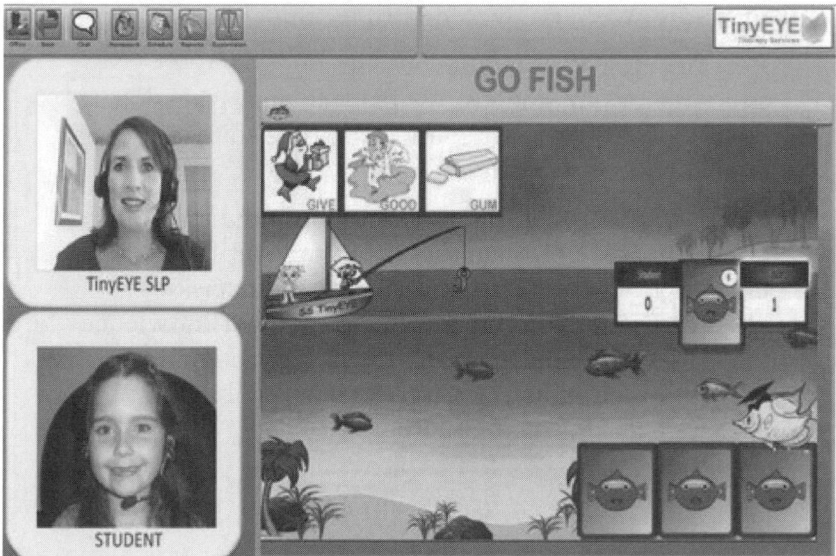

Figure 10–1. A screenshot of a typical TinyEye session.

We value ____." To identify a values trend, SLPs can brainstorm words or statements that describe their ideal qualities and commitments. The next step is to group similar ideas and then select one value from each group. Finally, the SLP should imagine using each value as a qualification for hiring a new SLP to the team. Which values would serve as a deal breaker if the teammate did not exude the quality or commitment? Although it can be difficult to remove value options from the brainstorm list, the goal is provide simple clarity and to drive the flow of a healthy business. This is accomplished by choosing a small set of core values and then explaining why each value is true for the company. Examples of core values that drive a service company are described in the following.

Our values lead our service. We are:

Family-focused: Our services are designed to be accessible and effective for families so that they can surround their children with a communication-enriched environment.

Friendly: We serve with gratitude, kindness, and joy.

Resourceful: We seek the best strategies and supports for our families. We balance our professional competencies with our spirit of learning so that our families experience triumphant results.

Honest: We provide families with clear and thorough communication throughout our partnership. We empower our families to make informed decisions about programming. We engage in a shared-knowledge platform, which means that families have ongoing access to their billing, session documentation, and success plans for their children."

Systems

Systems specifically delineate policies, procedures, and tools within any business. The purpose of systems is to produce clarity, accountability, and results. The private practitioner needs to consider both the service provider and the customer when creating the systems that govern business practices. To promote clarity, it is effective to provide a written explanation of systems that involve the customer and then verbally review the information together. This serves as an agreement and assists the SLP with addressing difficulties with the consumer. For example, if the patient or client has not forwarded payment when expected, it is helpful to have an agreement to refer to during the discussion. In start-up companies, these systems evolve with experience and growth.

Policies

Policies answer the question, "What is the expectation?" Companies commonly create policies for any topic that will require a decision. Policies often grow from recognizing potential problems. For example, a private practitioner may have a policy that customers will be billed for cancellations unless they provide a 24-hour prior notice.

Procedures

Procedures answer the question, "What steps do I take to make this happen?" Procedures are influenced by the policies and contribute to the standards. For example, the policy is that the company will bill the customer for missed sessions. However, because the SLP is committed to a family-focused approach, the procedure requires the service provider to e-mail a reminder to the families 24 hours before the sessions. This contributes to increased attendance, increased outcomes, and reduced billing for missed sessions. Companies require procedures for all aspects of operations from service delivery to business management.

Tools

Tools answer the question, "What can I use to streamline my systems so that I can work accurately and productively?" A first step is to imagine the ideal system for tracking and supporting the service for one patient or client from intake to discharge. Include the company accountabilities, such as file storage and accounts receivable. The next step is to make the systems scalable so that you could manage 10, 20, or 30 more clients with the same quality and efficiency. Today, there are ample online tools available for service tracking and client management.

Standards and Performance Indicators

Standards contribute to quality assurance and answer the questions, "What will make my services exceptional? What can customers expect when they partner with any SLP in my company? How will I make a difference for my clients every time we meet?" It is useful practice for the SLP to identify standards categories and then create service goals. Each goal should have a target feeling attached. The feelings define the customer's overall experience and impression, which can contribute to customer retention and referrals.

Standards Categories

Physical. Goals relate to the quality of the visual, auditory, and professional components of the presentation. Information is presented clearly by the SLP, while nurturing a partnership with the family. The family feels supported, trusted and relaxed because of this quality.

Family Focus. Goals relate to the ease of accessing your service and the relevance of your coaching. The SLP is transforming the approach based on family interests, goals, and ability. The family feels capable and excited.

Client Outcomes. Goals relate to introducing achievable objectives, providing effective strategies, tracking performance, and facilitating progress. The SLP is purposefully helping the client move forward by using engaging and relevant approaches. The family feels amazed at its own impact and confident about the SLP's services.

Service Tracking. Goals contribute to customer and company achievement through timely communication, documentation, and billing. The SLP is proactive and accountable with the responsibilities. The family feels grateful, peaceful, and prepared. They know they are in the company of a caring, capable professional who really is going to help their children grow to tell their own stories.

Customer Loyalty. Goals contribute to creating customer loyalty. The SLP actively provides differentiated, value-driven services that engage and retain the customer's loyalty. The customer feels enthusiastic about the services and comfortable with providing testimonials or referrals.

To confirm that the standards are effective and valued, SLPs should regularly ask the customers about their perception of services and suggestions for improvement. Finally, the private practitioner could ask the customer to complete a survey or provide a testimonial about his or her experience. Both positive and negative feedback can be used to improve and grow the company.

Tjan (2011) describes a simple customer feedback process called the Net Promoter Score System. It asks customers one question, "How likely is it that you would recommend this company to a friend or colleague?" Customers respond on a 0 to 10 point rating scale and are categorized into three groups: (a) Promoters (score 9–10) are loyal enthusiasts who will keep buying and refer others, fueling growth; (b) Passives (score 7–8) are satisfied but unenthusiastic customers who are vulnerable to competitive offerings; and (c) Detractors (score 0–6) are unhappy customers who can damage your brand and impede growth through negative word-of-mouth. To calculate the company's score, note the percentage of customers who are Promoters and subtract the percentage who are Detractors.

Key Performance Indicators

Key performance indicators are objective measurements that reflect the critical success factors of an organization and gauge the health of the company. Key performance indicators might include target productivity ratio, billable hours, number of visits, and service outcomes.

Developing and Growing a Customer Base

To become a sustainable company, SLPs need to constantly replenish their customer base and forecast how they will attract new clients. Private practitioners should be prepared to make decisions on four key marketing components (Mullins, Walker, Boyd, & Larreche, 2005): (a) Product—What is the service? Who will it serve? How will the service bring value? (b) Pricing—What is the rate for the services? Do the rates differ based on time or service components? When pricing a product, SLPs need to consider reimbursement from insurance companies and third-party payers (DeRuiter, 2010). DeRuiter (2010) directs private practitioners to ASHA's online resources on reimbursement. (c) Placement—Where will the services take place? (d) Promotion—Who is the target audience of the promotional tools? Where will the target audience be looking for information? How and where should the promotion be placed so it will be received?

Moving forward, the SLP needs to continuously analyze opportunities, build relationships, remain accessible, and clarify the value of the services. The goal is to attract ideal customers toward the business (Grodzki, 2000).

Three strategies for developing a client base are growing through referrals, creating a presence, and building capacity.

Growing Through Referrals

Provide Valuable Resources

A referral source is a person or agency that directs business to a company. Private practitioners need to be visible, accessible, and relevant to the referral source. Extending useful resources and services to potential referral points promotes a system that naturally replenishes the client base. For example, regularly providing milestone charts to doctors and psychologists, making newsletters for preschools, leading a stroke support group, and offering in-services to schools demonstrates the SLP's value and accessibility to the potential clients. Building relationships that are founded in trust is a valuable investment into the sustainability of the practice.

Cycles and Accessibility

Planning for the upcoming year in 3-month intervals encourages the SLP to seek and create opportunities based on predictable cycles. Reaching out to other SLPs about when they need support with their programs can facilitate referrals and create opportunities to market the company. For a company that serves children who are in need of speech and language services, the following are examples of cycles that can help start a referral base that is built on collaboration:

> **Vacation and Conference Peak Times:** Serve as a substitute SLP when a same location SLP is away.

Spring Screenings: Partner with a same location SLP or provide total services for preschool and kindergarten screenings. Offer parent information seminars about school readiness.

Fall Waitlists: Once services start for the school year, clients may find themselves on a waitlist and eagerly await their turn for support.

Blocks: When students have short bursts of therapy blocks, there is an opportunity to continue the care between their blocks.

Compensatory Services in the Summer: When students did not access all of their IEP minutes during the school year, there is an opportunity to provide supplemental programming.

Accessible Services All Year: Clients face scenarios where they have been assessed in an urban center; however, they cannot feasibly return on a regular basis for therapy. There is an opportunity to provide consistent services between intermittent visits to the urban center. Simultaneously, collaborating with other professionals on the client support team provides a new network for referral points.

Creating a Presence

A professional, helpful, and relatable presence influences customers and referral sources to make a favorable impression of the company, its services, and its owner. There are many cost-effective strategies to creating a presence that will grow a customer base:

Obtain a professional email address and e-mail signature.

Establish a simple and appealing setup for the logo, Web appearance, and forms.

Drive a Web presence that delivers compelling content (Meerman-Scott, 2007).

With today's technology, consumers frequently complete an Internet search to learn more about a topic. Grodzki (2013) reported that 78% of consumers look online first when seeking a professional service. Private practitioners have an opportunity to present themselves as the go-to resource for information and support. To make the Web presence effective, SLPs should recall the purpose of their company and then drive the content and image to serve that goal. A carefully designed presence will ultimately place a lot of marketing power into the hands of the online community. Meanwhile, existing customers will appreciate the user-friendly access to their service provider's resources. Helpful platforms are a website, Facebook page, LinkedIn, and a blog that are regularly updated with valuable and interesting information. Because every page should serve as an invitation for a potential customer to become a paying customer, content and contact information needs to be organized, searchable, and clearly presented.

Extend the reach of the Web presence.

SLPs can increase the number of people who see information about the company. The goal is to turn viewers into customers (Grodzki, 2009).

- Buy a domain name from a Web-hosting company. A domain name is a Web address, such as http://www.tinyeye.com. Grodzki (2009) reported that .com endings are more effective than .net or .biz.
- Inquire if other professionals, such as occupational therapists, would like to participate in cooperative marketing. For example, two professionals share each other's links and help to promote services.
- Participate in online discussions by commenting on blogs and sharing relevant Facebook posts.
- Tag blogs with words that people are likely going to use when searching for a service or information.

- Update blog postings regularly to keep them relevant to search engines.
- Plant a word-of-mouth seed by sending a "grand-opening" message to a network of colleagues, peers, and family. Repeatedly post interesting information that will invite others to gravitate toward the company.
- Seek associations that promote and support private practitioners. Corporate Speech Pathology Network (CORSPAN), American Academy of Private Practice in Speech Pathology and Audiology (AAPPSPA), ASHA, and regional associations are helpful connections.

Building Capacity

It is in the best interest of the private practitioner to pursue strategies for enriching skills, systems, and services. Below are seven considerations to strengthen the functions of a company to promote profit and growth.

The private practitioner should continue to develop skill sets for driving the company's success. Seek continuing education materials and courses with a focus on business management, marketing, sales, and human resources topics. Participate in ASHA's Business Institute, which provides coaching for private practitioners.

Study the revenue and reimbursement timeline provided by different payment sources, such as private pay, insurance, or Medicaid. The SLP should also track revenue generated by different types of clients. Information from these sources helps private practitioners build and balance caseloads to proactively generate more revenue (Foehl, 2009).

Forecast and develop a scalable organizational structure that would contribute to quality growth. Consider future functions and the related personnel, such as team leaders and administrative support.

Attract and retain exceptional colleagues who serve a specific purpose in the company.

Hiring an SLP who can meet the needs of the target population or bringing in an assistant who can execute all the nonclinical tasks can help the practice owner invest time in activities that will bring the most value to the company. To avoid extraneous employment expenses, consider starting new hires as subcontractors on a casual basis. Having the right person serve in the right role is considered the most essential aspect of successful companies (Erling, 2011). Establish hiring and training protocols that support the company culture and facilitate competency within the telepractice model.

Balance creative thinking about growth with analytical thinking about profit.

Identify methods for reducing expenses, without sacrificing quality. Grodzki (2009) suggests reviewing all expenses and then negotiating to reduce costs. Increase productivity by analyzing how much time and effort is invested into nonbillable tasks. Consider changes in tools or systems that will increase output, while decreasing input. Strive to delegate, automate, streamline, and clarify tasks so that everyone involved in the company is contributing to a highly productive system that will ultimately improve service and profits. From this healthy profit point, the private practitioner will have room to dream about incorporating the next set of inspired ideas that will drive the achievement of the company's vision.

Study the leadership and company culture. Recognize the unbreakable core principles that drive decisions, actions, and determination. On the hardest days, these principles become the guiding medium for moving through change, setbacks, and obstacles.

Create a buzz about the service platform and highlight the exceptional outcomes that result from giving clients access to quality therapy services. Help to normalize the telepractice medium so consumers can recognize the value of the service, rather than fearing the unknown.

With just one client, SLPs transition from starting a private practice to operating a private practice. Welcoming the first client to the practice is a monumental event that will serve a large purpose in building a customer base and making improvements. When approaching referral sources about serving through a telepractice platform, a common question for the SLP is, "How does that work?" The SLP needs to provide clarity about the tools, process, and experience. This information helps others recognize the ease of the platform and the quality of the service. Once the SLP has provided service excellence to one client and has refined the related systems, there is a valuable story to share with potential referral sources. While highlighting positive points, it is valuable to share examples of working through challenges as well.

Professional Considerations

"Private practice and self-regulation go together, and one fundamental responsibility for clinicians is to adhere to the ASHA Code of Ethics" (Denton, 2009). The profession of speech-language pathology upholds precise standards in terms of qualifications, best practice, and ethics. In addition to building a strong business base, the SLP must infuse his or her practice with professional principles. Telepractice enables SLPs to serve clients in or outside of the immediate region. It is the responsibility of the SLP to learn about the professional requirements of the region where the client is living. From the beginning, SLPs should commit to a decision-making framework that considers the welfare of the client as paramount while upholding the standards of the profession (Cohn, 2012).

Regional and National Information

Before working in a state, SLPs must investigate regional and national requirements for providing ethical, professional services. ASHA's website provides speech-language pathologists with detailed information about telepractice, private practice, and related responsibilities. Specifically, ASHA's policies (http://www.asha.org/policy) and ASHA's State by State pages (http://www.asha.org/advocacy/state/) offer extensive information. Ten important topics for review include:

1. Licensing and credentials
2. Code of ethics
3. Position on telepractice
4. Informed consent process
   When services are delivered through a telepractice platform, the informed consent process must include additional information, such as a description of the equipment and how services may differ from same location services (ASHA Telepractice Working Group, 2005).
5. The Health Insurance Portability and Accountability Act and Privacy Protection
   Professionals who submit claims or share health care information in an electronic format must follow HIPAA requirements and have a National Provider Identifier (Lusis, 2008). To comply with privacy regulations, practitioners should incorporate encryption, which is a technique for transforming information into an unreadable format to protect it from wrongful access. The American Medical Association (2010) compiled valuable information for encryption in its publication entitled HIPAA Security Rule: Frequently Asked Questions Regarding Encryptions of Personal Health Information.
6. Preferred practice guidelines
7. Continuing education and other requirements to maintain the credentials
8. Malpractice insurance

9. Reimbursement and billing guidelines
10. Client rights.

Quality of Service Delivery Platform

Service provided through telepractice has the same standards as same location or "in person" service. Quality, security, and treatment outcomes should not decrease for clients who access services through a telepractice platform. Face-to-face, online communication is growing in familiarity due to tools such as Skype and Facetime. SLPs have quality options for choosing a telepractice service delivery platform.

Top of the line or "business class" teleconferencing equipment, such as the Polycom model, provide secure videoconferencing and information-sharing capabilities. There are various options depending on the targeted use. Costs associated with these systems can be discouraging to SLPs who are starting a private practice. It is helpful to do a cost-benefit analysis to determine the value of the investment over time.

Online Web conferencing systems, such as GoToMeeting, offer cost-effective, easily accessible options for videoconferencing, screen sharing, and material presentation. There are several online options that SLPs can research. Tools such as a document camera, screen sharing, and document scanners enable clinicians to include meaningful resources into the sessions.

Fully integrated online systems, such as TinyEYE, provide SLPs with a comprehensive service platform. All tools, activities, documentation, and videoconferencing are housed within the secure system that connects the SLP with the client for therapy services.

Key questions for determining the potential quality of services include:

1. How can I predict and impact the quality of my connection?
2. What are the security features? Will the system support my HIPPAA compliance? Who will help me with technical quality?

3. What tools would I need to purchase?
4. What standards will I commit to for my clients and how will I uphold these standards through my service?
5. What training will I need to provide effective and engaging sessions through my model?
6. How will I build a relationship with my customer and provide a clear presence, even though I am at a different location?

Private practitioners can access ASHA's (2005) document on quality indicators for professional service programs to establish a platform that meets professional standards. The document serves as a self-assessment tool and contributes to a professionally sound company.

Conclusion

This chapter outlined strategies for starting a private practice that incorporates a telepractice platform into its core business. SLPs who are skilled at melding preferred practices in both business management and speech-language pathology will bring the greatest value to the clients they serve. Similarly, helping SLPs to develop quality telepractice services can promote retention in the profession, and telepractice allows SLPs to extend their geographic service delivery to clients who otherwise would have been underserved or not served at all. Building a business, incorporating telepractice delivery models, and ensuring clients receive needed services can be challenging; however, by following the advice outlined in the chapter, SLPs will at least have a roadmap to establishing and growing a successful private practice that is both professionally rewarding and inspiring.

References

Alvares, R., Gable, R., Grogan-Johnson, S., Rowan, L., Taylor, J., & Schenker, J. (2011). A pilot exploration of speech sound disorder intervention delivered by telehealth to school-age children. *International Journal of Telerehabilitation, 3*, 31–42.

American Medical Association. (2010). *HIPAA Security Rule: Frequently Asked Questions Regarding Encryption of Personal Health Information.* Retrieved from http://www.ama-assn.org/resources/doc/psa/hipaa-phi-encryption.pdf.

American Speech-Language-Hearing Association. (2005). *Knowledge and skills needed by speech-language pathologists providing clinical services via telepractice.* Retrieved from http://www.asha.org/policy.

American Speech-Language-Hearing Association. (2005). *Quality indicators for professional service programs in audiology and speech-language pathology.* Retrieved from http://www.asha.org/policy.

Brown, J. (2011). ASHA and the evolution of telepractice. *Perspectives on Telepractice, 1*(1), 4–9.

Cohn, E. (2012). Tele-ethics in telepractice for communication disorders. *Perspectives on Telepractice, 2, 3–15*(1), 4–9.

Cope Grand, L., & Stout, C. (2005). *Getting started in private practice: The complete guide to building your mental health practice.* Hoboken, NJ: John Wiley & Sons.

Denton, D. R. (2009, August 11). Watch out for these ethical traps in private practice. *ASHA Leader.* Retrieved from http://www.asha.org/Publications/leader/2009/090811/090811j/.

DeRuiter, M. (2010). Business: Developing a marketing plan: Initial considerations. *Perspectives on Administration and Supervision, 20*, 248–253.

Dunbar, I., & McDonald, M. (2004). *Market segmentation: How to do it, how to profit from it.* Burlington, MA: Elsevier Butterworth-Heinemann.

Erling, D. (2011). *Match: A systematic, sane process for hiring the right person every time.* Hoboken, NJ: John Wiley & Sons Inc.

Finch, B. (2010). *How to write a business plan.* India: Replika Press PVT Ldt.

Foehl, A. Payer and patient mix: Keys to a healthy private practice. *ASHA Leader.* Retrieved August 11, 2009, from http://www.asha.org/Publications/leader/2009/090811/090811i/.

Grodzki, L. (2000). *Building your ideal private practice: A guide for therapists and other healing professionals.* New York, NY: W.W. Norton & Company, Inc.

Grodzki, L. (2009). *Crisis proof your practice: How to survive and thrive in an uncertain economy.* New York, NY: W.W. Norton & Company, Inc.

Lusis, I. Bottom line: Private practice and HIPAA. *ASHA Leader.* Retrieved September 2, 2008, from http://www.asha.org/Publications/leader/2008/080902/bl080902/.

MacDonald, L. (2006). *Start and market a successful private practice.* San Francisco, CA: Chronical Books LLC.

Meerman-Scott, D. (2007). *The new rules of marketing and PR: How to use news releases, blogs, podcasting, viral marketing, and online media to reach buyers directly*. Hoboken, NJ: John Wiley & Sons, Inc.

Theodoros, D. (2012). A new era in speech-language pathology practice: Innovation and diversification. *International Journal of Language Pathology, 3,* 189–199.

Tjan, A. (2011). Strategy on one page. *Harvard Business Review Blog Network.* Retrieved April, 15, 2013, from http://blogs.hbr.org/tjan/2011/06/strategy-on-one-page.html.

11

International Applications of Telepractice in Speech-Language Pathology

Gabriella Constantinescu and Dimity Dornan

Introduction

The current era is one of radical transition in health care in all countries regardless of wealth, as they face comparable challenges to health care delivery such as access to, equity, quality, and cost-effectiveness of services (World Health Organization, 2010). These challenges are exerting intense pressure for change across all disciplines, including speech-language pathology. Telepractice is a viable service delivery option for navigating this transition in heath care, and speech-language pathologists (SLPs) worldwide will need to become adaptive lifelong learners to keep pace with the continual advances in information and communication technologies and their application in service delivery. It has been predicted that as early as 2016, almost 45% of the world will have access to the Internet (Dean et al., 2012), making it readily accessible to SLPs and our clients worldwide. If the last two centuries were the centuries for power, this century must be devoted to empowerment, particularly of our clients in all countries, by ensuring access to optimal services that meet their individual needs. This can only be achieved by sharing what we know. To aid knowledge sharing, this chapter will provide some of the global perspectives on the benefits and barriers to telepractice uptake, and focus on research studies conducted internationally that have demonstrated the potential of telepractice, along with clinical considerations for SLPs.

Benefits of Telepractice to Clients

In looking broadly at the benefits to clients, telepractice has the potential to assist with the timely access to specialized services that may otherwise be inaccessible or reduced due to the distance from the service, difficulties with transport, travel, cost, and travel time. For clients, such issues can pose real barriers to accessing traditional speech-language pathology services. For instance, access to regular sessions in the early years is an integral part of many early intervention programs for young children. Families living outside of metropolitan areas may find it difficult to meet the requirements of weekly or fortnightly face-to-face sessions for a period of at least 3 years due to the excessive cost of travel, the large distances, and the overall disruption to family life. In the adult population, clients with progressive neurodegenerative disorders such as Parkinson's disease may experience debilitating physical symptoms that make it difficult for them to commit to regular sessions, thus compromising outcomes. These issues can be further magnified for older individuals who may no longer drive and rely on their spouses, who may also be elderly, for assistance with transportation. Access issues due to geographic constraints are also significant in countries such as Australia and Canada where potential clients live outside of metropolitan areas. In Australia for instance, approximately one third of the population lives in regional and remote areas of the country (Australian Bureau of Statistics, 2011), and the country land area is only somewhat smaller than that of the United States (USA). Telepractice, as a model of service delivery, can help overcome the barriers to clients. Furthermore, by providing services directly to clients in their community or home environment, there is the likelihood of better outcomes from higher retention in treatment programs and generalization of treatment effects to their everyday environment, as well as improved quality of life, higher involvement of family members/caregivers, and less risk of further isolation in their community.

Benefits of Telepractice to Speech-Language Pathologists

There are also numerous benefits of telepractice to SLPs. For instance, this modality allows for improved access to clients and delivery of quality services with the reduced need for travel and associated costs. With the use of distance learning tools, telepractice can provide greater access to quality education for SLPs. It also allows for professional connectivity though mentoring, support, development opportunities, and knowledge sharing that may also assist with the retention of SLPs in sole positions and/or in rural and remote areas. SLPs in developed countries may also be provided with opportunities to work with clients in developing countries such as those with cleft lip and/or palate, which they may seldom see untreated in their own clinical caseloads. Moreover, telepractice may open up new channels for communication between SLPs and other health professionals, with the ability to augment collaboration and networking, benefiting not only professionals and clients, but also the health system.

Global Benefits of Telepractice

In the global arena, telepractice, as illustrated in Figure 11-1, has the potential to assist in improving the quality of life of individuals in developing countries and in addressing some of the United Nations' Millennium Development Goals such as achieving universal primary education, promoting gender equality and empowering women, and eradicating extreme poverty and hunger (United Nations, 2005). Timely access to speech-language pathology services can reduce the impact that a communication disorder may have on individuals, thus allowing them to be active participants in

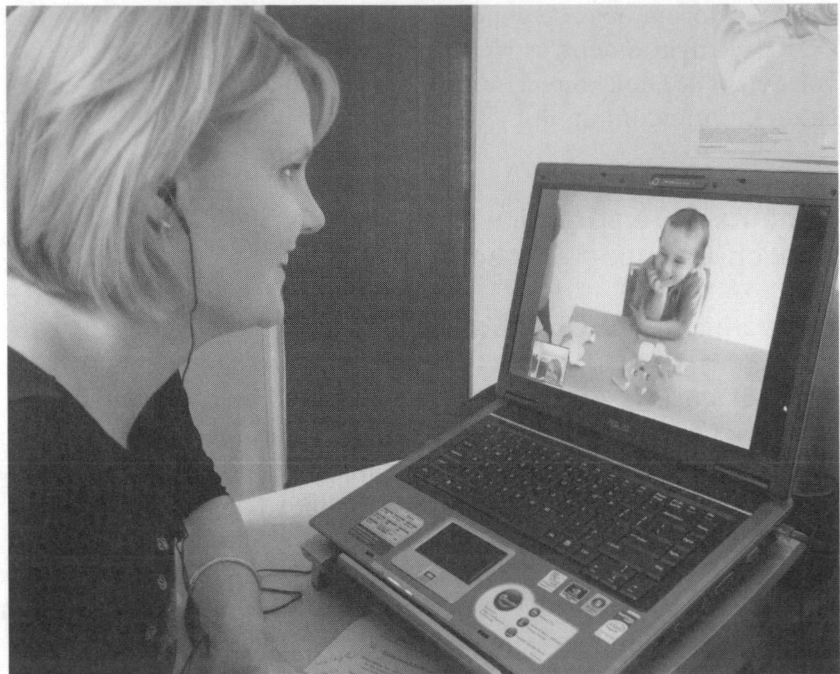

Figure 11–1. LSLS Cert AVT Michelle Ryan delivering an eAVT lesson to Coden and his mum who live 800 miles from the Brisbane Hear and Say Centre.

their community. For example, children with hearing loss in developing countries accessing early intervention services via telepractice will benefit directly by receiving services that can help them reach their spoken language potential. This can lead to greater participation in mainstream schooling and more effective learning, higher participation in further education, and improved long-term earnings and well-being.

For girls in general, being able to access education means that they are more likely to access medical care later during pregnancy, and be better educated about immunization, nutrition, and sanitation practices that will help to improve the survival rate, health, and nutrition of their children (The World Bank, 2012). Telepractice also has the potential to address the additional goal of developing global partnerships, on which other health and educational programs can be built and peace relationships developed. As professionals moving into the era of precision medicine, telepractice can also provide the scale and range of client data to the SLP, allowing for the unique tailoring of effective treatments to clients worldwide (Darzi, Mirnezami, Macdonnell, & Nicholson, 2012).

Barriers to the Adoption of Telepractice and Moving Forward

In moving forward with telepractice, SLPs must be aware of the potential challenges to the successful integration of telepractice into mainstream services and how to advocate for this modality. The universal barriers identified across health care disciplines and also relevant to speech-language pathology include: (1) the cost of equipment, maintenance, transport, and training, particularly in developing countries, with little work currently undertaken on the cost-effectiveness of services; (2) the ethical and legal aspects relating to medical malpractice and liability and service provision between different states and countries; (3) issues surrounding patient privacy, confidentiality, and consent; (4) patient and professional satisfaction with the modality; and (5) the limited evaluation of the effectiveness of this modality (World Health Organization, 2010).

The World Health Organization (WHO) has recommended a number of strategies to facilitate the uptake of telemedicine into health care including: (1) establishing governance mechanisms such as national agencies for the promotion and development of telemedicine; (2) establishing policies and strategies for planning, developing, and evaluating services and addressing relevant ethical and legal issues; (3) involving scientific institutions such as universities, hospitals, health, and technology agencies and dedicated research institutions in assessing a range of programs; as well as (4) undertaking rigorous evaluation of projects with timely dissemination of outcomes. Furthermore, based on the recent Global Observatory for eHealth survey of WHO Member States, the four greatest information needs required to support the development of telemedicine were identified as the cost of the service, clinical uses, infrastructure needs, and evaluation on the effectiveness of the service (World

Health Organization, 2010). The previously mentioned strategies and information needs also have application to telepractice. At the grassroots level, SLPs can advocate for telepractice by sharing information about their programs and undertaking evidence-based research in this area. The following section explores the telepractice research conducted internationally in speech-language pathology outside of the United States and report on the research outcomes and lessons learned, as outlined by leaders in the field. To ensure the information is most relevant to SLPs and captures current activities, the studies reviewed here are published works in peer-reviewed journals since 2009.

International Telepractice Research

Telepractice as a mode of service delivery is still in its infancy and relatively few studies have validated this approach within speech-language pathology. As with the medical disciplines that adopted the use of telemedicine, the initial pioneering work in telepractice was primarily undertaken in the United States and influenced by the information and communication technologies available at the time. The earlier use of the telephone (Helm-Estabrooks & Ramsberger, 1986; Vaughn, 1976) and closed-circuit television systems (Mashima et al., 2003; Wertz et al., 1992) were replaced by satellite- and now PC-based videoconferencing as the preferred method, more closely resembling the face-to-face modality. Telepractice research has been completed internationally, with the most proactive countries outside of the United States being Australia, the United Kingdom, Canada, and the Netherlands. Studies have been conducted in the assessment and treatment of various motor speech, language, voice, literacy, and fluency disorders, as well as dysphagia in pediatric and adult cases.

Australia

A recent survey of telepractice activity across Australia revealed promising findings about the adoption of this modality in clinical practice (Hill & Miller, 2012). The 52 respondents reported providing telepractice services from a number of settings representing typical clinical practice such as public health facilities (majority), private practice, public education settings, community service, and some specialist services. The most commonly utilized form of information and communication technology was the telephone, followed by email and videoconferencing, with a higher number of SLPs utilizing videoconferencing in regional than in metropolitan areas. In relation to the types of services provided using telepractice, 40% were assessments and 86% were treatments. For the latter, consultations were by far the majority, with follow-up, support services, and direct therapy making up the rest. Pediatric services were provided more often than adult services. The top five types of direct therapy most frequently delivered to pediatric clients included expressive language, fluency, speech, receptive language, and literacy. For adults, direct therapy included fluency, dysarthria, voice, expressive language, and dysphagia. In general, telepractice was utilized in up to 30% of caseloads and clients were able to access services from their home (majority), medical center, school, or work (the technology utilized was not described). Overall, these findings are encouraging, and it is anticipated that telepractice services will continue to increase over the coming years. A number of facilitators for telepractice uptake were identified in the survey including professional development, demonstrations by clinicians, access to electronic resources, funding to establish services, and formal training (Hill & Miller, 2012). Together with evidence-based research, these facilitators will assist SLPs in advocating for telepractice use. The following sections review the current research conducted in Australia.

The University of Queensland Research

In the last few years, the Telerehabilitation Research Unit has been leading the research in telepractice on the international scene. Here, a number of laboratory-based clinical validation trials have been conducted. These have spanned a wide range of disorders, including adult dysarthria, apraxia of speech, aphasia, voice, dysphagia, and pediatric language and literacy. The common element to these studies has been the use of a custom-made PC-based videoconferencing system to meet the specific requirements of clinical face-to-face management. The requirements included the ability to: (1) deliver assessment and treatment in real-time with the SLP and participant able to adequately view and hear each other during the sessions and to establish appropriate rapport. This was achieved via videoconferencing using a 128 kbit/s Internet connection over the PC, which at the time of the studies was the minimum speed used in Queensland's public health systems. To assist with the clarity of the audio signal and to minimize distortion, both the participant and online SLP wore a headset microphone; (2) perceptually rate speech, voice and oro-motor parameters during assessments in real time and, where necessary, to be able to record and store video and audio assessment data for review off-line at a later date. Store-and-forward capabilities were incorporated within the system, allowing for the capture of high-quality video and audio recordings; and (3) provide the participant with appropriate reading materials and stimuli during assessment and treatment. The remote display of text and prerecorded audio and video demonstrations at the participant site were incorporated in the system design; and (4) the system must be easy to operate and follow a similar approach to face-to-face management. The system was designed to be used intuitively by the SLP, without technical knowledge or extensive training. Furthermore, to simplify operations from the perspective of the participant, the system enabled the online SLP to remotely control all aspects of the sessions, including adjusting the web cameras at the participant site remotely for maximum viewing of the participants at all times (Constantinescu, 2010).

Dysarthria, apraxia of speech, and aphasia. Hill and colleagues (2009a, 2009b, 2009c), utilized the videoconferencing system with 24 participants with dysarthria resulting primarily from cerebrovascular accident (CVA) and traumatic brain injury (TBI) (severity levels not stated); 11 participants with acquired apraxia of speech following CVA (severity levels not stated) and with concomitant mild to moderate aphasia and/or dysarthria; and 32 participants with mild to severe aphasia following CVA and TBI and with concomitant mild to moderate dysarthria. For the aphasia study, a touch screen facility was added to the videoconferencing system to enable participants to point to images as they would have in the paper-based stimulus book. Participants traveled to the university or hospital laboratory for the studies. As per the assessment protocol established at the university, participants were assessed simultaneously by two SLPs, one in the face-to-face environment (i.e., located within the same room as the participant), and the second SLP online, conducting the assessment through videoconferencing. The SLPs were randomized to lead the assessment (online or face-to-face), and the second SLP acted as the silent rater and did not interact with the participant. The simultaneous assessment ensured that participant test-retest variability was eliminated. For the dysarthria study, the assessments included an informal oro-motor and perceptual speech assessment, sections of the Assessment of Intelligibility of Dysarthric Speech (Yorkston & Beukelman, 1981), and determining an overall dysarthria diagnosis for each participant. The apraxia study utilized the Apraxia Battery for Adults-2 (Dabul, 2000), while the aphasia study included the use of the Boston Diagnostic Aphasia Examination-3 (Goodglass, Kaplan, & Barresi, 2001) and the Boston Naming Test (Kaplan, Goodglass, & Weintraub, 2001). The telepractice modality was found to be: (1) valid and reliable for all assessment types, with outcomes of good strength of agreement in the dysarthria study between all ratings in the online and face-to-face environments, high intra- and interrater reliability for all parameters, as well as high participant satisfaction with the online-led assessments; (2) no significant differences and moderate to very good agreement between the online and face-to-face ratings of apraxia of speech, reasonable intra- and interrater reliability, and high participant satisfaction with the online-led assessments; and (3) no significant differences between the online and face-to-face ratings and high agreement between ratings for all severity levels on the aphasia study, and high participant satisfaction with the online-led assessments.

Clinical considerations for SLPs. It was acknowledged that certain aspects of the online environment did make it more difficult at times to rate some assessment tasks and these considerations may be useful for the practicing SLP. For instance, even with sufficient background lighting and contrast to enhance visualization of the participants online, the fixed web camera positioning and focus still made it difficult at times to view some of the participants' facial features. Additionally, the occasional audio break-up and difficulties with clearly viewing participants due to the Internet connection made it more challenging at times to assess aspects of aphasia such as naming and paraphasia, as well as apraxia of speech (parameters not specified). It was suggested that for individuals with more severe apraxia of speech, evaluations conducted face-to-face may be better suited as they may provide a greater understanding of the participant's severity level and performance (Hill et al., 2009a, 2009b).

Voice. Research was conducted in the assessment and treatment of the speech and voice disorder associated with Parkinson's disease (PD). Here, the videoconferencing system incorporated the additional use of an external acoustic speech processor connected to the system that allowed for sampling of real-time, calibrated average measures of vocal sound pressure level, fundamental frequency, and duration via the participant headset microphone. In the assessment study, 61 participants with PD and mild to severe hypokinetic dysarthria were assessed at the university on a battery of acoustic and perceptual measures. The battery consisted of an instrumental evaluation of mean sound pressure level, maximum duration of sustained vowel phonation, and maximum fundamental frequency range. The perceptual measures included ratings of voice and nonspeech oro-motor parameters, overall articulatory precision, and speech intelligibility in reading and conversation. The SLPs were randomized to the environment, with only one administering the assessment. There were 30 online-led assessments conducted in total. The results indicated that the telepractice modality was valid and reliable, with comparable measures within the clinical criterion (≥80%) obtained for online and face-to-face ratings of all acoustic parameters, the majority of perceptual parameters, and for intra- and interrater reliability. Participant satisfaction was also high (80% satisfied or very satisfied) with the online-led environment (Constantinescu, 2010; Constantinescu et al., 2010a).

In the treatment study, a randomized controlled noninferiority trial was conducted with 34 participants with idiopathic PD and mild to moderate hypokinetic dysarthria that had taken part in the assessment study. Seventeen participants received the Lee Silverman Voice Treatment (LSVT®LOUD) in either the online or face-to-face environments at the university. The LSVT®LOUD is the most effective and evidence-based treatment for PD and hypokinetic dysarthria and promotes increased respiratory drive, vocal fold adduction, and carryover of the louder voice into functional communication. The treatment was delivered intensively, 1 hour a day, 4 days a week over a 4-week period, in accordance with the LSVT®LOUD program (Ramig, Bonitati, Lemke, & Horii, 1994). Daily sessions consisted of repetitive speech loudness drills and hierarchical tasks that were performed at high intensity and maximum effort. During the treatment tasks, the SLP monitored the participant's vocal loudness (dB) and quality, and aided calibration (i.e., the participant's ability to self-monitor and consistently use their louder voice in everyday communication). In the online environment, the videoconferencing system was used by the online SLP to view and sample acoustic measures in real time and display reading material. Statistical analyses confirmed the validity of online LSVT®LOUD delivery with noninferiority of the online modality for the primary outcome measure of mean change in sound pressure level in conversation. No significant main effects for treatment environment, dysarthria severity, and interaction effects were noted for all acoustic measures, and participants in both groups showed statistically significant improvements with treatment on the majority of measures. Moreover, there were no failed treatment sessions, all sessions were conducted within the necessary 1-hour time frame, and participants who received online LSVT®LOUD were overall more than satisfied or very satisfied (more than 80%) with online treatment (Constantinescu, 2010; Constantinescu et al., 2011).

A final feasibility trial was conducted of home-based online delivery of LSVT®LOUD for a participant with idiopathic PD and mild hypokinetic dysarthria, located at a distance of 90 km from the university. A 128 kbit/s Internet connection over the public network was established between the two sites. This was achieved using a 128 kbit/s Internet connection at the SLP end that limited the bandwidth of the Asynchronous Digital Line broadband Internet connection used by the participant. On the whole, the study demonstrated the suitability of home-based LSVT®LOUD, with the participant showing substantial improvements on most of the acoustic and perceptual parameters and high satisfaction with the approach. There were no failed treatment sessions and the majority of sessions ran very smoothly, with sufficient audio and video quality for treatment delivery (Constantinescu, 2010; Constantinescu et al., 2010b). A large-scale randomized controlled study is currently underway investigating the home-based delivery of the LSVT®LOUD.

Clinical considerations for SLPs. In the voice studies, a number of challenges unique to the online environment were identified and solutions were put in place to appropriately manage these. In relation to the audio quality, occasional delays of up to 3 seconds resulted from the Internet connection and were managed by SLPs and participants actively waiting until the other had finished speaking before replying. Where necessary during treatment, the SLPs also adopted further strategies to help minimize the effects of the audio delay including: (1) using shorter and more precise instructions to facilitate the flow of the conversation and to minimize the likelihood of talking on top of each other; (2) waiting until the task was completed before providing feedback; and (3) using obvious and easy to detect hand cues rather than verbal feedback for quick input, such as "stop" to terminate the task, hand raising to indicate the need to increase loudness, or "thumbs-up" for appropriate performance and to continue with the task. The SLPs were able to quickly adopt the use of such strategies, and the majority of participants were also able to easily follow this routine. Some of the participants with moderate dysarthria and a level of cognitive difficulty required greater prompting from the SLPs for shaping the desired vocal responses, especially during the first few treatment sessions. For these participants, the SLPs successfully utilized as many verbal and nonverbal strategies as necessary. The predictable nature of the LSVT®LOUD sessions in general greatly aided the uptake of the online modality for all participants and minimized any difficulties that potentially related to the audio quality.

In relation to the video quality, the frame rate and pixelated image especially during movement made it more difficult for the participants and SLPs to clearly view each other during the sessions. In the assessment study, the store-and-forward function was a valuable addition to the videoconferencing system as it helped with ratings of perceptual speech and voice parameters. It also allowed for better visual discrimination of oro-motor parameters. For treatment, the SLPs utilized the store-and-forward function in situations where clearer viewing of participants was needed such as to detect: (1) whether participants were phonating effectively at the top of the breath with an open-mouth position; (2) the presence of muscle tension in the head and neck regions (contraindicated for treatment); and (3) the optimal participant positioning and posture during the sessions. In general, as the assessment and treatment sessions did not require a lot of physical movement, the participants and SLPs were able to sit relatively still in front of the PC during the sessions, which allowed for the least image pixelation with videoconferencing. Telepractice applications with high-bandwidth videoconferencing and Web cameras with greater zoom and focus capabilities would help to improve the real-time audio and video quality.

Despite the videoconferencing system being very user friendly, on occasion the difference in establishing eye contact online presented a unique challenge for the SLPs. Unlike face-to-face where eye contact was achieved naturally, the online SLPs needed to actually look up at the web camera on top of the monitor rather than at the participant on the screen in order to be perceived as making eye contact. This process, and the need to operate the videoconferencing system at the same time, made the interaction with the participants somewhat unnatural for the SLPs. However, the SLPs' growing experience in the use of the videoconferencing system during the course of the studies and the prescriptive nature of the LSVT®LOUD enabled quick uptake of skills and proficiency, with minimal impact on delivery. In future, the repositioning of the web camera closer to the participant image would allow the

SLP to maintain eye contact more easily, while at the same time conducting the session. Finally, to ensure the smooth delivery of home treatment, sessions were conducted in a quiet room of the participant's home, which reduced any household distractions and noise, and telephone calls were not taken during the sessions (Constantinescu, 2010; Constantinescu et al., 2010a, 2010b; Constantinescu et al., 2011).

Dysphagia. The videoconferencing system was further utilized in a number of dysphagia studies. An earlier trial assessed the swallowing and communication function of 10 participants postlaryngectomy (Ward et al., 2009). The additional features of the videoconferencing system included the use of: (1) videoconferencing via a commercial 3G phone network (maximum throughput 3.5 Mbit/s); (2) a freestanding camera with built-in autofocus and high video capture resolution; (3) an external light source for improved viewing of the stoma; and (4) a local participant view to assist the participant with positioning themselves in front of the SLP camera for better viewing of the stoma. Simultaneous assessments were conducted by two SLPs, one face-to-face in Brisbane, and another leading the online sessions in a regional city, approximately 1,700 km away. Assessment measures included swallowing, communication, visual inspection of the stoma and voice prosthesis (where applicable), stoma care, and recommendations for management. The results showed the feasibility of online assessment, with high agreement within the clinical criteria (>80%) obtained between the SLPs on the majority of measures, as well as complete agreement on recommendations for management. Some difficulties with the wireless connection were encountered for a few sessions, resulting in disconnections and intermittent audio and video breakup. However, all sessions were able to be completed and high participant and SLP satisfaction was obtained with the online assessment.

In looking at dysphagia management in more detail, a clinical trial explored the validity and reliability of online assessment (Ward, Sharma, Burns, Theodoros, & Russell, 2012a). Here, 40 participants with mild to severe dysphagia resulting from a range of neurological, surgical, and nonsurgical conditions were assessed simultaneously in the face-to-face and online environments. The same procedures as the initial pilot study (Sharma, Ward, Burns, Theodoros, & Russell, 2011) were adopted including: (1) randomizing the two SLPs to the assessments (the online SLP leading the assessments remotely); (2) utilizing an assistant at the participant site; and (3) administering the clinical swallowing examination to determine participant orientation, alertness, posture, oral hygiene, dental status, oro-motor and laryngeal function, performance on food and fluid trials, and recommendations for management. The additional features of the videoconferencing system included: (1) fixed and freestanding Web cameras for close-up and lateral viewing of participants; (2) free-field combined microphone and speaker with echo-canceling features; and (3) a lapel microphone worn by the participant for improved vocal clarity. Prior to the assessment, the assistant set up the videoconferencing system and prepared the food and fluid trials. During the sessions, the assistant helped participants with: (1) their positioning in front of the web cameras to ensure optimal viewing by the online SLP; (2) placing the lapel microphone on the participant's collar, the pulse oximeter on their finger, and surgical tape over the thyroid notch for improved viewing of laryngeal movement during swallowing; (3) providing support to the participant where needed; (4) administering the food and fluid trials; and (5) relaying any necessary information to the online SLP such as pulse oximeter readings, oro-motor function, and clarifying observations where needed. The study findings helped establish the validity and reliability of online dysphagia assessment, with agreement within the clinical criteria (>80%) on the majority of measures including clinical management decisions, high intra- and interrater reliability, and high SLP satisfaction with the online modality.

Clinical considerations for SLPs. The occasional audio and video delays encountered during the assessments were appropriately managed using the store-and-forward function of the videoconferencing system. It was noted that the assistant played an integral role in the successful delivery of sessions and should be considered a necessary addition to future online assessments. Furthermore, the delivery modifications such as the use of white laryngeal tape, clear plastic cups and spoons, and food dye added to the water should be utilized to enhance the visualization of laryngeal movement, water intake, and spillage respectively (Sharma et al., 2011; Ward et al., 2012a).

The team also explored the potential impact of participant factors on the delivery of the online assessment (Ward, Sharma, Burns, Theodoros, & Russell, 2012b). From the clinical trial, 10 participants were selected based on the online SLP ratings of their sessions as being less efficient than face-to-face. SLP notes on the participants from the time of the assessments revealed a number of participant factors that impacted the SLP ratings. These included: speech and/or voice disorders; hearing impairments; movement disorders; and behavioral and/or emotional issues. The speech and voice difficulties made it more difficult for the online SLP to understand participants during conversation, and to note changes in vocal quality on the food and fluid trials, as a potential sign of aspiration. In these situations, the assistant was relied upon more heavily to relay information to the SLP. For participants with unaided hearing difficulties, the SLP needed to simplify instructions to make them easier to understand, and the assistant was also relied upon to increase the speaker volume at the participant end and where necessary, to repeat instructions. Finally, the assistant was integral in assisting with the positioning of the freestanding camera for the participant with dyskinesia, and in managing behavioral issues such as impulsivity that occurred for some participants during the food and fluid trials.

Pediatric Language, Literacy, and Speech. Three pediatric assessment studies were also undertaken at the University of Queensland. One study looked at the language ability of 25 children aged between 5 to 9 years with diagnosed or suspected language impairment. Assessments were conducted simultaneously in the face-to-face and online environments using the Concepts and Following Directions, Word Structure, Recalling Sentences and Formulated Sentences core language subtests of the Clinical Evaluation of Language Fundamentals-4 (Semel, Wiig, & Secord, 2003). The SLPs and participants were randomly assigned to the environment. A touch screen facility was also incorporated into the videoconferencing system for recording of participant responses on one of the subtests. The study showed the validity and reliability of online language assessment for young children with no significant differences between ratings for the total raw and scaled scores on all subtests, very good agreement for individual items on all subtests, core language score and severity level, as well as very good intra- and interrater reliability (Waite, Theodoros, Russell, & Cahill, 2010a).

An assessment of literacy was undertaken with 20 children aged 8 to 13 years and previously diagnosed or suspected delays in reading and/or spelling (Waite, Theodoros, Russell, & Cahill, 2010b). The children were assessed on a battery of standardized assessments including subtests of the Queensland University Inventory of Literacy (QUIL; Dodd, Holm, Oerlemans, & McCormick, 1996), the South Australian Spelling Test (Westwood, 2005), and the Neale Analysis of Reading Ability-3 (Neale, 1999). Like the previous study, assessments were conducted simultaneously by two SLPs with the same system architecture. The study also demonstrated the validity and reliability of telepractice for assessing literacy, with very good agreement and within the clinical criteria (≥80%) between the online and face-to-face SLPs on the raw and scaled scores for the majority of parameters and very good intra- and interrater reliability on all parameters.

The final study investigated the speech intelligibility, and oro-motor structure and function of 20 children aged 4 to 9 years with identified or suspected speech disorders (Waite, Theodoros, Russell, & Cahill, 2012). The children were simultaneously assessed by the two SLPs on an informal oro-motor assessment and conversational speech sample that was rated for intelligibility. A high level of agreement was obtained between the online and face-to-face ratings of speech intelligibility, oro-motor function, and intra- and interrater reliability, indicating that online speech assessment is valid and reliable.

Clinical considerations for SLPs. The videoconferencing system was appropriate for use in the assessments, and the online SLPs felt able to interact with the participants during the assessments, monitor their concentration levels throughout and make clinical judgments about their capabilities. However, the audio delay, break-up, and occasional echo that occurred during the reading assessment of the Neale-3 made it more difficult for the online SLPs to provide timely prompts and corrections as part of the assessment protocol, making it distracting for some of the participants or influencing their reading rate. Some future considerations as reported by the team to facilitate online assessment administration with children included using: (1) child-sized headphones; (2) child-sized seats to improve positioning; (3) multipoint touch screens that allow for recording of two or more simultaneous responses as per assessment task requirements; (4) prerecorded stimuli to prevent interference due to audio breakup; (5) applications using higher bandwidth as a possible solution to the audio; (6) system modifications allowing recordings of SLPs and participants without echo; as well as (7) video instead of audio recordings of participant responses to aid the intelligibility of responses for the online SLPs.

Overall future directions and recommendations. The studies conducted at The University of Queensland have provided validation for telepractice in the assessment and treatment of a number of adult and pediatric client populations. Common future directions and recommendations reported in the studies that can assist with advancing the knowledge base of telepractice in speech-language pathology and the uptake into clinical practice are listed here. These include large-scale studies involving: (1) greater numbers of SLPs of varying degrees of proficiency in order to determine the possible effects of proficiency on outcomes; (2) participants with a wide range of communication and swallowing disorders; (3) a wide range of assessment parameters; (4) comprehensive analyses of participant and SLP satisfaction with the online modality; (5) recommendations for videoconferencing system requirements to meet client needs for assessment and treatment; (6) in-depth cost benefit analyses from the perspectives of the client and service provider; and (7) home-based delivery of assessment and treatment in order to fully understand the benefits and challenges of this modality. Home-based delivery of the LSVT®LOUD is currently being investigated.

Hear and Say, Queensland

Hear and Say provides an example of the clinical application of telepractice for children with hearing loss—as seen in Figure 11-2.

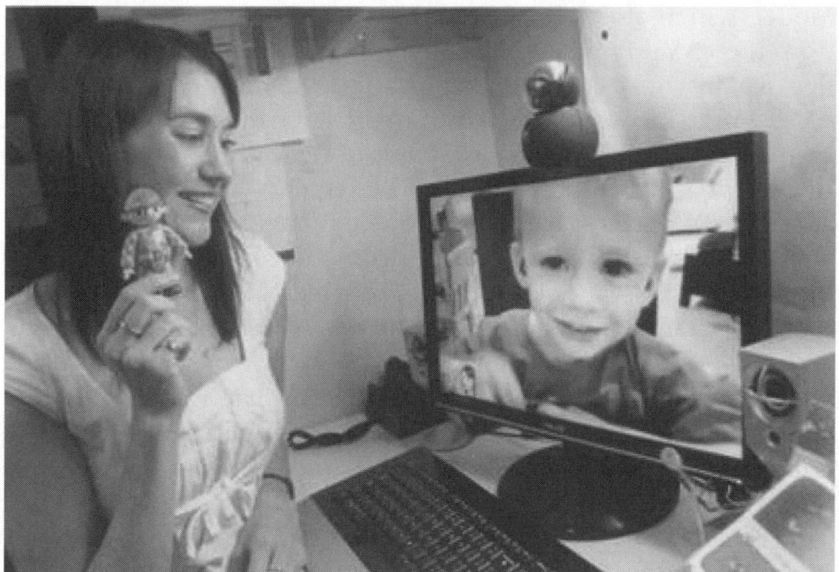

Figure 11–2. Young Tommy in his home in Dubai interacting via eAVT with LSLS Cert AVT Lynda Close in Brisbane, Australia.

Hear and Say is an early intervention and pediatric implantable technologies (including cochlear implants) center. Early intervention is provided through auditory-verbal therapy (AVT), an effective parent-based program that promotes one-to-one therapy with active parental participation, aggressive audiological management, and modern hearing technology (e.g., hearing aids and cochlear implants). The approach guides parents to develop their child's spoken language through listening, with the end goal of allowing children with hearing loss to reach their full potential in the hearing world (AG Bell Academy for Listening and Spoken Language, 2013). At Hear and Say, families typically enroll in the AVT program following identification of their newborn's hearing loss via newborn hearing screening, and sessions are provided from this point until school entry, as need requires. The traditional face-to-face AVT service is currently provided to 172 children and families across Queensland through the metropolitan center in Brisbane and four regional centers. Under the banner of the Hear and Say eMPOWER

Model, which also includes eAudiology and eTraining and Education, the eAVT Program currently supports 41 children and families, making up 19% of the organization's clinical population. The eAVT Program was developed to meet the needs of children with hearing loss and their families living in regional and remote areas of Queensland. For these families, the regular weekly or fortnightly access to the face-to-face service for a minimal of 3 years cannot be achieved due to the large distances from the centers, excessive cost of travel, and disruption to family life. Over the past 15 years, the eAVT Program has evolved from the use of the telephone, e-mail, and two-way videoconferencing, to the formalized program using webcam videoconferencing via the Internet that has been in place since 2005. The eAVT Program has also supported a number of families living in other states of Australia, as well as in Dubai, Papua New Guinea, Singapore, China, and Abu Dhabi.

The AVT delivery for both the face-to-face and eAVT Programs conforms to the 10 AVT principles (AG Bell Academy for Listening and Spoken Language, 2013). In each 1-hour session, parents teach their child specific concepts through listening under the guidance of an auditory-verbal therapist. Individual goals for each child are planned on a 6-month basis, incorporating listening, early communication, language, speech, cognition, social interaction (i.e., communicative competence), and fine and gross motor skills that are expected for children with normal hearing of the same age. Goals from each category are integrated into each session and taught through activities from themed "lesson boxes." All face-to-face sessions are conducted in-person at one of the Hear and Say centers on a weekly, biweekly, or monthly basis, depending on the child's needs. The eAVT Program is conducted in the same manner as face-to-face, with the following alterations: (1) sessions delivered between the therapist in Brisbane and the parent and child at home via PC-based videoconferencing; (2) planning sessions involving the therapist and parent held via videoconferencing on alternate weeks, to enable planning and discussion of session goals and carryover into the child's everyday environment; (3) themed lesson boxes with materials to support lessons and carryover are mailed out to families on a monthly rotation to ensure that all families have access to the appropriate learning activities; (4) biannual therapist visits to the child's home and educational setting (if applicable) for face-to-face contact, lessons, standardized speech and language assessments, and monitoring of progress; and (5) biannual family visits to the Brisbane center for face-to-face contact, lessons, assessment, and attendance at auditory-verbal playgroup and parent education. Therapy sessions are delivered using Skype for Windows on PCs via high-speed broadband. This platform has been chosen as it is readily available and provides videoconferencing at no additional cost to the families or the center. Therefore, it is a sustainable method for providing the eAVT Program. The additional equipment used by the therapist and family to enhance the audio-visual quality during videoconferencing is a web camera, external speakers, and a desktop microphone.

The feasibility of the eAVT Program has previously been described in a satisfaction study (Constantinescu, 2012). Here, the five therapists providing eAVT services at the time and 13 of the 17 parents completed satisfaction questionnaires. The questions related to: (1) the audio and video quality; (2) equipment use (Skype, Web camera, desktop microphone); (3) general interaction and communication; (4) service delivery access and convenience; and (5) overall satisfaction. The outcomes were promising, with therapists and parents showing high satisfaction on the majority of sections. Parents also found the eAVT Program to be a better alternative than the necessary regular travel to receive face-to-face sessions, and were satisfied or very satisfied with the program overall. Moreover, all parents would recommend the eAVT Program to others, suggesting that the need is being appropriately met by the eAVT Program (Constantinescu, 2012).

A later study demonstrated the effectiveness of the eAVT Program by comparing the language outcomes of a group of seven children in the eAVT Program to a matched group of children receiving face-to-face AVT (Constantinescu et al., submitted). No significant differences in language scores were obtained between the two groups on the Preschool Language Scale-4 (Zimmerman, Steiner, & Pond, 2002) at approximately 2 years postoptimal amplification (i.e., hearing aids or cochlear implants). Another promising finding was that the mean standard score for the children in the eAVT group was within the average range for hearing peers on all measures of Total Language, Auditory Comprehension, and Expressive Communication. A larger validation study is currently underway to further quantify these outcomes. The findings will inform clinical practice at Hear and Say and help to establish clinical benchmarks for spoken language development and progress for children in the eAVT Program, all important factors for the long-term success and sustainability of the program.

Clinical considerations for SLPs. As outlined in the satisfaction study (Constantinescu, 2012), the audio quality over Skype was compromised on occasion due to the Internet connection and this resulted in some audio delays, echo/static, and audio fading in and out. For the therapists, these issues made it more difficult at times to identify the more subtle aspects of the child's speech productions, particularly for the younger children. However, as AVT is a parent-based program, the audio quality was not seen as a barrier to online delivery, as therapists could rely on the parents for clarification of their child's speech. Similarly, although difficulties were encountered by therapists when engaging directly with the younger children, this did not hamper the session quality or delivery as interaction/rapport was achieved online between parents and therapists, as well as adequate coaching of parents. The video quality during videoconferencing did cause some pixelation and delays and it was suggested that prerecorded strategies and therapy tasks could be used in situations where the video quality is compromised.

As part of Hear and Say's eMPOWER Model, telepractice is also being utilized clinically in one of the regional centers, for the remote MAPping of cochlear implants for children with hearing loss. This eAudiology Program will soon be provided to all regional centers and where necessary, on accompanying therapist visits to families enrolled in the eAVT Program. The eAudiology Program has recently been validated (Rushbrooke, 2012) and together with eAVT, the programs are providing comprehensive services in line with the face-to-face services that are meeting the needs of children with hearing loss and their families in rural and remote Queensland. Additionally, the eTraining and Education Program is supporting professionals in teaching listening and spoken language to their clients worldwide. Since 2010, 55 professionals from across Australia and New Zealand, Singapore, the Philippines, India, Indonesia, the United Kingdom, and Zimbabwe have taken part in the courses offered through the program. The courses are delivered using a collaborative learning platform with videoconferencing facilities and interactive whiteboard capacity using an Internet protocol (IP) on the Internet (Chen & Ko, 2010; Hastie, Hung, Chen, & Kinshuk, 2010; Wang, Chen, & Levy, 2010). For the purpose of the courses, the platform is utilized for self-paced learning and live tutorials with professionals at Hear and Say.

> The opportunities afforded by telepractice are empowering parents by improving access to specialized services such as AVT for their children with hearing loss. The potential for the use of technology in audiological management is also exciting and the advances will continue to guide our Hear and Say eMPOWER service delivery model. By demonstrating the effectiveness of telepractice, we hope that this will also increase confidence in using this service delivery for clinicians and parents, enabling children to reach their full potential.
> —Emma Rushbrooke, Clinical Director, Hear and Say

First Voice and VidKids, Australia

First Voice is the national voice for member organizations in Australia providing listening and spoken language early intervention. The centers are located throughout the nation and include Hear and Say, The Shepherd Centre in New South Wales and the Australian Capital Territory, Taralye in Victoria, Cora Barclay Centre in South Australia, and Telethon Speech and Hearing in Western Australia. There is also an affiliate organization, The Hearing House, in New Zealand. In 2012, First Voice centers and Vision Australia, a leading national provider of blindness and low vision services in Australia, formed the consortium known as VidKids Alliance and received Australian Federal Government funding for the implementation of the project "Remote Hearing and Vision Services for Children with Vision and/or Hearing Impairment in Australia." Over the next 3 years, the project will assist more than 125 children, and AVT will be provided to children with hearing loss and their families via broadband videoconferencing. It is anticipated that the services provided as part of the telepractice program will be sustainable long term.

The Royal Institute for Deaf and Blind Children (RIDBC), Sydney

RIDBC also provides services to children with hearing and/or vision loss and their families across Australia. The organization has been using telepractice approaches to reach families since the late 1990s, and in 2004 the national program, known as RIDBC Teleschool™, was founded with the funding assistance of the Australian Federal Government. RIDBC Teleschool supported 171 Australian families in 2011 (including speech-language pathology services for children with hearing loss), and also some families living in Dubai, Singapore, India, Samoa, and Fiji (McCarthy, 2012). RIDBC Teleschool utilizes a dedicated videoconferencing system using PC or television monitors to deliver sessions between the therapist and family sites. The system features include: (1) videoconferencing over a private network; (2) a high-quality camera at both ends with pan, tilt, and zoom function that is controlled remotely by the therapist; and (3) the ability to record sessions, share data, and involve multiple participant sites. A number of multimedia resources are also utilized by families to enhance and complement lessons such as print, video, Web-based, and iPad applications, and a private password-protected website aimed at connecting parents in the program and sharing information. Parent and professional courses are also delivered via telepractice. RIDBC Teleschool offers an early intervention program for children with hearing loss, and their families and children are eligible for support until they reach the age of 18 years (McCarthy, 2012). RIDBC Teleschool has been noted to be an effective service for children with hearing loss, achieving high parent satisfaction and family engagement (McCarthy, Muñoz, & White, 2010). Outcomes data are needed to quantify these findings.

Clinician considerations for SLPs. It was suggested that the initial solid foundation in face-to-face delivery and the use of technology will facilitate the successful delivery of telepractice services for children with hearing loss. Being flexible and creative in the delivery of services, adaptable to change, and having good time management and organizational skills will also benefit the SLP working in this modality (McCarthy, 2012).

The University of Sydney

The Lidcombe Program. The Australian Stuttering Research Centre has been leading fluency research in telepractice internationally in both the adult and pediatric fields. Telepractice has been utilized in the delivery of the Lidcombe Program (Onslow, Packman, & Harrison, 2003), an efficacious parent-based treatment for children who stutter. The program requires weekly clinic visits where parents are taught to administer verbal contingencies for their child's stutter-free and unambiguous stuttered speech, promoting the maintenance of treatment outcomes. Earlier studies have demonstrated the success of the program delivery over the telephone (Lewis, Packman, Onslow, Simpson, & Jones, 2008; Wilson, Onslow, & Lincoln, 2004). More recently, a case study described the program delivery via Skype between the SLP in Melbourne and a 4-year-old child and family in South Africa (Erickson, 2012). With this approach, it was noted that the child was able to make substantial improvements in reducing his stuttering from 20% syllables stuttered pretreatment (severity rating of 7), to current 0.7% syllables stuttered (severity rating of 2) posttreatment, and on his way to stutter-free speech.

Clinical considerations for SLPs. The parent's view of telepractice was very positive, describing the approach as convenient, stress free, and even better than face-to-face. The parent felt a sense of trust and connectedness with the SLP, despite being located in different countries. From the SLP's point of view, the approach allowed for a supportive relationship between the SLP and parent. It was recommended that SLPs should be aware of possible Internet connection difficulties that may occur with this approach and to be able to implement strategies to minimize difficulties such as effectively communicating therapy instructions. Furthermore, it was suggested that it would benefit SLPs to first have a strong foundation in face-to-face treatment delivery and confidence in the use of technology before undertaking telepractice, to ensure the best outcomes for clients. The overall benefits of telepractice were recognized as the timesaving factor, greater access to evidence-based treatments, and comfort for families as they receive treatment in their own homes, as well as greater insight for SLPs into the child's everyday environment. A larger validation study using Skype delivery for the Lidcombe Program is currently underway to quantify these findings.

The Camperdown Program. Recent studies in adult fluency have been very promising in demonstrating the benefits of telepractice using the Camperdown Program (O'Brian, Onslow, Cream, & Packman, 2003). This behavioral treatment is based on the control of stuttering using prolonged speech and consists of weekly individual sessions and a group practice day. The program uses recorded training material to teach clients prolonged speech through imitation. There is no programmed instruction and clients use whatever features they find useful from the training material to control their stuttering. Clients also use a 9-point severity rating scale to rate their stuttering and speech naturalness as part of self-management. A randomized controlled noninferiority trial was undertaken of the Camperdown Program delivery via telepractice (Carey et al., 2010). In this study, 40 participants were randomly assigned to the traditional face-to-face or telepractice groups and received treatment. For participants in the telepractice group, (1) treatment via the telephone replaced face-to-face sessions; (2) training materials were mailed out as audiotapes; (3) a designated telephone voicemail line was used for participants to record speech samples for evaluation by the SLP; and (4) home practice replaced the group practice day. The study validated the use of telepractice for the Camperdown Program, with no significant differences between face-to-face and telepractice for the primary outcome measure of percent syllables stuttered at 9 months postrandomization. Furthermore, no significant differences were also found in percent syllables stuttered immediately posttreatment, 6 and 12 months, with treatment effects maintained at the 12-month follow-up. The telepractice delivery also reduced SLP contact time by an average of 3.7 hours compared to face-to-face, and was considered to be clinically and statistically significant. Participants in both groups rated talking on the telephone and learning the speech restructuring pattern as extremely easy and building rapport with the SLP as easy. Interestingly, only the participants in the telepractice group found the treatment delivery as extremely convenient. The authors concluded that the use of the telephone as a low-technology telepractice application has great potential in addressing access and inequity issues for clients who stutter.

Clinical considerations for SLPs. The benefits outlined in the earlier pilot study of the Camperdown Program delivery via the telephone are also applicable here (O'Brian, Packman, & Onslow, 2008). The treatment via the telephone allowed for the retention of participants in the program who due to changes in work circumstances, illness, or moving interstate, would have been unable to continue with the treatment if it was delivered face-to-face. There was also the additional benefit to participants of having the phone contact time with the SLP scheduled at convenient times that did not require them to take time off work.

Two further telepractice applications have been utilized in the delivery of the Camperdown Program by the team at the Australian Stuttering Research Centre. The program delivery via webcam videoconferencing was trialed with three adolescent participants diagnosed with moderate-severe stuttering (Carey, O'Brian, Onslow, Packman, & Menzies, 2012). The participants received weekly individual sessions over Skype and emailed recorded speech samples to the SLP for later review. The study findings were promising, with a mean group reduction of 83% in the percentage of syllables stuttered from pretreatment to entry to maintenance, and high retention of results at 12 months postentry to maintenance. Parents and participants found the modality to be easy and convenient and would prefer this approach to face-to-face management if future treatment was required.

Finally, the stand-alone Web-based delivery of the Camperdown Program has been investigated (Erickson et al., 2012). Here, all aspects of the program were incorporated into the linked administration website and treatment phases became available to participants once they had completed the required goals of the previous phases. The website was also able to store participant responses and provide problem-solving strategies to the participants on their speech problems. The two participants in this study showed improvements in their speech, with reduced percentage of syllables stuttered by 59% and 61% respectively compared to pretreatment, as well as reduced self-reported stuttering severity and situational avoidance. The authors suggested that the web-based program is feasible for reducing stuttering and presents a possible solution for clients in overcoming clinic fees, travel costs, time away from work, and allowing for self-paced management. It was proposed that a service delivery that combines SLP input and the web-based program may be a suitable option for some clients, as well as for generalist SLPs with less experience in working with this clinical population, where the Web-based program can guide treatment.

> The Camperdown Program is now offered via phone or Internet Webcam. The choice to receive treatment will depend on a number of factors including lifestyle, distance from the clinic, client familiarity with the technology, and of course client preference for one method of delivery compared to another. I see ultimately that clients will have a much broader range of choices on how to receive therapy. For some clinicians and clients, in-clinic treatment delivery will remain a first preference. However, as clients have greater access to information about a range of therapies, they will want to seek access to the therapy of their choice. Sometimes that will mean accessing it from a different therapist, a different city, or a different country. Technology will facilitate this. I see the day when clients will also be able to access group therapy from their home or work place, and treatment programs that are clinician free. And as a clinical researcher, I see exciting times ahead as we develop new methods and trial them with various technologies.
> —Dr Brenda Carey, Speech Pathologist and Clinical Research, Australian Stuttering Research Centre

The United Kingdom

In the United Kingdom, a proof-of-concept study by Howell and colleagues (2009) investigated the home-based delivery of the LSVT®LOUD using a PC-based videoconferencing system, a broadband Internet connection, and Skype. Three participants with idiopathic PD and mild to moderate hypokinetic dysarthria were treated online within their homes. Participants were required to have a computer with a broadband Internet connection, web camera, headset microphone, and a Skype and email account in order to take part in treatment. Due to the complexity of the LSVT®LOUD program that requires the live viewing of acoustic data by the SLP during each session, one treatment session a week (4 of the 16 sessions) needed to be conducted face-to-face in order to objectively monitor this data, which could not be done online. The authors acknowledged that the treatment delivery could therefore not be classified as online, rather a mixed treatment modality. Posttreatment improvements were noted in mean sound pressure level for maximum sustained vowel phonation, reading, and monologue tasks. Although this study touched on the feasibility of online LSVT®LOUD delivery, there is a need for online applications to closely replicate face-to-face assessment and treatment delivery in order to be seen as an alternative/additional mode of service delivery.

Canada

The University of Sherbrooke, Québec

Some telepractice studies have been undertaken in Canada. In adult rehabilitation, a pilot study was conducted in Québec to investigate the feasibility of online delivery of anomia therapy (Dechêne et al., 2011). In this study, three participants with poststroke aphasia took part and were treated in the home setting. The telepractice application utilized included the following features: (1) videoconferencing using a high-speed Internet connection; (2) wide angle camera and omnidirectional microphone; and (3) touch screen tablet PC in the home to assist with the writing tasks. Participants received

12 sessions to improve their confrontation naming skills. The sessions included baseline assessment, lexical training, circumlocution training, and postassessment of trained stimuli. The study demonstrated the feasibility of online treatment of anomia with clinically relevant improvements noted for all participants on confrontation naming of trained items and to a lesser extent, untrained items. Participant satisfaction with the approach was also high for all.

Clinical considerations for SLPs. Certain areas for consideration regarding the study design were noted: (1) the use of two screens at the participant site for videoconferencing and display of printed material was found to impact on concentration for some participants; (2) some issues with eye contact were encountered by the SLP due to the positioning of the Web camera; (3) audiodelays affected turn-taking during some sessions; and (4) it may be necessary to consider the larger display of stimuli to assist participants with vision difficulties.

Children's Hearing and Speech Centre, British Columbia

Richardson (2012) described the telepractice programs offered through Children's Hearing and Speech Centre in British Columbia. Here, two programs were established to provide services for children with hearing loss outside of metro Vancouver. Children from birth to 3 years have access to AVT in the home (five children supported to date), and those from kindergarten to grade 12 receive speech, language, and listening intervention and other support in the school setting (14 children from seven schools supported to date). Both programs are conducted using a videoconferencing system via a dedicated high-speed Internet connection. The author noted that the programs have been embraced by the families and students, and that telepractice has eliminated the geographical barrier that would have impacted on parent choices for these children regarding their early intervention. Further objective data are needed to support these findings.

Clinical considerations for SLPs. The cost of equipment upgrades has been identified as a potential challenge in maintaining the high level of service, as the technology currently utilized has been discontinued. Ongoing training is also needed as a result of staffing changes, and for the school program, session planning and preparation (often by telephone or email) is integral as information technology support is variable.

The Netherlands

In addition to telepractice applications closely resembling face-to-face services and requiring the presence of an SLP, stand-alone web-based applications in the absence of an SLP are starting to be utilized. As noted earlier with the Web-based delivery of the Camperdown Program for adults who stutter, such applications have the advantage of allowing clients to receive treatment in their homes, and also to support and intensify therapy and to maintain outcomes once discharged from traditional face-to-face therapy. In the case of the latter, an E-learning based Speech Therapy (EST) web application was developed for speakers with dysarthria to help improve their vocal loudness (Beijer, Rietveld, Hoskam, et al., 2010; Beijer, Rietveld, van Beers, et al., 2010). The application allows the SLP to tailor make the speech training by selecting audio files from the hierarchy of vowels to sentences containing the target pitch and loudness levels for the client to listen to and practice. The client then uploads his or her recorded speech files and receives automatic feedback about their pitch and loudness. SLPs can further analyze the samples as needed. In a case study, Beijer, Rietveld, Hoskam and colleagues (2010) trialed EST with a participant diagnosed with PD (severity level of hypokinetic dysarthria not specified). The participant followed a 4-week home program and improved in speech intelligibility immediately posttreatment, with some maintenance at 11 weeks follow-up. The participant found the EST easy to use and the home treatment as convenient. An auditory discrimination test has also been developed for use in conjunction with the EST. The test has largely been shown to be a sensitive tool in determining client suitability for EST based on auditory discrimination skills, as it has been suggested that clients with difficulties discriminating their own speech from the target may have less than optimal outcomes with the EST, user dissatisfaction, or lower treatment retention (Beijer, Rietveld, & van Stiphout, 2011).

Speech-Language Pathologists and the Future of Telepractice

The studies reviewed in this chapter have provided the groundwork for telepractice research internationally and highlighted the benefits of this modality in the delivery of services to adult and pediatric clients with a range of communication and swallowing disorders. Future research will only strengthen the evidence base for this modality and support uptake into clinical practice. SLPs will also continue to play an integral role in advocating for this uptake through knowledge sharing of their programs and by providing clear information on the cost of services, which is currently lacking in all telepractice studies, the clinical uses of the service, infrastructure requirements and usability, and the undertaking of rigorous research studies to evaluate the effectiveness of telepractice. SLPs need to become adaptive lifelong learners and embrace the use of information and communication technology in teaching and learning opportunities. Investment in professional education will also be required to achieve this. At the same time, governing bodies, policies, and strategies around telepractice need to be established to further address issues surrounding malpractice and liability, privacy, confidentiality, and consent, and to assist with future funding. Some strategies for SLPs on knowledge sharing and reducing barriers to telepractice delivery are provided in Tables 11–1 and 11–2.

Table 11–1. Speech-Language Pathologists as Advocates for Telepractice Knowledge

Sharing of telepractice work should include detailed information on:
■ Technology requirements, setup, and procedures for running the service ■ Useability and SLP and client requirements ■ Infrastructure requirements (e.g., equipment, connectivity, and bandwidth specifications) ■ Cost of equipment and service (e.g., equipment, installation, maintenance, connectivity charges) ■ Cost-benefit of service to the organization and client ■ Licensure, reimbursement, and funding requirements (where applicable) ■ Clinical uses of telepractice in the management of clients with a wide range of communication and swallowing disorders

Table 11–1. *(continued)*

- Useful strategies for SLPs to facilitate successful service delivery
- User satisfaction from the perspective of the SLP and client, covering areas such as the audio and video quality, rapport, useability, and overall service delivery
- Rigorous research study designs investigating the effectiveness of telepractice (feasibility, validity, and reliability, with large-scale randomized controlled trials being the gold standard)
- Directions and recommendations for future research and uptake of telepractice

Table 11–2. Speech-Language Pathologists as Advocates for Telepractice

Strategies to Assist in Reducing Current Barriers
■ Take an interest in new technology and proactively incorporate this into clinical practice
■ Set direction for change and commit to it
■ Empower clients by providing them with optimal services to meet their individual needs
■ Motivate and support clients and colleagues with the transition into telepractice
■ Mentor and train colleagues in the use of new technology in clinical practice
■ Improve learning by undertaking professional education
■ Share knowledge through publications, presentations, and workshops
■ Advocate for telepractice at the community, institutional, and government level by sharing knowledge on the benefits of telepractice as a service delivery method
■ Become active members of professional associations with an interest in telepractice to enable further knowledge sharing at the clinical and research level
■ Get involved at the policy level and provide solutions for addressing current barriers

As greater resources are available to them, the developed countries continue to lead the research in telepractice and can assist with the uptake in developing countries by providing the evidence base for telepractice with a wide range of clinical services and client populations. Telepractice offers great prospects for addressing some of the toughest challenges for the world today in relation to access, equity, quality, and cost-effectiveness of health services. We need to embrace telepractice wholeheartedly as we devote this century to the empowerment of our clients.

> The empowerment contemplated in this insightful and ambitious statement can be found in the rapidly growing and increasingly accessible Internet. Conventional computers, desktops, and laptops have been joined by tablets and smart phones. Wired and wireless access to the Internet and its World Wide Web is transforming our ability to reach everyone online. About one third of the world's population has access to the Internet and more will join as long as infrastructure continues to grow and speeds increase. Soon these devices will be joined by an "Internet of Things" (appliances, office equipment, sensor networks, entertainment equipment, security and environmental monitoring systems). There is no end in sight.
>
> —Vint Cerf, Internet Pioneer

References

AG Bell Academy for Listening and Spoken Language. *The AG Bell Academy for Listening and Spoken Language*. Retrieved January 1, 2013, from http://www.listeningandspokenlanguage.org/AGBellAcademy/.

Australian Bureau of Statistics. (2011). *Regional population growth, Australia 2009–10.* (Cat. No. 3218). Canberra, ACT, Australia: Author.

Beijer, L. J., Rietveld, T. C. M., Hoskam, V., Geurts, A. C. H., & de Swart, B. J. M. (2010). Evaluating the feasibility and the potential efficacy of e-Learning-Based Speech Therapy (EST) as a Web application for speech training in dysarthric patients with Parkinson's disease: A case study. *Telemedicine and e-Health, 16*(6), 732–738.

Beijer, L. J., Rietveld, T. C. M., van Beers, M. M. A., Slangen, R. M. L., van den Heuvel, H., de Swart, B. J. M., et al. (2010). E-learning-based speech therapy: A Web application for speech training. *Telemedicine and e-Health, 16*(2), 177-180.

Beijer, L. J., Rietveld, A. C. M., & van Stiphout, A. J. L. (2011). Auditory discrimination as a condition for e-learning based speech therapy: A proposal for an auditory discrimination test (ADT) for adult dysarthric speakers. *Journal of Communication Disorders, 44*, 701-718.

Carey, B., O'Brian, S., Onslow, M., Block, S., Jones, M., & Packman, A. (2010). Randomized controlled non-inferiority trial of a telehealth treatment for chronic stuttering: The Camperdown Program. *International Journal of Language and Communication Disorders, 45*, 108-120.

Carey, B., O'Brian, S., Onslow, M., Packman, A., & Menzies, R. (2012). Webcam delivery of The Camperdown Program for adolescents who stutter: A Phase I trial. *Language, Speech, and Hearing Services in Schools, 43*, 370-380.

Chen, N-S., & Ko, L. (2010). An online synchronous test for professional interpreters. *Educational Technology and Society, 13*(2), 153-165.

Constantinescu, G. (2010). *The assessment and treatment of disordered speech and voice in Parkinson's disease using a PC-based telerehabilitation system*. Unpublished doctoral thesis, The University of Queensland, Brisbane, QLD, Australia.

Constantinescu, G. (2012). Satisfaction with telemedicine for teaching listening and spoken language to children with hearing loss. *Journal of Telemedicine and Telecare, 18*, 267-272.

Constantinescu, G., Theodoros, D., Russell, T., Ward, E., Wilson, S., & Wootton, R. (2010a). Asscssing disordered speech and voice in Parkin son's disease: A telerehabilitation application. *International Journal of Language and Communication Disorders, 45*(6), 630-644.

Constantinescu, G. A., Theodoros, D. G., Russell, T. G., Ward, E. C., Wilson, S. J., & Wootton, R. (2010b). Home-based speech treatment for Parkinson's disease delivered remotely: A case report. *Journal of Telemedicine and Telecare, 16*, 100-104.

Constantinescu, G., Theodoros, D., Russell, T., Ward, E., Wilson, S., & Wootton, R. (2011). Treating disordered speech and voice in Parkinson's disease online: A randomised controlled non-inferiority trial. *International Journal of Language and Communication Disorders, 46*, 1-16.

Constantinescu, G., Waite, M., Dornan, D., Rushbrooke, E., Brown, J., McGovern, J., Ryan, M., & Hill, A. (manuscript submitted for publication). *The effectiveness of telemedicine for teaching listening and spoken language to children with hearing loss*.

Darzi, A., Mirnezami, R., Macdonnell, M., & Nicholson, J. (2012). *Preparing for precision medicine*. Geneva, Switzerland: World Economic Forum.

Dean, D., DiGande, S., Field, D., Lundmak, A., O'Day, J., Pineda, J., & Zwillenberg, P. (2012). *The Internet economy in the G-20: The $4.2 trillion opportunity.* Boston, MA: Boston Consulting Group, Inc.

Dechêne, L., Tousignant, M., Boissy, P., Macoir, J., Héroux, S., Hamel, M., ... Pagé, C. (2011). Simulated in-home teletreatment for anomia. *International Journal of Telerehabilitation, 3*(2), 3–10.

Dodd, B., Holm, A., Oerlemans, M., & McCormick, M. (1996). *Queensland University Inventory of Literacy*. Brisbane, Australia: Department of Speech Pathology and Audiology, The University of Queensland.

Erickson, S. (2012). No boundaries: Perspectives of international Skype delivery of the Lidcombe Program. *Journal of Clinical Practice in Speech-Language Pathology, 14*(3), 146–148.

Erickson, S., Block, S., Menzies, R., Onslow, M., O'Brian, S., & Packman, A. (2012). Stand-alone Internet speech restructuring treatment for adults who stutter. *Journal of Clinical Practice in Speech-Language Pathology, 14*(3), 118–123.

Goodglass, H., Kaplan, E., & Barresi, B. (2001). *Boston Diagnostic Aphasia Examination* (3rd ed.). Philadelphia, PA: Lippincott, Williams & Wilkins.

Hastie, M., Hung, I-C., Chen, N-S., & Kinshuk. (2010). A blended synchronous learning model for educational international collaborations. *Innovations in Education and Teaching International, 47*, 9–24.

Helm-Estabrooks, N., & Ramsberger, G. (1986). Aphasia treatment delivered by telephone. *American Journal of Physical Medicine and Rehabilitation, 67*, 51–53.

Hill, A. J., & Miller, L. (2012). A survey of the clinical use of telehealth in speech-language pathology across Australia. *Journal of Clinical Practice in Speech-Language Pathology, 14*(3), 110–117.

Hill, A. J., Theodoros, D. G., Russell, T. G., & Ward, E. C. (2009a). The redesign and re-evaluation of an Internet-based telerehabilitation system for the assessment of dysarthria in adults. *Telemedicine and e-Health, 15*(9), 840–850.

Hill, A. J., Theodoros, D., Russell, T., & Ward, E. (2009b). Using telerehabilitation to assess apraxia of speech in adults. *International Journal of Language and Communication Disorders, 44*(5), 731–747.

Hill, A. J., Theodoros, D. G, Russell, T. G., Ward, E. C., & Wootton, R. (2009c). The effects of aphasia severity on the ability to assess language disorders via telerehabilitation. *Aphasiology, 23*(5), 627–642.

Howell, S., Tripoliti, E., & Pring, T. (2009). Delivering the Lee Silverman Voice Treatment (LSVT) by Web camera: A feasibility study. *International Journal of Language and Communication Disorders, 44*(3), 287–300.

Kaplan, W., Goodglass, H., & Weintraub, S. (2001). *Boston Naming Test* (2nd ed.). Baltimore, MD: Lippincott, Williams & Wilkins.

Lewis, C., Packman, A., Onslow, M., Simpson, J., & Jones, M. (2008). A phase II trial of telehealth delivery of the Lidcombe Program of early stuttering intervention. *American Journal of Speech-Language Pathology, 17*, 139–149.

Mashima, P. A., Birkmire-Peters, D. P., Syms, M. J., Holtel, M. R., Burgess, L. P., & Peters, L. J. (2003). Telehealth: Voice therapy using telecommunications technology. *American Journal of Speech-Language Pathology, 12*(4), 432–439.

McCarthy, M. (2012). RIDBC Teleschool™: A hub of expertise. *Volta Review, 112*(3), 373–381.

McCarthy, M., Muñoz, K., & White, K. R. (2010). Teleintervention for infants and young children who are deaf or hard-of-hearing. *Pediatrics, 126*(Suppl. 1), 52–58.

Neale, M. D. (1999). *Neale Analysis of Reading Ability: Manual and reader* (3rd ed.). Camberwell, Australia: Australian Council for Educational Research.

O'Brian, S., Onslow, M., Cream, A., & Packman, A. (2003). The Camperdown Program: Outcomes of a new prolonged-speech treatment model. *Journal of Speech, Language, and Hearing Research, 46*, 933–946.

O'Brian, S., Packman, A., & Onslow, M. (2008). Telehealth delivery of the Camperdown Program for adults who stutter: A phase I trial. *Journal of Speech, Language, and Hearing Research, 51*, 184–195.

Onslow, M., Packman, A., & Harrison, E. (2003). *Lidcombe Program of Early Stuttering Intervention: A clinician's guide*. Austin, TX: Pro-Ed.

Ramig, L. O., Bonitati, C. M., Lemke, J. H., & Horii, Y. (1994). Voice treatment for patients with Parkinson's disease: Development of an approach and preliminary efficacy data. *Journal of Medical Speech-Language Pathology, 2*(3), 191–209.

Richardson, L.L. (2012). Children's Hearing and Speech Centre—Telepractice programs. *Volta Review, 112*(3), 429–433.

Rushbrooke, E. (2012). *Remote MAPping for children with cochlear implants.* Unpublished master's thesis, The University of Queensland, Brisbane, QLD, Australia.

Semel, E., Wiig, E. H., & Secord, W. A. (2003). *Clinical evaluations of language fundamentals* (4th ed.). San Antonio, TX: Psychology Corporation.

Sharma, S., Ward, E. C., Burns, C., Theodoros, D., & Russell, T. (2011). Assessing swallowing disorders online: A pilot telerehabilitation study. *Telemedicine and e-Health, 17*(9), 688–695.

The World Bank. (2012). *Millennium development goals: Goal 2: Achieve universal primary education by 2015.* Retrieved December 15, 2012, from http://www.worldbank.org/mdgs/education.html.

United Nations. (2005). *The millennium development goals report.* New York, NY: Author.

Vaughn, G. R. (1976). Tel-communicology: Health-care delivery system for persons with communicative disorders. *American Speech-Language-Hearing Association, 18,* 13–17.

Waite, M. C., Theodoros, D. G., Russell, T. G., & Cahill, L. M. (2010a). Internet-based telehealth assessment of language using the CELF-4. *Language, Speech and Hearing Services in Schools, 41,* 445–458.

Waite, M. C., Theodoros, D. G., Russell, T. G., & Cahill, L. M. (2010b). Assessment of children's literacy via an Internet-based telehealth system. *Telemedicine and e-Health, 16*(5), 564–575.

Waite, M. C., Theodoros, D. G., Russell, T. G., & Cahill, L. M. (2012). Assessing children's speech intelligibility and oral structures, and functions via an Internet-based telehealth system. *Journal of Telemedicine and Telecare, 18,* 198–203.

Wang, Y., Chen, N-S., & Levy, M. (2010). The design and implementation of a holistic training model for language teacher education in a cyber face-to-face learning environment. *Computers and Education, 55*(2), 777–788.

Ward, E., Crombie, J., Trickey, M., Hill, A., Theodoros, D., & Russell, T. (2009). Assessment of communication and swallowing post-laryngectomy: A telerehabilitation trial. *Journal of Telemedicine and Telecare, 15,* 232–237.

Ward, E. C., Sharma, S., Burns, C., Theodoros, D., & Russell, T. (2012a). Validity of conducting clinical dysphagia assessments for patients with normal to mild cognitive impairment via telerehabilitation. *Dysphagia, 27,* 460–472.

Ward, E. C., Sharma, S., Burns, C., Theodoros, D., & Russell, T. (2012b). Managing patient factors in the assessment of swallowing via telerehabilitation. *International Journal of Telemedicine and Applications, Early online article,* 1–6.

Wertz, R. T., Dronkers, N. F., Berstein-Ellis, E., Sterling, L. K., Shubitowski, R. E., Shenaut, G. K., et al. (1992). Potential of telephonic and television technology for appraising and diagnosing neurogenic communication disorders in remote settings. *Aphasiology, 6,* 195–202.

Westwood, P. (2005). *Spelling: Approaches to teaching and assessment* (2nd ed.). Camberwell, Australia: Australian Council for Educational Research.

Wilson, L., Onslow, M., & Lincoln, M. (2004). Telehealth adaptation of the Lidcombe Program of early stuttering intervention: Five case studies. *American Journal of Speech-Language Pathology, 13*, 81-93.

World Health Organization (2010). *Telemedicine: Opportunities and Developments in Member States: Report on the Second Global Survey on eHealth.* Geneva, Switzerland: Author.

Yorkston, K. M., & Beukelman, D. R. (1981). *Assessment of intelligibility of dysarthric speech.* Austin, TX: Pro-Ed.

Zimmerman, I. L., Steiner, V. G., & Pond, R. E. (2002). *Preschool language scale* (4th ed.). San Antonio, TX: Psychological Corporation.

12

Future Directions in Telepractice and Service Delivery

K. Todd Houston, Anne M. Fleming, and Kelly J. Brown

Introduction

The renowned writer and futurist, Alvin Toffler, has been credited as stating, "the illiterate of the 21st century are not those who cannot read and write but those who cannot learn, unlearn, and relearn" (Toffler, n.d.). Today, society continues to adapt to rapid technological adoption in almost every aspect of work and home life and even health care, which is affecting how individuals relate to each other and to professionals who provide specialized services. New technologies, usually enabled by broadband Internet connectivity, are eliminating barriers caused by distance and bringing like-minded people together to connect, to share information, to learn, and to advocate. Not surprisingly, Americans are connecting to the Internet in the largest numbers in history, with 85% of all U.S. adults reporting frequent Internet use (Fox, 2012). High-speed, broadband Internet availability continues to grow with a reported 66% of U.S. homes now having this level of connectivity (Smith, 2010). Through federal efforts, such as those funded by the U.S. Department of Agriculture, and other localized state initiatives, rural and underserved areas of the country are gaining broadband Internet connectivity (IOM, 2012). Likewise, Internet habits are changing as well. When adults who report using the Internet were asked about their usage, 59% responded that they seek out health information—often from peer-to-peer interactions (Fox, 2012). These new levels of connectivity, coupled with tablet and notebook computers and smartphones, create a rich virtual environment for continued expansion of telepractice service delivery models and mobile health applications within speech-language pathology. Although some barriers may still exist, those will be eliminated in time. For speech-language pathologists, knowledge of the prevailing trends in technology, health care, and practice standards will allow a more proactive approach to telepractice and will help ensure that more children and adults have access to the vital speech and language services they are seeking.

Changes in Technology

Mobile Technology

Mobile phones and tablet computers have revolutionized the way that people send and receive information, making it possible for consumers to share audio, video, and text data through a cellular or wireless Internet (i.e., wifi) data connection. In 2013, an estimated 87% of Americans have a cell phone, with 45% of these individuals owning a smartphone (i.e., Internet connectivity capability and features beyond basic text and phone service). More significantly, 55% of Americans are using a smartphone to access the Internet and almost one-third report that they use their smartphone as their primary device to access the Internet (Brenner, 2013).

Many smartphones allow users to connect using face-to-face video calling. There are free "voice over internet protocol" (VoIP) software programs (e.g., Skype, ooVoo, WiCall, Fring, MobileVoip, Tango, etc.) that offer applications supported by a variety of smartphones. These applications allow users to make videophone calls to another user by signing up for a free username and agreeing to terms and conditions. FaceTime, an Apple product, is built-in software that allows the same functionality. As was mentioned in previous chapters, the current limitations to these free software applications include privacy and encryption concerns, and practitioners must ensure that these services adhere to appropriate standards.

Usage of mobile devices (e.g., smartphones, tablet computers) is expected to continue to grow over the next decade. It is predicted that sales of these devices will increase to 215 million by 2016, which is a 25% increase in 5 years (Greenspun & Coughlin, 2012). In addition, it is estimated that there will be 10 billion mobile devices in use worldwide by 2016 (Fox, 2012). The highest rates of tablet computer ownership occur with adults age 35 to 44 with almost half (49%) now owning such a device, which is significantly more than any other age group (Zickuhr, 2013). As well, an expected 1.4 billion mobile health and fitness apps (i.e., mobile software applications) will be downloaded by 2017, with health apps increasing the fastest over the next 5 years (Slabodkin, 2013). Current data trends indicate that as more people gain access to mobile devices that have broadband connectivity, the potential for using this technology to seek medical information, monitor health conditions, or participate in telepractice services will increase. More importantly, consumers will demand this level of connectivity from their health care service providers, which will increase the information flow from the practitioner to the patient.

Prevailing trends indicate that hospitals, medical centers, and physician practices are greatly expanding their use of mobile technology and social media to connect with their patients. Although some physicians are embracing this new level of connectivity, others argue that health care providers are just starting to comprehend the potential that these technologies, when appropriately utilized, can do to improve patient outcomes. In his book, *The Creative Destruction of Medicine: How the Digital Revolution Will Create Better Health Care* (Topol, 2012), Dr. Eric Topol describes the biggest innovations of the past 30 years to be:

1. Internet, broadband
2. personnel computer and laptop
3. mobile phones

4. e-mail
5. DNA testing and sequencing.

Topol acknowledges that the typical smartphone now incorporates the first four of these innovations. In time, he predicts that the fifth, DNA testing and sequencing, will be added to mobile devices. Topol states, "these extraordinary accomplishments . . . have set up a profound digital disruption of medicine. Until now we did not have the digital infrastructure to even contemplate such a sea change in medicine. And until now the digital revolution has barely intersected the medical world. But the emergence of powerful tools to digitize human beings with full support of such infrastructure creates an unparalleled opportunity to inevitably and forever change the face of how health care is delivered," (Topol, 2012, p. 5). Thus, the evolution of these technologies will continue to impact health care, how practitioners will communicate and interact with their patients, and how diagnostic and treatment services are delivered across disciplines, including speech-language pathology.

Mobile Health

The convergence of broadband Internet connections, ease of technology use, and patients' access to mobile devices (e.g., smartphones, tablet computes, portable monitoring devices, etc.) has facilitated a rich environment for the rapid adoption of mobile health or mHealth applications. In short, mHealth is a range of health care services supported by mobile devices. In more specific terms, mobile telemedicine may be defined as the communication or consultation between health care professionals and patients using voice, text, data, imaging, or video functions of a mobile device (World Health Organization, 2011). Whereas other health care disciplines have adopted mHealth platforms and support a range of services, the potential for its use in speech-language pathology is just now being realized.

Mobile health technology has the potential to generate substantial cost savings through remote health monitoring and reporting. One study estimated the savings could near $197 billion over

25 years in the United States (Fox, 2012). Remote monitoring technology uses mobile devices to transmit health information taken in real time from patients, reducing the need for them to visit their health care provider to obtain comparable data. One such use could be "gluco phones" (i.e., smartphones with an app used to measure glucose levels in the blood) that transmit these results to physicians for monitoring.

Beyond fitness and wellness monitoring, the possibilities for remote monitoring devices and mobile device applications that cater to health care needs are endless. In speech-language pathology, various applications—such as those designed for tablet computers—are available to clinicians to use as tools to deliver specific interventions, treatments, counseling, and to track patient outcome data. For many speech-language pathologists, their tablet computer and its range of apps have become an essential tool that is utilized daily.

Through a combination of mHealth tools and telepractice, treatment has the potential to be more individualized, functional, and community-based. For example, using a smartphone or tablet and an encrypted connection, a clinician may be able to coach a patient who has suffered a traumatic brain injury by seeing and hearing him attempt the memory strategies in a more natural, community setting. The clinician may be in her office while the patient visits his favorite coffee shop, and the clinician can easily monitor how the patient is using his learned strategies and could even provide coaching and feedback in real time. These technologies may free both the patient and the clinician from the sterile treatment rooms that often result in contrived scenarios and reduced carryover and generalization of targeted skills.

The potential for remote monitoring in speech-language pathology is feasible as well. That is, a smartphone with an app could be designed to monitor patient performance in various situations. For example, for a patient who is attempting to improve his fluency, the app could measure how many dysfluencies occurred under various conditions, the number of communication partners, the time of day they occurred, and the geographic location of the patient at the time. This performance data could be monitored, collected, and uploaded automatically to a secure database for later analysis by the speech-language pathologist. Collecting this type of functional outcome data will allow for more individualized and focused treatment and intervention for both pediatric and adult patients with a range of communication delays and disorders.

Although not an app used with a smartphone or tablet computer, an innovative system has been developed to collect data about parent-child language interactions. The Language Environment Analysis (LENA) system allows a clinician to monitor the language input given to a child during daily interactions as well as an analysis of conversational turns taken between a caregiver and a child (LENA, 2013). The child wears a device that records the interactions and is later analyzed by specialized software on a computer. The system provides estimations of adult words, conversational turns, child vocalizations, and TV and electronic sounds (i.e., background noise) in a child's natural language environment, and a breakdown of the composition of the audio environment. The system also includes Automatic Vocalization Assessment (AVA) and LENA Developmental Snapshot assessments that measure expressive and receptive language skills (LENA, 2013). The clinician can use this information to give feedback to parents and caregivers about the language environment in the home. By using this remote monitoring device and the accompanying software, clinicians are able to obtain a more detailed understanding of the daily interactions between the parent and child, which can lead to more tailored interventions that foster improved communication development and outcomes. The LENA system can be a useful tool and is just one example how mobile technology is shaping clinical practice.

Digital and Social Media

The terms digital media and social media frequently are used interchangeably. However, purists would argue that the term "digital" refers to the *medium* in which information is conveyed (i.e., Internet, online). Social media, more specifically, represents those channels or outlets that allow users, such as speech-language pathologists and their patients, to make connections. Defining it more specifically, Kaplan and Haenlein (2010) refer to social media as the use of web-based and mobile devices (e.g., smartphones, tablet computers) to turn communication into an interactive dialogue that allows for the creation and exchange of user-generated content. To clarify the various forms of social media, the researchers developed a classification scheme to describe each:

- collaborative projects (e.g., Wikipedia)
- blogs and microblogs (e.g., WordPress, Twitter, Tumblr)
- content communities (e.g., YouTube, Vimeo, Flickr)
- social networking sites (e.g., Facebook, LinkedIn, Google+)
- virtual game worlds (e.g., World of Worldcraft)
- virtual social worlds (e.g., Second Life)
  (Kaplan & Haenlein, 2010)

Recently, Duggan and Brenner (2013) found that 67% of Internet users report using a social networking site, and whereas other sites continue to attract users, Facebook continues to be the dominant online destination. To illustrate, by the end of year in 2004, 1 million active users were on Facebook. This number was quickly eclipsed and has grown exponentially since, capping over 1 billion users by the end of 2012 (facebook.com). On a variety of social networking sites, individuals are logging on to like, comment, connect, share, tweet, repost, pin, blog, and follow areas of interest ranging from celebrities to grassroots causes and everything in between. Many national product chains have turned to social media to help promote their brand and to connect with new consumers. Increasingly, social media is becoming a tool for health care providers, including speech-language pathologists, to connect with and interact with patients and attract new ones.

A survey of 1,060 U.S. adults by the Health Research Institute (2012) profiled their health care-related social media activities. The following results represent the growing connection between social media and health care.

- 42% of responders have used social media to access health-related consumer reviews (e.g., of treatments or physicians);

- Nearly 30% of responders have supported a health-related cause;
- 25% of responders have posted online about a health-related experience;
- 20% of responders have joined a health forum or community;
- 61% of responders say they would trust information posted by a health care provider;
- 41% of responders say they are likely to share with providers via social media;
- More than 80% of people aged 18 to 24 are likely to share health care information through social media websites; and
- Nearly 90% of individuals would engage in health care activities or trust information found via social media.

Social Networks

More specifically, Masic, Sivic, Toromanovic, Borojevic, & Pandza (2011) define a social network as a social structure made of individuals or organizations associated with one or more types of interdependence (friendship, common interests, work, knowledge, prestige) that can be organized to exchange information, knowledge, or financial assistance. When analyzing the current use of online social networking within health care, the authors propose dividing these networks into several groups, depending on methods, field of operations, or expertise of those who participate in specific networks:

- Social networks with personal connectivity (e.g., transplant networks, individuals with specific diagnoses, etc.);
- Global Internet social networks (e.g., Facebook, LinkedIn);
- Specific Internet health-related social networks (e.g., Health Care Forums, group pages where topics are discussed through postings);
- Medial social Internet networks for nonprofessionals (e.g., DailyStrength, CaringBridge, CarePages, etc.);
- Scientific Internet social networks (e.g., BiomedExperts, ResearchGate, iMedExchange, etc.);

- Social Internet networks supported by professionals (e.g., the American Speech-Language Hearing Association's ASHA Community); and
- Scientific networks in the world's biomedical literature databases (e.g., Current Contents, ISI Web Knowledge, PubMed/Medline, EBSCO, etc.).

As Masic et al. (2012, p. 52) state, "social networks today have a very significant impact on health promotion and allow millions of users fast, easy and concise access to the most important and useful medical information." For many speech-language pathologists, the typical means of connecting with other practitioners or with their patients most likely is through more traditional tools: a static website, phone calls, or e-mail. Although useful in some contexts, these methods are proving to be time consuming, inefficient, and no longer match the expectations of today's health consumers—which are our patients. Social media and online social networking are supporting direct ways of connecting, communicating, and collaborating with other practitioners and with new and potential patients. Simply relaying information is no longer adequate; basic information should be provided as a starting point that facilitates deeper engagement and prolonged interaction. Moving forward, it will be imperative for speech-language pathologists to establish a digital presence for their respective programs. Some professionals may choose to become "curators" of information and use their social networking sites as a collection of resources for patients—thus becoming a professional seen as a source of reliable information. Articles of interest to a particular health demographic could be pooled together by the practitioner and shared with current and prospective patients. This model allows for the rapid distribution of material as well as possible person-to-person interactions. Other speech-language pathologists may choose to produce their own unique user-generated material that can be distributed through social networking. For example, a short video detailing how to do a listening check with a child with hearing loss could be produced and shared across multiple social media sites. With the click of a mouse, patients could access this instructional video and gain valuable information from a respected professional. A combination of both approaches would create a database of both original and collected material. More importantly, as patients increasingly search for information and resources, speech-language pathologists must have a presence in these digital communities. As Howard Luks, MD, states, "At its heart, digital media is about people, it is about relationships, it is about communication. A social media presence is about educating, engaging and growing your audience, improving outcomes, and compliance" (Luks, 2011).

Gamification and Simulated Clinical Experiences

Gamification is the use of game mechanics and game design techniques in nongame contexts, (Mashable, 2013), such as health care or even speech-language pathology. Typically, gamification applies to nongame applications and processes, in order to encourage people to adopt them, or to influence how they are used. Gamification works by making technology more engaging, by encouraging users to engage in desired behaviors, by showing a path to mastery and autonomy, by helping to solve problems and not being a distraction, and by taking advantage of humans' psychological predisposition to engage in gaming. The technique can encourage people to perform chores that they ordinarily consider boring, such as completing surveys, shopping, filling out tax forms, or reading Web sites (Mashable, 2013).

Gamification is just beginning to play a role in the field of speech-language pathology. When developed with a specific desired educational or clinical outcome, gaming can be engaging, highly motivating, and can function to reinforce specific communication behaviors that may be difficult to otherwise practice consistently in more traditional "therapy" settings. More importantly, games have been shown to foster greater transfer of newly learned skills from an educational or clinical setting to a real-world setting (Gibson, Aldrich, & Prensky, 2007). As Williams (2013) describes, "Imagine being able to offer clients the opportunity to complete an online simulation for any everyday scenario, such as ordering at a fast food restaurant or interacting with peers in a school cafeteria setting. SLP professionals would be able to observe real-time client behaviors in a variety of simulated settings."

Cloud Computing

As technology continues to evolve, a shift toward *cloud computing* has already started to occur. Simply put, a cloud-based system allows users to upload information into a Web server that functions as a virtual hard drive (i.e., the cloud). The information stored in the cloud can then be accessed by multiple users and/or by different devices (e.g., notebook or tablet computer, smartphone). Applying cloud computing to speech-language pathology—and especially to telepractice—will allow clinicians and clients to share information easily and from multiple devices. In an asynchronous telepractice service delivery model, the clinician could upload a video recording of the session into the cloud that could be accessed later by the client on a smartphone, tablet, or laptop. Likewise, virtual games with built-in simulations of speech and language targets could be played within the cloud, and the patient's outcome data could be reviewed simultaneously or at a later time by the clinician.

In a synchronous telepractice service delivery model, the session could take place through the cloud using multiple systems and continue to access the same information. For example, Polycom has released software that utilizes cloud technology to allow users of various software programs, such as Facebook, Skype, and Google Talk, to connect and interact in real time. That is, multiple users are able to connect simultaneously without requiring dedicated videoconferencing hardware systems at multiple locations. Similarly, Cisco, the company that now manufactures the Tandberg videoconferencing systems, also has entered the cloud computing arena. A relatively new software called Cisco Jabber (formally known as Movi) allows users to connect from multiple locations through a range of devices to participate in a teleconferencing session.

Thus, cloud-based computing will continue to evolve and various applications that support telepractice service delivery models and gamification will be developed and/or refined. Going forward, cloud-based computing will continue to affect various aspects of speech-language pathology, and because most mobile devices, such as tablet computers and smartphones, are manufactured to interact seamlessly with "the cloud," the opportunity exists for further expansion of telepractice models and gamification that have not yet been realized.

Pre-service and In-service Training: Increasing Capacity in the Delivery of Telepractice

To ensure that telepractice becomes a more standard service delivery model, university training programs will need coursework, supervised practica, and field-based experiences that provide graduate students in speech-language pathology with the foundational training for them to become competent telepractitioners. Presently, at least three universities—Kent State University, the University of Maine, and the University of Akron—are considered among the earliest adopters of telepractice-related coursework and clinical practicum for students in speech-language pathology.

Through the School of Speech-Language Pathology and Audiology at the University of Akron, students have the opportunity to take coursework on topics related to telepractice and are assigned to participate in clinical practica through the Telepractice and eLearning Laboratory (TeLL). The TeLL is an on-site telepractice clinic in which graduate students treat patients at a distance under the supervision of faculty who are certified speech-language pathologists and have extensive experience providing services through telepractice. Through the TeLL, graduate students learn how to troubleshoot the telecommunications equipment, how to remotely collect patient outcome data, how to effectively deliver speech and language services at a distance to both children and adults, and how to coach parents when the child is a preschooler or younger. In addition, the graduate students evaluate their own performance and receive feedback from an experienced faculty member. The program is growing and currently allows a select number of graduate students to leave the university with the knowledge and skills to implement telepractice into their future practice.

For practicing professionals, the American Speech-Language-Hearing Association (ASHA) continues to expand its advocacy, resources, and training opportunities for its members. Its most recent Special Interest Group (SIG) is devoted to telepractice in speech-language pathology and audiology (SIG 18), and one of the fastest growing SIGs within the association. Furthermore, ASHA has developed a preferred practice portal devoted to telepractice, which is becoming an invaluable resource for practitioners. And, as any interested attendee would notice, the number of short courses and general sessions devoted to telepractice service delivery continues to rise with each annual convention.

Outside of ASHA, other organizations continue to be leaders in training, policy development, and advocacy. Most notably, the American Telemedicine Association (ATA) has its own SIG devoted to telerehabilitation, which includes membership from a range of allied health disciplines (please see Appendix C for the ATA's "A Blueprint for Telerehabilitation Guidelines"). Organizations that support specific interventions or causes and have large professional memberships, such as the Alexander Graham Bell Association for the Deaf and Hard of Hearing (AG Bell), also can provide opportunities for training and produce scholarly publications that support telepractice (Stedler-Brown, 2012). And finally, professional learning communities devoted to telepractice service delivery models, such as the one hosted by the National Center for Hearing Assessment and Management (NCHAM) at Utah State University, have proved to be effective outlets to share knowledge, resources, and other materials among professionals who are interested in telepractice service delivery models (Behl, Houston, & Stedler-Brown, 2012). The availability of these professional training and networking opportunities are encouraging, and as telepractice models are more widely adopted, practitioners will need a range of professional development opportunities from short courses and workshops to more in-depth residences in facilities that can host extensive in-service training.

Conclusion

The field of speech-language pathology has arrived at an exciting point in its history. Changes in telecommunications technology, the availability of broadband Internet connections, the widespread use of mobile devices such as smartphones and tablet computers, the growth in social media and social networking, new federal health care policies, and increasing consumer demand for technology-enabled interactions with health care providers have all combined to create exciting opportunities for the use of telepractice service delivery models and mobile health applications. Although issues related to professional licensure and insurance reimbursement continue to affect practice, these challenges will be resolved through ongoing professional and consumer advocacy. Technological advances are changing how speech-language pathologists practice, and as President John F. Kennedy said, "Change is the law of life. And those who look only to the past or present are certain to miss the future." As speech-language pathologists, we should embrace the future and leverage these new opportunities to ensure that more children and adults who need our services are able to receive them. The only limitation we have is our imagination.

References

American Speech-Language-Hearing Association. (2005). *Speech-language pathologists providing clinical services via telepractice: Technical report* [Technical report]. Available from http://www.asha.org/policy.

American Telemedicine Association. (2010). *Telemedicine in the Patient Protection and Affordable Care Act*. Retrieved from http://www.americantelemed.org/docs/default-source/policy/telehealth-provisions-within-the-patient-protection-and-affordable-care-act.pdf.

Behl, D. D., Houston, K. T., & Stedler-Brown, A. (2012). The value of a learning community to support telepractice for infants and toddlers with hearing loss. *Volta Review, 112*(3), 313–327.

Brenner, J. (2013, Jan. 31). *Pew Internet: Mobile. Pew Research Center's Internet and American Life Project.* Retrieved from http://pewinternet.org/Commentary/2012/February/Pew-Internet-Mobile.aspx.

Duggan, M., & Brenner, J. (2013). *The demographics of social media users–2012. Pew Research Center's Internet and American Life Project.* Retrieved from http://www.pewinternet.org/~/media//Files/Reports/2013/PIP_SocialMediaUsers.pdf.

Fox, S. (2012, Nov. 8). *Mobile health 2012. Pew Research Center's Internet and American Life Project.* Retrieved from http://www.pewinternet.org/~/media//Files/Reports/2012/PIP_MobileHealth2012.pdf.

Gibson, D., Aldrich, C., & Prensky, M. (2007). *Games and simulations in online learning: Research and development frameworks*. Hershey, PA: Information Science Publishing.

Greenspun, H., & Coughlin, S. (2012). *mHealth in an mworld: How mobile technology is transforming health care.* Retrieved from http://www.deloitte.com/assets/Dcom-UnitedStates/Local%20Assets/Documents

/us_chs_2012_mHealth_HowMobileTechnologyIsTransformingHealthcare_032213.pdf.

Health Research Institute. (2012). *Social media "likes" healthcare: From marketing to social business*. PricewaterhouseCoopers. Retrieved from http://www.pwc.com/us/en/health-industries/publications/health-care-social-media.jhtml.

Institute of Medicine. (2012). *The role of telehealth in an evolving health care environment: Workshop summary.* Washington, DC: National Academies Press.

Kaplan, A. M., & Haenlein, M. (2010). Users of the world, unite! The challenges and opportunities of social media. *Business Horizons*, *53*, 59–68.

LENA. (2013). *Lena: Every word counts.* Retrieved from http://www.lenababy.com/LenaHome/why-use-lena-home.aspx.

Luks, H. (2011). *Establishing a digital media presence. Mayo Clinic.* Retrieved from http://socialmedia.mayoclinic.org/.

Mashable (2013). *Gamification.* Retrieved from http://mashable.com/category/gamification/.

Masic, I., Sivic, S., Toromanovic, S., Borojevic, T., & Pandza, H. (2012). Social networks in improvement of health care. *Materia Socio Medica*, *24*(1), 48–53.

Slabodkin, G. (2013). *Report: 1.4 billion mobile health, fitness app downloads by 2017.* FierceMobile Healthcare. Retrieved from http://www.fiercemobilehealthcare.com/story/report-14-billion-mobile-health-fitness-app-downloads-2017/2013-06-03.

Smith, A. (2010, Aug. 11). *Home broadband 2010.* Retrieved from http://www.pewinternet.org/~/media//Files/Reports/2010/Homebroadband2010.pdf.

Stedler-Brown, A. (Ed.). (2012). Current knowledge and best practices for telepractice [Monograph]. *Volta Review, 112*(3), 191–447.

Topol, E. (2012). *The creative destruction of medicine: How the digital revolution will create better health care*. New York, NY: Basic Books.

Williams, S. (2013). Telepractice: New and emerging technologies that promise change. *Perspectives on Telepractice*, *3*(1), 23–30.

World Health Organization. (2011). mhealth: New horizons for health through mobile technologies. *Global Observatory for eHealth Series*, *3*, 1–112. Retrieved from http://www.who.int/goe/publications/goe_mhealth_web.pdf.

Zickuhr, K. (2013). *Tablet ownership 2013. Pew Research Center's Internet and American Life Project.* Retrieved from http://pewinternet.org/Reports/2013/Tablet-Ownership-2013.aspx.

APPENDIX A

School-Based Telepractice Needs Assessment

Based on Crutchley, S., Dudding, C., Grogan-Johnson, S., and Alvares, R. (November 2010).

Category	Needs	Challenges	Associated Cost?	Solutions
Infrastructure & Equipment				
1. What room/space is available for telepractice services at SLP and student locations? 2. Are the room characteristics adequate at each site? (Consider: door/privacy, phone connection, sufficient electrical outlets, adequate lighting, room acoustics, handicap accessibility, proximity to printer, scanner, fax machine) 3. What equipment is needed? (May include: dedicated videoconferencing equipment, computer, wide-screen monitor, Web camera, document camera, headsets, microphone, audio splitter, scanner, printer, fax, telephone, desk, table, chairs) 4. What equipment is already available? 5. Do you have adequate Internet access? (Consider: available bandwidth during peak usage, potential need to reconfigure firewalls to allow telepractice, availability of hard wired vs. wireless access)				

Category	Needs	Challenges	Associated Cost?	Solutions
Personnel & Training				
1. Do you have SLP(s) with required state credentials? 2. Do you have a paraprofessional to assist at the student site? 3. Define the roles and responsibilities for the SLP and the assistant in telepractice. 4. How will these roles and responsibilities be communicated to the SLP and assistant? 5. How will you train the SLP and assistant on correct use and troubleshooting of telepractice equipment? 6. Is there CE available to provide the SLP with skills needed to be successful in providing telepractice? 7. Are IT personnel available for initial set up and ongoing support at both sites? 8. Who will supervise the paraprofessional? 9. Will substitutes be trained and available for the SLP and the paraprofessional?				
Intervention Program				
1. How will you select your clients? 2. How will you determine that telepractice is suitable for your clients? 3. What alternatives are available if a client is not able to participate in telepractice?				

Category	Needs	Challenges	Associated Cost?	Solutions
Intervention Program				
4. How will you consider Least Restrictive Environment? 5. Will your students be seen individually or in groups? 6. Is the selected technology adequate to support group intervention? (Consider the need for multiple headsets, wide-angle Web camera, seating arrangements, student distance from microphone) 7. What student-related services will be available? (Consider IEP and MFE meetings, parent meetings, open house, team meetings, CE) 8. How will you gather student data (electronically vs. physical data recording)? 9. Where will student data be stored? 10. How will documentation be completed? (Consider access to district software or online services) 11. What therapy materials are needed? (Consider software, online resources, permission to scan and use copyrighted therapy materials, books, materials for use with a document camera) 12. What is the procedure for troubleshooting and assistance with technology glitches?				

Category	Needs	Challenges	Associated Cost?	Solutions
Integration & Collaboration				
1. Do you have support from the building principal, special education director, IT coordinator, and other district decision makers? 2. How will you introduce the project to faculty, parents, and students? 3. How will you integrate the project with other services in the district? 4. What mechanisms are in place to provide ongoing communication to parents and faculty regarding student progress? 5. How will you establish collaborative relationships with general education teachers? 6. What mechanism is in place to respond to parent and faculty concerns? 7. How will you integrate your services with the general curriculum? 8. What is the role of the SLP and the paraprofessional in communicating with faculty and parents 9. Have you identified and considered cultural and/or diversity issues? (Consider traditional practices, idiosyncratic words, views on technology)				

Category	Needs	Challenges	Associated Cost?	Solutions
Continuous Improvement/Evaluation				
1. How will you measure faculty, parent, and student satisfaction? 2. How will you measure student success? 3. How will you be aware of new advances in telepractice technology? 4. How will you measure reliability of technology?				
Funding/Reimbursement/Cost of Service Delivery				
1. Will the service be provided by a district employee or by contracted services? 2. Who will purchase and maintain the necessary equipment? 3. Is Medicaid reimbursement available? 4. Can the paraprofessional accept additional school-related responsibilities in addition to working with the telepractice project? 5. Will a time study be completed to determine increased efficiency? 6. Are grants or donations available to help fund the program?				
Safeguards				
1. How will student data and records be maintained? 2. Have you completed a risk analysis to ensure necessary HIPPA and IDEA compliance? 3. Do you have a copy of the district regulations for maintaining student confidentiality?				

Category	Needs	Challenges	Associated Cost?	Solutions
Safeguards Continued				
4. Do you need to develop security and privacy guidelines specifically for this project? 5. How will you communicate the privacy and security guidelines to parents? 6. Are the security and privacy guidelines included in the training for the telepractice SLP and paraprofessional?				

APPENDIX B

American Speech-Language-Hearing Association's Practice Portal: Telepractice

The goal of the American Speech-Language-Hearing Association's (ASHA) Practice Portal is to assist audiologists and speech-language pathologists in their day-to-day practices by making it easier to find the best available evidence and expertise in patient care, identify resources that have been vetted for relevance and credibility, and increase practice efficiency. Our goal is not to provide a practice "recipe" but to make available to you the information and resources you need to guide your decision-making. The Practice Portal site and the content of the clinical and professional issues topics are in "beta" mode and will evolve in response to user feedback.

To view the Practice Portal, visit the link at: http://www.asha.org/practice-portal/

Overview

Telepractice is the application of telecommunications technology to the delivery of speech-language pathology and audiology professional services at a distance by linking clinician to client/patient or clinician-to-clinician for assessment, intervention, and/or consultation.

Supervision, mentoring, and preservice and continuing education are other activities that may be conducted through the use of technology. However, these activities are not included in ASHA's definition of telepractice and are best referred to as telesupervision/distance supervision and distance education. (See Clinical Supervision in Speech-Language Pathology: Technical Report [ASHA, 2008] for information related to the use of technology in clinical supervision in speech-language pathology.)

ASHA adopted the term *telepractice* rather than the frequently used terms telemedicine or telehealth to avoid the misperception that these services are used only in health care settings. Other terms such as teleaudiology, telespeech, and speech teletherapy may be used in addition to telepractice. Services delivered by audiologists and speech-language pathologists are also included in the broader generic term telerehabilitation (American Telemedicine Association, 2010). The use of telepractice does not remove any existing responsibilities in delivering services, including adherence to the Code of Ethics, Scope of Practice in Audiology, and Scope of Practice in Speech-Language Pathology, state and federal laws (e.g., licensure, HIPAA), and ASHA policy.

Telepractice venues include schools, medical centers, rehabilitation hospitals, community health centers, outpatient clinics, universities, clients'/patients' homes, residential health care facilities, child care centers, and corporate settings. There are no inherent limits to where telepractice can be implemented, as long as the services comply with national, state, institutional, and professional regulations and policies.

The two most common terms describing types of telepractice are synchronous (client/patient interactive) and asynchronous (store and forward). Synchronous services are conducted with interactive audio and video connection in real time to create an in-person experience similar to that achieved in a traditional encounter. Synchronous services may connect a client/patient or group of clients/patients with a clinician, or they may include consultation between a clinician and a specialist (Department of Health and Human Services, n.d., 2012). In asynchronous services, images or data are captured and transmitted (i.e., stored and forwarded) for viewing or interpretation by a professional. Examples include transmission of voice clips, audiologic testing results, or outcomes of independent client/patient practice. Hybrid applications of telepractice include combinations of synchronous, asynchronous, and/or in-person services. Clinicians and programs should verify state licensure and payer definitions to ensure that a particular type of service delivery is consistent with regulation and payment policies.

Expert Opinion

- Telepractice is an appropriate model of service delivery for the professions of audiology and speech-language pathology (ASHA, 2005a, 2005b).
- The quality of services delivered via telepractice must be consistent with the quality of services delivered in-person (ASHA, 2005a, 2005b).

Roles and Responsibilities

ASHA's position statements for audiologists and speech-language pathologists providing clinical services via telepractice (ASHA, 2005a, 2005b) affirm that telepractice is an appropriate model of service delivery for audiologists and speech-language pathologists. ASHA requires that individuals who provide telepractice abide by the ASHA Code of Ethics, including Principle of Ethics II, Rule B, which states, "Individuals shall engage in only those aspects of the profession that are within their competence, considering their level of education, training, and experience" (ASHA, 2010).

Roles and responsibilities for audiologists and SLPs in the provision of services via telepractice include:

- understanding and applying appropriate models of technology used to deliver services;
- understanding the appropriate specifications and operations of technology used in delivery of serviccs;
- calibrating and maintaining clinical instruments and telehealth equipment;
- selecting clients who are appropriate for assessment and intervention services via telepractice;
- selecting and using assessments and interventions that are appropriate to the technology being used and that take into consideration client/patient and disorder variables;
- being sensitive to cultural and linguistic variables that affect the identification, assessment, treatment, and management

of communication disorders/differences in individuals receiving services via telepractice;
- training and using support personnel appropriately when delivering services;
- being familiar with the available tools and methods and applying them to evaluate the effectiveness of services provided and to measure outcomes;
- maintaining appropriate documentation, including informed consent for use of telepractice and documentation of the telepractice encounter;
- being knowledgeable and compliant with existing rules and regulations regarding telepractice including security and privacy protections, reimbursement for services and licensure, liability and malpractice concerns;
- collaborating with physicians for timely referral and follow-up services (Hofstetter, Kokesh, Ferguson, & Hood, 2010);
- using Web-based technology to engage clients through virtual environments and other personally salient activities (Towey, 2012).

Telepractice is constantly evolving. Ongoing education and training is required to maintain expertise and familiarity with changes in technology and potential clinical applications (Cohn, 2012).

Licensure

A growing number of states have legal provisions regarding telepractice. (See State Provisions for Telepractice [ASHA, 2012].) Clinicians should verify state licensure requirements and policies regarding telepractice, both in the states where they are licensed and where they wish to telepractice, prior to initiating services.

Current guidance in medical and legal practices indicates that the client's/patient's location determines the site of service. As a result, telepractitioners must be licensed in both their home states and in the states in which the clients/patients reside. Recognizing that this can be a burden to practitioners and a barrier to the growth of telepractice, ASHA is encouraging state licensure boards to consider less restrictive alternative models of licensure. Civilian employees of the Department of Defense and the Department of Veterans Affairs may not be bound by the same licensing requirements. Confirm the specific licensing requirements for your circumstances. ASHA is also working with a coalition of other provider organizations to address the issue of licensure portability for the use of telepractice (Brannon, Cohn, & Cason, 2012; Cason & Brannon, 2011; Cohn, Brannon, & Cason, 2011).

International Considerations

ASHA-certified audiologists and speech-language pathologists who deliver telepractice services to individuals in other countries are bound by the ASHA Code of Ethics and other official ASHA policy documents that guide ethical and appropriate practice. Prior to providing international telepractice services, it is important to confirm requirements, if they exist, for the practice of audiology or speech-language pathology in the specific countries (see Audiology and Speech-Language Pathology Associations Outside of the United States for a list of international associations);

- consult additional resources on providing services with cultural and linguistic sensitivity.

Reimbursement

Before initiating services verify that funding source(s) will cover services delivered via telepractice. (See FAQs on Telepractice Reimbursement and Licensure at http://www.asha.org/Practice/telepractice/TelepracticeFAQs/.) Telepractice providers should be prepared to educate payers about how telepractice services are delivered and the benefits to clients/patients and payers. Education materials include research articles, organization policies and procedures to assure provider training and quality services, educational/informed consent materials for clients/patients, video clips, and testimonials.

Private Health Insurance

There is a trend for states to pass legislation mandating coverage of telepractice. Generally, the mandates require health insurers, subscription plans, and health maintenance organizations to cover the cost of health care services provided through telepractice on the same basis as those provided through in-person visits. Insurers may reimburse for telepractice in states without mandates; however, given the variability of state requirements, the practitioner should first check with the payer.

Medicare

Medicare reimburses some telemedicine providers for specific services under specified conditions, but audiologists and speech-language pathologists and other rehabilitation professionals are not currently included in legislation as eligible providers. ASHA and other organizations have been actively lobbying for legislation to expand eligibility to include audiologists and speech-language pathologists among others.

Medicaid

Medicaid is a federal/state entitlement program for low-income individuals and families. Each state:

- administers its own programs,
- establishes its own eligibility standards,
- chooses the type, amount, duration, and scope of services,
- sets the rate of payment for services.

Some states have explicitly authorized reimbursement for telepractice by audiologists or speech-language pathologists or have established a general trend for reimbursement of telehealth. Practitioners should contact the appropriate state Medicaid office to verify how a telepractice service should be reflected in the billing code and documentation.

Self-Pay

Services that are not covered by private insurance or public payers may be paid for out of pocket by the client/patient, provided the services meet all other relevant legal and ethical standards.

Client/Patient Selection

Because clinical services are based on the unique needs of each individual client/patient, telepractice may not be appropriate in all circumstances or for all clients. Candidacy for receiving services via telepractice should be assessed prior to initiation of services. The client's/patient's culture, education level, age, gender, and other characteristics may influence the appropriateness of audiology and speech-language services provided via telepractice.

Consider the potential impact of the following factors on the client's/patient's ability to benefit from telepractice:

- physical and sensory characteristics, including
- hearing ability,
- visual ability (e.g., ability to see material on a computer monitor),
- manual dexterity (e.g., ability to operate a keyboard if needed),
- physical endurance (e.g., sitting tolerance);
- cognitive, behavioral, and/or motivational characteristics, including
  - level of cognitive functioning,
  - ability to maintain attention (e.g., to a video monitor),
  - ability to sit in front of a camera and minimize extraneous movements to avoid compromising the image resolution,
  - willingness of the client/patient and family/caregiver (as appropriate) to receive services via telepractice;
- communication characteristics, including
  - auditory comprehension,
  - literacy,

  - speech intelligibility,
  - cultural/linguistic variables,
  - availability of an interpreter;
- client's/patient's support resources, including
  - availability of technology,
  - access to and availability of resources (e.g., telecommunications network, facilitator),
  - appropriate environment for telepractice (e.g., quiet room with minimal distractions),
  - ability of the client/patient, caregiver, and/or facilitator to follow directions to operate and troubleshoot telepractice technology and transmission.

Environmental Considerations

Attention to environmental elements of care is important to ensure the comfort, safety, confidentiality, and privacy of clients/patients during telepractice encounters. Room location, design, lighting, and furniture should optimize the quality of video and audio data transmission and minimize ambient noise and visual distractions in all participating sites. Advance planning and preparation is needed for optimal positioning of the client/patient, test and therapy materials, and for placement of the video monitor and camera (Jarvis-Selinger, Chan, Payne, Plohman, & Ho, 2008).

Practice Areas

The growing body of research on the use of telepractice for communication disorders includes many studies demonstrating the comparability of telepractice and in-person services.

Audiology

Computer-based clinical applications are common in audiology today (Choi, Lee, Park, Oh, & Park, 2007; Kokesh, Ferguson, Patricoski, & LeMaster, 2009). For example, audiometers; auditory brainstem response (ABR), otoacoustic emissions (OAEs), and immittance testing equipment; and hearing aid systems are frequently computer peripherals, which can be interfaced to existing telepractice networks. Manufacturers are now promoting equipment with synchronous or store-and-forward capabilities.

Practice areas where teleaudiology is being used include:

- aural rehabilitation (Polovoy, 2009; Yates & Campbell, 2005)
- cochlear implant fitting (Wasowski et al., 2012)
- hearing aid fitting (Campos & Ferrari, 2012)
- infant and pediatric hearing screenings (Krumm, Huffman, Dick, & Klich, 2007; Krumm, Ribera, & Schmiedge, 2005; Lancaster, Krumm, Ribera, & Klich, 2008)
- pure tone audiometry (Krumm, Ribera, & Klich, 2007)
- speech in noise testing (Ribera, 2005)
- videootoscopy (Burgess et al., 1999; Eikelboom, Atlas, Mbao, & Gallop, 2002; Heneghan, Sclafani, Stern, & Ginsburg, 1999; Sullivan, 1997).

Speech-Language Pathology

Telepractice is being used in the assessment and treatment of a wide range of speech and language disorders, including:

- articulation disorders (Crutchley, Dudley, & Campbell, 2010; Waite, Cahill, Theodoros, Busuttin, & Russell, 2006)
- autism (Parmanto, Pulantara, Schutte, Saptono, & McCue, 2013)
- dysarthria (Hill et al., 2006)
- fluency disoders (Carey, O'Brian, Onslow, Packman, & Menzies, 2012; Lewis, Packman, Onslow, Simpson, & Jones, 2008)
- language and cognitive disorders (Brennan, Georgeadis, Baron, & Barker, 2004; Waite, Theodoros, Russell, & Cahill, 2010)
- dysphagia (Malandraki, McCullough, He, McWeeny, & Perlman, 2011; Perlman & Witthawaskul, 2002)

- voice disorders (Halpern et al., 2012; Mashima et al., 2003; Theodoros et al., 2006; Tindall, Huebner, Stemple, & Kleinert, 2008; Towey, 2012).

Modification of Assessment and Treatment Techniques and Materials

Clinicians who deliver telepractice services must possess specialized knowledge and skills in selecting assessments and interventions that are appropriate to the technology and that take into consideration client/patient and disorder variables. Hence, assessment and therapy procedures and materials may need to be modified and adapted to accommodate the lack of physical contact with the client/patient. These modifications should be reflected in the interpretation and documentation of the service.

School Setting Considerations

Stimulated by shortages or maldistribution of clinicians in some school districts, distances between schools in rural districts, and opportunities to offer greater specialization of services within a district, schools are currently the most common setting in which telepractice services are delivered. Telepractice contracts may be developed with the local education agency or school district, or the services may be provided by audiologists and speech-language pathologists employed by the district. Some states authorize Medicaid reimbursement for eligible students in schools.

The effectiveness of telepractice as a service delivery model in the schools is well documented (Grogan-Johnson, Alvares, Rowan, & Creaghead, 2010; Grogan-Johnson et al., 2011; Lewis et al., 2008; McCullough, 2001; Scheideman-Miller et al., 2002; Waite et al., 2006). In addition, parents, clients, and clinicians report satisfaction with telepractice as a mode of service delivery (Crutchley, Dudley, & Campbell, 2010; McCullough, 2001; Rose et al., 2000; Scheideman-Miller et al., 2002).

The administrative body responsible for defining telepractice-based services in a school or school district should:

- ensure that telepractice clinicians (who may not reside in the state where the school is located) meet all state requirements to practice in the school,
- make certain that telepractice clinicians have knowledge, skills, and training in the use of telepractice,
- recognize that every student may not be best served by a telepractice model and give students the opportunity to receive traditional in-person services,
- inform parents that they have the right to decline telepractice services for their child,
- provide parents with an informed consent, satisfaction survey, or other feedback option and opportunities to discuss concerns about their child's progress or the telepractice program,
- document service delivery via telepractice on the Individualized Education Plan (IEP) and during the IEP meeting,
- formulate policies that ensure protection of privacy during the services as well as documentation of the services,
- provide on-site support for the telepractice sessions, including the assignment of an individual to accompany the student to the session and provide support during the session,
- develop a plan for in-servicing staff, training on-site facilitators, and maintaining ongoing contact and collaboration with teachers, parents, and other school personnel, thereby ensuring that state standards are met,
- develop a system of program evaluation to measure the effectiveness of the service and satisfaction of stakeholders.

Telepractice Technology

The use of technology is an inherent element of telepractice. Specifications and selection of the appropriate equipment and connectivity vary according to the telepractice application. Technical support and training in the use of telepractice equipment are essential for success; furthermore, these needs will be ongoing as technology continues to evolve.

Videoconferencing Equipment (hardware, software, and peripheral devices)

Video communication can be accomplished through the use of personal videophones, videoconferencing software, and dedicated videoconferencing hardware and computer-based secure web-based programs. Factors/options in the selection of videoconferencing equipment include:

- camera capabilities (e.g., pan-tilt-zoom [PTZ] and resolution), display monitor capabilities (e.g., size, resolution, and dual display), microphone and speaker quality, and multisite capability;
- peripheral devices, such as recording devices or auxiliary video input equipment for computer interfacing, document cameras, or other specialized cameras with high resolution (e.g., fiberoptic videoendoscopes);
- additional modes of real-time interaction through applications such as screen sharing, whiteboards, online presentations, or text chat.

Connectivity

During telepractice, information is transmitted across a telecommunications connection (e.g., point-to-point, dedicated line, Web-based) between participants at different sites. Consider the following factors in determining appropriate connection strategy:

- Network connection speed impacts overall quality of video and audio clarity. A review of 225 articles on videoconferencing in clinical contexts, including speech-language pathology, revealed that a minimum bandwidth of 384 Kbps was needed to establish adequate audio and visual clarity (Jarvis-Selinger et al., 2008).

- Available bandwidth may be reduced by the number of users on the communication network, for example, during peak usage times in schools.
- Higher connection speeds may be required for high-definition (HD), dual-streaming video presentation, or hosting multipoint calls. Lower bandwidth may result in delays, jitter, and loss of data and may interfere with quality of signals for clinical decision-making or normal turn taking in conversational discourse.
- Establishing an alternative connection (e.g., telephone, e-mail) enables participants to troubleshoot connection problems or to reschedule the session.
- Lack of technological compatibility may be a barrier to connecting sites with different hardware, software, and bandwidth speeds. A financial investment may be required to upgrade the infrastructure to ensure the interoperability of equipment at all participating sites.
- Secure transmission during telepractice may be obtained through the use of encryption, unique passwords, unique meeting numbers, secure connection via virtual private network (VPN), and hardware/software firewalls.

Facilitators in Telepractice for Audiology and Speech-Language Services

Although only certified and/or licensed audiologists and speech-language pathologists can provide professional services via telepractice, appropriately trained individuals may be present at the remote site to assist the client/patient. Unless restricted by institutional or state policies or regulations, the facilitator may be a teacher's aide, nursing assistant, audiology assistant, or speech-language pathology assistant, teleaudiology clinical technician, telepresenter or other type of support personnel, interpreter, family member or caregiver, among others.

The type of paraprofessional required at the remote site may vary depending on the type of service being provided. It is the responsibility of the audiologist or speech-language pathologist to direct the session and ensure that the facilitator is adequately trained to assist. Adequate training includes knowledge of and sensitivity to cultural and linguistic differences of clients/patients, as well as the ways such differences may influence participation in telepractice. The hierarchy for preferred interpreters in telepractice is consistent with that used for interpreters during in-person practice. Practitioners must also be aware of applicable state policies and regulations on the use of facilitators.

State and Federal Laws and Regulations

Practitioners should be aware of federal and state regulations relating to privacy and security, including those pertaining to storage and transmission of client information.

Privacy and Security

Clinicians providing services via telepractice are bound by federal and state regulations as they would be when providing in-person services. Federal legislation about privacy and security for covered entities include the Health Insurance Portability and Accountability Act of 1996 (HIPAA; U.S. Department of Health and Human Services [HHS], n.d.), the Health Information Technology for Economic and Clinical Health Act of 2009 (HITECH; HHS, n.d.), and the Family Educational Rights and Privacy Act of 1974 (FERPA; U.S. Department of Education, n.d.). States may also have privacy or security requirements that are more stringent than federal requirements. (See Health Insurance Portability and Accountability Act for general information about HIPAA. See also HIPAA Security Rule: Frequently Asked Questions, HIPAA: Electronic Data Interchange (EDI) Rule, and HIPAA Security Technical Safeguards.)

Determining how to be compliant with these regulations is complex. There are no absolute standards that dictate which software programs meet all requirements. For example, a vendor cannot guarantee that a product is HIPAA-compliant, because the policies of the provider and how a program is implemented are variables that help determine the effectiveness of the program's privacy and security measures. Consulting an expert who specializes in these issues is advisable. Further discussion of the complexities of privacy is provided by Cohn and Watzlaf, 2011.

Security of treatment rooms and remote access to electronic documentation must be considered to protect client/patient privacy and confidentiality at both sites. Clients/patients should be given an opportunity to decide who should be present at their locations when they receive services, and a camera may be used to scan the clinician's environment to ensure privacy. All persons in rooms at both sites should be identified prior to each session or when the individual(s) enters the session.

To manage risk, clinicians are advised to obtain documentation of informed consent from the client/patient. This may include a description of the equipment and services to be delivered, how services via telepractice may differ from services delivered in person, any modifications that will be made in assessment protocols, and potential confidentiality issues. Documentation may also include the type of equipment used, the identity of every person present, the location of the client/patient and the clinician, and the type and rate of transmission.

It is the clinician's role to ensure client/patient confidentiality when telepractice services are used. In order to do so, clinicians must have knowledge of:

- state and federal regulations pertaining to electronic storage of consumer information for local computer servers and local area networks, servers shared by wide area networks, and servers accessible by Internet users;
- types of technologies with privacy protections, including new or evolving forms of software and hardware solutions to ensure consumer privacy (e.g., encryption, virtual private networks [VPN], firewalls);
- the need for telepractice software and hardware applications to be configured for use with encryption, VPN, or firewall applications;

- applications of VPN software, including downloading and configuring VPN software for modem, backbone, and satellite connections;
- principles for training support and professional personnel concerning appropriate local standards for privacy of health care information of consumers;
- breach notification policy.

Enlisting Stakeholder Support

It is essential for practitioners to gain the support of stakeholders—including clinicians, administrators, sponsors/payers, technical and support staff, teachers, multidisciplinary team members, students and parents, and clients and family members/caregivers—when implementing a telepractice program. Without understanding, planning, collaboration, and a receptive attitude toward telepractice on the part of all stakeholders, a program that has been launched can fail.

Methods for enlisting support include:

- adding telepractice to the organization's strategic plan to ensure administrative support and allocation of resources;
- integrating telepractice program needs into existing organizational processes, personnel networks, and training activities;
- conducting preimplementation planning with technical support staff to troubleshoot firewall and bandwidth issues;
- learning about and advocating for reimbursement mechanisms to sustain telepractice programs;
- educating staff on roles and responsibilities and the organization's plan for provider training, quality assurance, provider and client/caregiver/student/parent satisfaction, and ongoing program development;
- conducting outreach to the community, including satisfaction surveys.

Resources

American Telemedicine Association http://www.americantelemed.org/

Center for Connected Health Policy http://cchpca.org/

Center for Telemedicine Law http://ctel.org/

Office for the Advancement of Telehealth http://www.hrsa.gov/ruralhealth/about/telehealth/

State Licensure Telepractice Provisions http://www.asha.org/Practice/telepractice/StateProvisionsUpdateTelepractice/

Telepractice: Frequently Asked Questions http://www.asha.org/Practice-Portal/Professional-Issues/Telepractice/Telepractice-Frequently-Asked-Questions/

VHA Office of Telehealth Services http://www.telehealth.va.gov/

References

American Speech-Language-Hearing Association. (2005a). *Audiologists providing clinical services via telepractice* [Position statement]. Retrieved from http://www.asha.org/policy.

American Speech-Language-Hearing Association. (2005b). *Speech-language pathologists providing clinical services via telepractice* [Position statement]. Retrieved from http://www.asha.org/policy.

American Speech-Language-Hearing Association. (2010). *Code of ethics* [Ethics]. Retrieved from http://www.asha.org/policy.

American Speech-Language-Hearing Association. (2012). *State provisions update for telepractice.* Retrieved from http://www.asha.org/Practice/telepractice/StateProvisionsUpdateTelepractice/.

American Speech-Language-Hearing Association. (n.d.). *Audiology and speech-language pathology associations outside of the United States*. Retrieved from http://www.asha.org/members/international/intl_assoc/.

American Speech-Language-Hearing Association. (n.d.). *FAQs on telepractice reimbursement and licensure*. Retrieved from http://www.asha.org/Practice/telepractice/TelepracticeFAQs/.

American Speech-Language-Hearing Association. (n.d.). *Health Insurance Portability and Accountability Act*. Retrieved from http://www.asha.org/practice/reimbursement/hipaa/.

American Speech-Language-Hearing Association. (n.d.). *HIPAA: Electronic Data Interchange (EDI) Rule*. Retrieved from http://www.asha.org/practice/reimbursement/hipaa/hipaa_edi_faq/.

American Speech-Language-Hearing Association. (n.d.). *HIPAA Security Rule: Frequently asked questions*. Retrieved from http://www.asha.org/practice/reimbursement/hipaa/securityrule/

American Speech-Language-Hearing Association. (n.d.). *HIPAA security technical safeguards*. Retrieved from http://www.asha.org/Practice/reimbursement/hipaa/technicalsafeguards/.

American Telemedicine Association. (2010). *A blueprint for telerehabilitation guidelines*. http://www.americantelemed.org/docs/default-source/standards/a-blueprint-for-telerehabilitation-guidelines.pdf?sfvrsn=4.

Brannon, J., Cohn, E. R., & Cason, J. (2012). Making the case for uniformity in professional state licensure requirements. *International Journal of Telerehabilitation, 4*(1), 41–46.

Brennan, D. M., Georgeadis, A. C., Baron, C. R., & Barker, L. M. (2004). The effect of videoconference-based telerehab on story retelling performance by brain injured subjects and its implication for remote speech-language therapy. *Telemedicine Journal and e-Health, 10*(2), 147–154.

Burgess, L., Holtel, M., Syms, M., Birkmire-Peters, D., Peters, L., & Mashima, P. (1999). Overview of telemedicine applications for otolaryngology. *Laryngoscope, 109*(9), 1433–1437.

Campos, P. D., & Ferrari, D. V. J. (2012). Teleaudiology: Evaluation of teleconsultation efficacy for hearing aid fitting. *Journal da Sociedade Brasileira de Fonoaudiologia, 24*(4), 301–308.

Carey, B., O'Brian, S., Onslow, M., Packman, A., & Menzies, R. (2012). Webcam delivery of the Camperdown Program for adolescents who stutter: A phase I trial. *Language, Speech, and Hearing Services in Schools, 43*, 370–380.

Cason, J., & Brannon, J. A. (2011). Telehealth regulatory and legal considerations: Frequently asked questions. *International Journal of Telerehabilitation, 3*(2), 15–18.

Choi, J. M., Lee, H. B., Park, C. S., Oh, S. H., & Park, K. S. (2007). PC-based tele-audiometry. *Telemedicine Journal and e-Health, 13*(5), 501–508.

Cohn, E. R. (2012). Tele-ethics in telepractice for communication disorders. *Perspectives on Telepractice, 2*(1), 3-15.

Cohn, E. R., Brannon, J., & Cason, J. (2011). Resolving barriers to licensure portability for telerehabilitation professionals. *International Journal of Telerehabilitation, 3*(2), 31-33.

Cohn, E. R., & Watzlaf, V. J. M. (2011). Privacy and Internet-based telepractice. *Perspectives on Telepractice, 1*(1), 26-37.

Crutchley, S., Dudley, W., & Campbell, M. (2010). Articulation assessment through videoconferencing: A pilot study. *Communications of Global Information Technology, 2*, 12-23.

Eikelboom, R., Atlas, M., Mbao, M., & Gallop, M. (2002). Tele-otology: Planning, design, development and implementation. *Journal of Telemedicine and Telecare, 8*(Suppl. 3), 14-17.

Grogan-Johnson, S., Alvares, R., Rowan, L., & Creaghead, N. (2010). A pilot study comparing the effectiveness of speech language therapy provided by telemedicine with conventional on-site therapy. *Journal of Telemedicine and Telecare, 16*, 134-139.

Grogan-Johnson, S., Gabel, R., Taylor, J., Rowan, L., Alvarex, R., & Schenker, J. (2011). A pilot exploration of speech sound disorder intervention delivered by telehealth to school-age children. *International Journal of Telerehabilitation, 3*(1), 31-42.

Halpern, A. E., Ramig, L. O., Matos, C. E. C., Petska-Cable, J. A., Spielman, J. L., Pogoda, J. et al. (2012). Innovative technology for the assisted delivery of intensive voice treatment (LSVT®LOUD) for Parkinson disease. *American Journal of Speech-Language Pathology, 21*, 354-367.

Heneghan, C., Sclafani, A., Stern, J., & Ginsburg, J. (1999). Telemedicine applications in otolaryngology. *IEEE Engineering in Medicine and Biology Society, 18*(4), 53-62.

Hill, A. J., Theodoros, D. G., Russell, T. G., Cahill, L. M., Ward, E. C., & Clark, K. M. (2006). An Internet-based telerehabilitation system for the assessment of motor speech disorders: A pilot study. *American Journal of Speech-Language Pathology, 15*, 45-56.

Hofstetter, P. J., Kokesh, J. A., Ferguson, A. S., & Hood, L. J. (2010). The impact of telehealth on wait time for ENT specialty care. *Telemedicine and e-Health, 16*(5), 551-556.

Jarvis-Selinger, S., Chan, E., Payne, R., Plohman, K., & Ho, K. (2008). Clinical telehealth across the disciplines: Lessons learned. *Telemedicine and e-Health, 14*, 720-725.

Kokesh, J., Ferguson, A. S., Patricoski, C., & LeMaster, B. (2009). Traveling an audiologist to provide otolaryngology care using store and forward telemedicine. *Telemedicine and e-Health, 15*, 758-763.

Krumm, M., Huffman, T., Dick, K., & Klich, R. (2007). Providing infant hearing screening using OAEs and AABR using telehealth technology. *Journal of Telemedicine and Telecare, 14*(2), 102–104.

Krumm, M., Ribera, J., & Klich, R. (2007). Providing basic hearing tests using remote computing technology. *Journal of Telemedicine and Telecare, 13*(8), 406–410.

Krumm, M., Ribera, J., & Schmiedge, J. (2005). Using a telehealth medium for objective hearing testing: Implications for supporting rural universal newborn hearing screening programs. *Seminars in Hearing, 26*, 3–12.

Lancaster, P., Krumm, M., Ribera, J., & Klich, R. (2008). Remote hearing screenings via telepractice in rural elementary school. *American Journal of Audiology, 17*(2), 114–122.

Lewis, C., Packman, A., Onslow, M., Simpson, J., & Jones, M. (2008). A Phase II trial of telehealth delivery of the Lidcombe Program of Early Stuttering Intervention. *American Journal of Speech-Language Pathology, 17*, 139–149.

Malandraki, G. A., McCullough, G., He, X., McWeeny, E., & Perlman, A. L. (2011). Teledynamic evaluation of oropharyngeal swallowing. *Journal of Speech, Language, and Hearing Research, 54*, 1497–1505.

Mashima, P. A., Birkmire-Peters, D. P., Syms, M. J., Holtel, M. R., Burgess, L., & Peters, L. J. (2003). Telehealth: Voice therapy using telecommunications technology. *American Journal of Speech-Language Pathology, 12*(4), 432.

McCullough, A. (2001). Viability and effectiveness of teletherapy for preschool children with special needs. *International Journal of Language and Communication Disorders, 36*(Suppl. 1), 321–326.

Parmanto, B., Pulantara, W., Schutte, J., Saptono, A., & McCue, M. (2013). An integrated telehealth system for remote administration of an adult autism assessment. *Telemedicine and e-Health, 19*(2), 88–94.

Perlman, A. L., & Witthawaskul, W. (2002). Real-time remote telefluoroscopic assessment of patients with dysphagia. *Dysphagia, 17*(2), 162–167.

Polovoy, C. (2009). Aural rehabilitation telepractice: International project links NY student clinicians, Bolivian children. *ASHA Leader, 14*(8), 20–21.

Ribera, J. (2005). Interjudge reliability and validation of telehealth applications of the Hearing in Noise Test. *Seminars in Hearing, 26*, 13–18.

Rose, D., Furner, S., Hall, A., Montgomery, K., Datsavras, E., & Clarke, P. (2000). Videoconferencing for speech and language therapy in schools. *BT Technology Journal, 18*(1), 101–104.

Scheideman-Miller, C., Clark, P., Smeltzer, S., Cloud, A., Carpenter, J., Hodge, B., ... Prouty, D. (2002). Two-year results of a pilot study delivering speech therapy to students in a rural Oklahoma school via telemedicine. *Proceedings of the 35th Annual Hawaii International Conference on System Sciences* (pp. 1–9). Retrieved July 5, 2011, from http://origin-http://www.computer.org/plugins/dl/pdf/proceedings/hicss/2002/1435/06/14350161b.pdf.

Servicemembers' Telemedicine and E-Health Portability Act. (2011). Retrieved from http://www.govtrack.us/congress/bills/112/hr1832.

Sullivan, R. (1997). Video-otoscopy in audiologic practice. *Journal of American Academy of Audiology, 8*, 447–467.

Theodoros, D. G., Constantinescu, G., Russell, T. G., Ward, E. C., Wilson, S. J., & Wootton, R. (2006). Treating the speech disorder in Parkinson's disease online. *Journal of Telemedicine and Telecare, 12*(Suppl. 3), 88–91.

Tindall, L. R., Huebner, R. A., Stemple, J. C., & Kleinert, H. L. (2008). Videophone-delivered voice therapy: A comparative analysis of outcomes to traditional delivery for adults with Parkinson's disease. *Telemedicine and e-Health, 14*(10), 1070–1077.

Towey, M. (2012a). Speech telepractice: Installing a speech therapy upgrade for the 21st century. *International Journal of Telerehabilitation, 4*(2). doi:10.5195/ijt.2012.6112. Retrieved from http://telerehab.pitt.edu/ojs/index.php/Telerehab/article/view/6112.

Towey, M. (2012b). Speech therapy telepractice for vocal cord dysfunction (VCD): MaineCare (Medicaid) cost savings. *International Journal of Telerehabilitation, 4*(1), 34–36. doi:10.5195/ijt.2012.6095.

U.S. Department of Education. (n.d.). *Family Educational Rights and Privacy Act.* Retrieved from http://www2.ed.gov/policy/gen/guid/fpco/ferpa/index.html.

U.S. Department of Health and Human Services. (n.d.). *Health Information Technology for Economic and Clinical Health Act.* Retrieved from http://www.hhs.gov/ocr/privacy/hipaa/administrative/enforcementrule/hitechenforcementifr.html.

U.S. Department of Health and Human Services. (n.d.). *Health Insurance Portability and Accountability Act.* Retrieved from http://www.hhs.gov/ocr/privacy/.

U.S. Department of Health and Human Services, Centers for Medicare and Medicaid Services. (2012). *Telehealth services: Rural health fact sheet series.* Retrieved from http://www.cms.gov/Outreach-and-Education/Medicare-Learning-Network-MLN/MLNProducts/downloads/telehealthsrvcsfctsht.pdf.

U.S. Department of Health and Human Services, Health Information Technology and Quality Improvement. (n.d.). *What is telehealth?* Retrieved from http://www.hrsa.gov/healthit/toolbox/RuralHealthITtoolbox/Telehealth/whatistelehealth.html

Waite, M., Cahill, L., Theodoros, D., Busuttin, S., & Russell, T. (2006). A pilot study of online assessment of childhood speech disorders. *Journal of Telemedicine and Telecare, 12*(Suppl. 3), S3:92–94.

Waite, M., Theodoros, D., Russell, T., & Cahill, L. (2010). Internet-based telehealth assessment of language using the CELF-4. *Language, Speech, and Hearing Services in Schools, 41*, 445–448.

Wasowski, A., Skarzynski, H., Lorens, A., Obycka, A., Walkowiak, A., Skarzynski, P., et al. (2012). The telefitting method used in the national network of teleaudiology: Assessment of quality and cost effectiveness. *Journal of Hearing Science*, *2*(2), 81–85.

Yates, J. T., & Campbell, K. H. (2005). Audiovestibular education and services via telemedicine technologies. *Seminars in Hearing, 26*, 35–42.

Content Disclaimer

The Practice Resource Project, ASHA policy documents, and guidelines contain information for use in all settings; however, members must consider all applicable local, state, and federal requirements when applying the information in their specific work setting.

Source: Reprinted with permission from the Practice Portal: Telepractice. Retrieved from http://www.asha.org/practice-portal/

APPENDIX C

A Blueprint for Telerehabilitation Guidelines

David Brennan, MBE[1], Lyn Tindall, PhD[2], Deborah Theodoros, PhD[3], Janet Brown, MA[4], Michael Campbell, MS[5], Diana Christiana, MAT[6], David Smith[7], Jana Cason, DHS[8] Alan Lee, DPT[9]

[1]National Rehabilitation Hospital, Washington, DC,[2] Department of Veterans Affairs Medical Center, Lexington, KY,[3] The University of Queensland, Queensland, Australia,[4] American Speech-Language-Hearing Association, Rockville, MD,[5] University of North Carolina at Greensboro, Browns Summit, NC,[6] Clinical Communications, Sugar Land, TX,[7] Telehealth Resource Center-Marquette General Hospital, Marquette, MI,[8] Auerbach School of Occupational Therapy, Spalding University, Louisville, KY,[9] Mount St. Mary's College, Los Angeles, CA

ABSTRACT

Telerehabilitation refers to the delivery of rehabilitation services via information and communication technologies. Clinically, this term encompasses a range of rehabilitation and habilitation services that include assessment, monitoring, prevention, intervention, supervision, education, consultation, and counseling. Telerehabilitation has the capacity to provide service across the lifespan and across a continuum of care. Just as the services and providers of telerehabilitation are broad, so are the points of service, which may include health care settings, clinics, homes, schools, or community-based worksites. This document was developed collaboratively by members of the Telerehabilitation SIG of the American Telemedicine Association, with input and guidance from other practitioners in the field, strategic stakeholders, and ATA staff. Its purpose is to inform and assist practitioners in providing effective and safe services that are based on client needs, current empirical evidence, and available technologies. Telerehabilitation professionals, in conjunction with professional associations and other organizations are encouraged to use this document as a template for developing discipline-specific standards, guidelines, and practice requirements.

Keywords: Telerehabilitation, telepractice, rehabilitation, American Telemedicine Association

Introduction

The Telerehabilitation Special Interest Group of the American Telemedicine Association is comprised of practitioners in health and education, and technology specialists who are engaged in applying telecommunications and health information technologies to improve access to rehabilitation and educational services, and to support independent living. This document was developed collaboratively by members of the Telerehabilitation SIG, with input and guidance from other practitioners in the field, strategic stakeholders, and ATA staff.

The purpose of this guide is to inform and assist practitioners in providing effective and safe services that are based on client needs, current empirical evidence, and available technologies. The material in this guide addresses general principles and not specific practice guidelines for telerehabilitation and is not intended to replace the primary practitioner's clinical, educational, or technology decision-making about the appropriate course of action/management of any client. Inherent within this document is the recognition that safe and effective telerehabilitation practice requires specific training, skills and techniques as documented below. Furthermore, the material in this guide should not be interpreted, nor used, as a legal standard of care.

Scope and Definitions

Telerehabilitation refers to the delivery of rehabilitation services via information and communication technologies. Clinically, this term encompasses a range of rehabilitation and habilitation services that include assessment, monitoring, prevention, intervention, supervision, education, consultation, and counseling. Telerehabilitation services are delivered to adults and children by a broad range of professionals that may include, but is not limited to, physical therapists, speech-language pathologists, occupational therapists, audiologists, rehabilitation physicians and nurses, rehabilitation engineers, assistive technologists, teachers, psychologists, and dieticians. As other personnel such as paraprofessionals, family members, and caregivers may assist during telerehabilitation sessions, for the purposes of this document, the term 'professionals' will be used to denote professional providers of telerehabilitation services. The term 'clients' will be used to refer to all recipients of telerehabilitation services and is intended to include both patients in medical settings, and children and adults who receive services outside the medical sphere, for example, in schools or at home.

Telerehabilitation has the capacity to provide service across the lifespan and across a continuum of care. Just as the services and providers of telerehabilitation are broad, so are the points of service, which may include health care settings, clinics, homes, schools, or community-based worksites. Terminology used to describe telerehabilitation is similarly broad. Some terms are used specifically to refer to individual rehabilitation disciplines, such as telespeech (speech-language pathology) or teleOT (occupational therapy). More generic terms, such as teletherapy and telepractice are also used, allowing for a broader focus on populations and activities, such as educational settings and wellness promotion in addition to rehabilitation. It is not the intent of this document to resolve the debate over terminology; rather the goal is to provide consistency across applications, regardless of the vocabulary used. For the purposes of this document, the term 'telerehabilitation' will be used, and the reader is reminded that terminology may differ according to the application and location.

Key Principles

The following information represents key administrative, clinical, technical, and ethical principles that should be considered in the course of providing telerehabilitation services. They are based primarily on the American Telemedicine Association's Core Standards for Telemedicine Operations, and describe additional considerations that are present across applications within telerehabilitation and its related fields. As education and advocacy are central to the continued growth of telerehabilitation, this document can and should be used as a tool to educate members of the medical and education professions, students, stakeholders, administrators, legislators, and community members. Telerehabilitation professionals, in conjunction with professional associations and other organizations, are encouraged to use this document as a template for developing discipline-specific standards, guidelines, and practice requirements. A bibliography of research in the field can be found on the webpage for the Telerehabilitation Special Interest Group of the American Telemedicine Association (http://www.americantelemed.org).

Administrative Principles:

- Organizations and/or professionals shall comply with national, state, local and other credentialing, privileging, and regulatory requirements for licensure, certification, and for the use of telerehabilitation.
- Organizations and/or professionals shall be aware of their locus of accountability and any requirements (including those for liability insurance) that apply when practicing telerehabilitation. This includes credentialing requirements at the site where the practitioner is located and the site where the client is located (which may be different states or jurisdictions), in compliance with regulatory and accrediting agencies.
- If required, organizations and/or professionals shall use billing and coding processes that designate that telerehabilitation services have been provided (e.g. through the use of a modifier) as required per guidelines of the payer.
- Organizations and/or professionals shall have traceable documentation that a telerehabilitation session occurred with a client. This documentation should be available to both the referring and consulting sites as appropriate.

- Organizations and/or professionals shall be aware of the advanced requirements for privacy and confidentiality associated with provision of services through telehealth technology at both the originating site and remote setting.
- Organizations and/or professionals shall determine requirements for documentation, storage, and retrieval of client records to protect the client's personal health information in accordance with federal and state regulations (e.g. HIPAA, FERPA, etc.). Specific guidelines shall be in place to address access to client records so as to ensure that unauthorized users cannot access, alter, tamper with, destroy or otherwise misuse client information.
- Organizations and/or professionals shall have a mechanism in place for ensuring that clients are aware of their rights and responsibilities with respect to accessing health care via telehealth technologies, including the process for communicating complaints.
- Organizations and/or professionals shall ensure that an appropriate facilitator is available when necessary to meet client and provider needs before, during, and after the telerehabilitation encounter.
- Organizations and/or professionals engaged in telerehabilitation research shall ensure the protection of participants in research protocols. Research protocols shall be approved by local Institutional Review Board(s) and be in compliance with relevant legislation, regulations, and other requirements for supporting participant decision-making and informed consent as well as safeguarding of Protected Health Information.
- Organizations and/or professionals shall ensure they have appropriate technology expertise during planning and start-up phases of a telerehabilitation program. Reasonable care and diligence shall be used when selecting equipment for evaluating or treating a client. Practitioners need to take appropriate measures to familiarize themselves with equipment and safety issues with client use. To help ensure success, it is essential that all telerehabilitation providers

use appropriate planning prior to delivering services and are fully aware of the capabilities and limitations of the equipment they intend to use, and the impact it may have on service delivery.

- Organizations and/or professionals shall have in place a systematic quality improvement and performance management process that complies with any organizational, regulatory, or accrediting, requirements for outcomes management.
- Organizations and/or professionals that engage in collaborative partnerships shall be aware of applicable legal and regulatory requirements for appropriate written agreements, memorandum of understanding, or contracts. Those contracts, agreements, etc., shall be based on the scope and application of the telerehabilitation services offered and shall address the administrative, clinical, technical, and ethical requirements outlined in this document, as relevant, for all parties named.

Clinical Principles:

- Professionals shall be guided by existing discipline and national clinical practice guidelines when practicing via telehealth. Where guidelines, position statements, or standards for telerehabilitation exist from a professional organization or society (e.g. American Speech-Language Hearing Association (ASHA), American Physical Therapy Association (APTA), and American Occupational Therapy Association (AOTA)), these shall be reviewed and appropriately incorporated into practice. Given the variability of rehabilitation clients, candidacy and appropriateness for telerehabilitation should be determined on a case-by-case basis with selections firmly based on clinical judgment, client's informed choice, and professional standards of care.
- As in all settings, professionals shall have the appropriate education, training/orientation, and ongoing continuing education/professional development to insure they possess

the necessary competencies for the safe provision of quality health services. Providers of telerehabilitation should have competence in the use of equipment, as well as considerations related to clients with cognitive, physical, or perceptual impairments.

- Delivery of services via telerehabilitation, whether interactive or store-and-forward, may require modifications to treatment material, techniques, equipment, and setting. Regardless of any modifications made, professionals shall deliver services in accordance with professional standards of care and the principles of evidence-based practice (i.e., current best evidence, clinical expertise, and client values and goals). In telerehabilitation encounters, these modifications may include: using additional support staff at the remote site to assist the client with a physical activity or perform a hands-on assessment, digitally reproducing treatment materials for delivery via data sharing or presentation tools, or temporary modification of client environment.
- Professionals shall ensure that all persons in the therapy room at both sites are identified to all participants prior to initiation of the telerehabilitation session. Disclosure of individuals attending the session may be accomplished by announcing their presence.

Technical Principles:

- Organizations and/or professionals shall ensure that equipment sufficient to support diagnostic and/or treatment needs is available and functioning properly at the time of clinical encounters. Beyond basic telehealth technology, additional equipment is often required to provide telerehabilitation services. This equipment will vary based on application and may include, for example, a sound level meter to measure intensity of speech, an audiometer for hearing assessment, or online measurement tools and sensors to measure force or position during a physical therapy assessment.

- Organizations and/or professionals shall comply with all relevant laws, regulations, and codes for technology and technical safety.
- Organizations and/or professionals shall comply with federal and state regulations for protection of client health information and to ensure the physical security of telehealth equipment and the electronic security of data storage, retrieval, and transmission. Methods for protection of health information include the use of authentication and/or encryption technology, and limiting access to need-to-know (availability for those people who do require access).
- Organizations and/or professionals shall ensure that all personnel who use telehealth equipment to deliver information or services are trained in equipment operation and troubleshooting. Procedures shall also be in place to ensure the safety and effectiveness of equipment through on-going maintenance. Providers of telerehabilitation must know how to operate videoconferencing peripherals, such as document cameras and data sharing tools, to incorporate other treatment materials into a session and configure audio/video signals so they are appropriate for clients with visual or hearing impairments.
- Organizations and/or professionals shall have strategies in place to address the environmental elements of care, including the physical accessibility of the treatment space as well as usability of equipment. This is essential in telerehabilitation applications as considerations must be made for clients who have a variety of impairments in areas such as fine/gross motor skill, cognition, speech, language, vision, or hearing.
- Organizations and/or professionals shall have infection control policies and procedures in place for the use of telehealth equipment and client peripherals that comply with organizational, legal, and regulatory requirements. In particular, mechanisms shall be in place for the cleaning/sterilization of equipment for re-use by multiple clients.

Ethical Principles:

- The use of telehealth technology to deliver rehabilitation services requires consideration of professional ethical principles. Organizations and professionals that adhere to ethical principles of telerehabilitation shall:
- Incorporate organizational values and ethics into policy and procedures documents for telerehabilitation
- Comply with professional codes of ethics
- Inform clients of their rights and responsibilities when receiving rehabilitation through telehealth technology, including their right to refuse

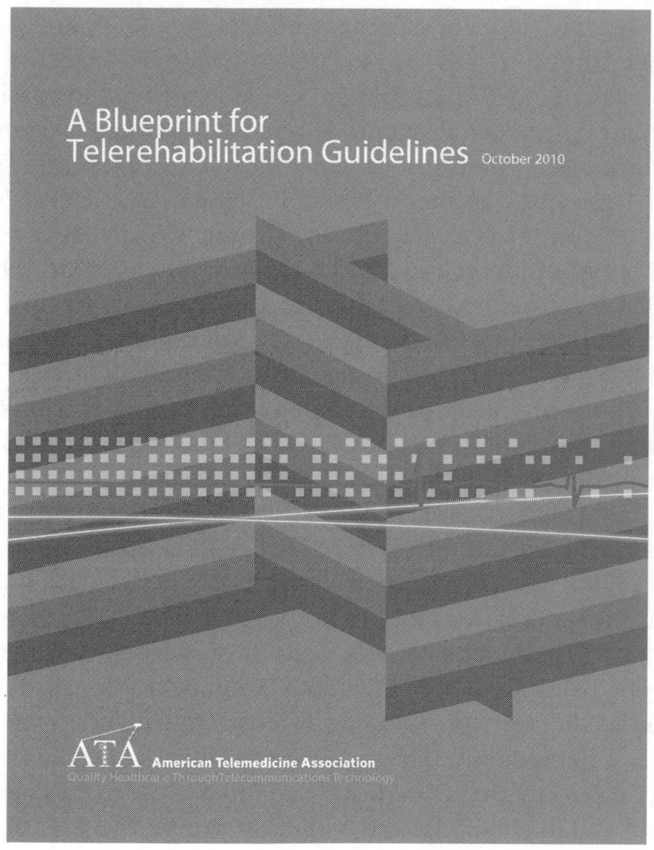

- Have in place a formal process for resolving ethical issues as well as policies that identify, eliminate, and reduce conflicts of interests associated with the provision of telerehabilitation services

Acknowledgments

This document was developed by a committee chaired by David Brennan, MBE and Lyn Tindall, PhD as part of the Telerehabilitation Special Interest Group of the American Telemedicine Association. The authors gratefully acknowledge the contributions of the following Working Group Members [WG], Consultants [C], Reviewers [R], Telerehabilitation Special Interest Group Chair [TR], ATA Standards and Guidelines Committee Member [SG], and ATA Staff [S]; Nina Antoniotti, RN, MBA, PhD, [Chair, SG], Director of Telehealth, Marshfield Clinic, Marshfield, WI; Jordana Bernard, MBA, [S], Senior Director, Program Services, American Telemedicine Association, Washington DC; Anne Burdick, MD, MPH, [SG], Associate Dean for Telemedicine and Clinical Outreach, Professor of Dermatology, Director, Leprosy Program, University of Miami Miller School of Medicine, Miami, FL; Jerry Cavallerano, PhD, OD, [SG], Staff Optometrist, Assistant to the Director, Joslin Diabetes Center, Beetham Eye Institute, Boston, MA; Ellen Cohn, PhD, CCC-SLP, [Chair, TR, WG], Associate Dean for Instructional Development, School of Health and Rehabilitation Sciences, University of Pittsburgh, Pittsburgh, PA; Paul Cox, MSEE, [WG], President, PERL Research, Huntsville, AL; Mary Fran Delaune, PT, MPT, [R], Director, Practice Department, American Physical Therapy Association, Alexandria, VA; Matt Elrod, PT, DPT, MEd, NSC, [R], Associate Director, Practice Department, American Physical Therapy Association, Alexandria, VA; Brian Grady, MD, [SG], VISN5 TMH Lead & Director, TeleMental Health, School of Medicine, University of Maryland, Baltimore, MD; Elizabeth Krupinski, PhD, [Vice Chair, SG], Associate Director, Program Evaluation, University of Arizona, Arizona Telemedicine Program, Department of Radiology, Research Professor, Department of Radiology Research, Tucson, AZ; Jonathan D. Linkous, MPA, [S], Chief Executive Director, American

Telemedicine Association, Washington, DC; Michael Pramuka, PhD, CRC, [WG], Rehabilitation Counselor, Walter Reed Medical Center, Washington, DC; Richard Schein, PhD, [WG], Postdoctoral Associate, School of Health and Rehabilitation Sciences, University of Pittsburgh, Pittsburgh, PA; Lou Theurer, [SG], Grant Administrator, Burn Telemedicine Program, University of Utah Health Sciences Center, Salt Lake City, UT; and Jill Winters, PhD, RN, [WG, SG], Dean and Professor, Columbia College of Nursing, Milwaukee, WI.

Index

Note: Page numbers in **bold** reference non-text material.

C

D

E

F

G

Q

R

S

U

V